Handbook of
Geriatric
Psychopharmacology

Handbook of Geriatric Psychopharmacology

Sandra A. Jacobson, M.D.
Ronald W. Pies, M.D.
David J. Greenblatt, M.D.

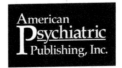

American Psychiatric Publishing, Inc.

Washington, DC
London, England

Copyright © 2002 American Psychiatric Publishing, Inc.
ALL RIGHTS RESERVED

Manufactured in the United States of America on acid-free paper
06   05   04   03   02   5   4   3   2   1
First Edition

American Psychiatric Publishing, Inc.
1400 K Street, N.W., Washington, DC20005
www.appi.org

Library of Congress Cataloging-in-Publication Data
Jacobson, Sandra A., 1953–
      Handbook of geriatric psychopharmacology / Sandra A.
  Jacobson, Ronald W. Pies, David J. Greenblatt.—1st ed.
         p. ; cm.
      Includes bibliographical references and index.
      ISBN 0-88048-823-9
      1. Geriatric psychopharmacology—Handbooks, manuals,
  etc. I. Pies, Ronald W., 1952–   II. Greenblatt, David J., 1945–
  III. Title.
      [DNLM: 1. Drug Therapy—Aged. 2. Aging—metabolism.
  3. Psychotropic Drugs—therapeutic use—Aged. WT 166 J17h 2002]
  RC451.4.A5 J334 2002
  615.78′0846—dc21

                                                          2001041366

British Library Cataloguing in Publication Data
A CIP record is available from the British Library.

Contents

PART 2

Treatment of Other Geriatric Syndromes and Disorders

About the Authors

Sandra A. Jacobson, M.D., is Assistant Professor of Psychiatry and Director of the Geriatric Psychiatry Fellowship Training Program at Tufts University School of Medicine in Boston, Massachusetts.

Ronald W. Pies, M.D., is Clinical Professor of Psychiatry at Tufts University School of Medicine in Boston, Massachusetts.

David J. Greenblatt, M.D., is Chairman of the Department of Pharmacology and Experimental Therapeutics at Tufts University School of Medicine in Boston, Massachusetts.

Preface

This handbook was written for residents, fellows, and colleagues in psychiatry and medicine who diagnose and treat psychiatric and neuropsychiatric conditions that can affect geriatric patients. It is intended as a practical, "how to" guide to clinical geriatric prescribing and, as such, represents something of a departure from hardbound reference texts published in this area. The information provided here comes from our own clinical experience and from our reading of the literature in geriatric psychopharmacology and is informed by a knowledge of pharmacological changes that occur with aging.

The handbook begins with an introduction focused on essentials of geriatric pharmacokinetics and a general approach to geriatric prescribing. Subsequent material is organized into two parts. In Part 1, each chapter covers a major psychotropic class, including information about pharmacology, clinical use, side effects, and treatment of selected syndromes and disorders. Summaries of prescribing data on selected drugs in each class appear at the end of each chapter.

Part 2 of the handbook covers several areas of geriatric psychopharmacology that do not fit well into the traditional organization of psychopharmacology books but are important enough to merit separate discussion: treatment of substance-related disorders, movement disorders, and dementias and other cognitive syndromes.

In the course of writing this handbook, it became even clearer to us that much of current practice in geriatric prescribing is based on anecdotal evidence and case report data. Controlled studies are sorely needed in most areas of geriatric psychopharmacology. We hope that this handbook provides some impetus for future research.

Introduction to Geriatric Psychopharmacology

Aging is associated with changes in function of various organ systems involved in drug distribution, metabolism, and elimination, and an understanding of these changes is essential to informed prescribing.

Pharmacokinetics and Aging

Pharmacokinetics involves the way a drug moves through the body. Figure 1–1 shows the disposition of a drug administered by various routes, from ingestion to elimination.

Absorption

A psychotropic drug taken orally passes from the stomach to the proximal small intestine, where most absorption takes place. The speed of absorption determines in part how quickly an oral drug takes effect, that is, its *onset of action.*

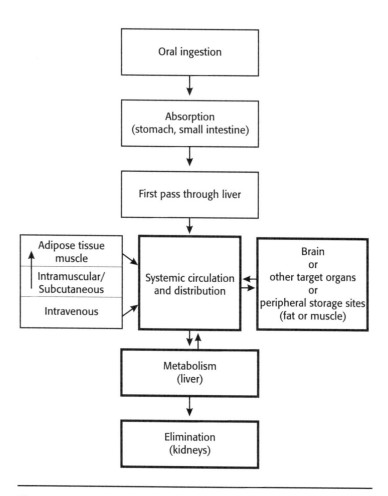

Figure 1–1.   Drug disposition: absorption, distribution, metabolism, and elimination.
Heavy-ruled boxes indicate processes most affected by aging.

Aging affects absorption the least of all pharmacokinetic processes, and, in general, psychotropic drugs are well absorbed by elderly patients. The presence of gastric pathology (e.g., hypochlorhydria) or drug interactions in the stomach (e.g., psychotropics with antacids or fiber supplements) can affect absorption, however, and in individual cases this effect can be clinically significant (Salzman 1998).

Parenteral administration of drugs (intramuscular [im] or intravenous [iv]) usually results in a faster onset of action because it circumvents gastrointestinal absorption and first-pass effects. This type of administration can be useful clinically, for example, in sedation of the dangerously agitated patient. It can also be hazardous, however, since side effects such as hypotension can develop rapidly.

Distribution

From the small intestine, the drug passes through the portal circulation to the liver. A proportion of the drug is passed on through the liver to the systemic circulation. For some psychotropic agents, a much larger proportion is metabolized in the liver (and, to a lesser extent, in the intestinal wall) before it enters the circulation, a process known as *first-pass metabolism* (Salzman 1998). Ingestion of grapefruit juice has been found to inhibit first-pass metabolism of drugs metabolized by the cytochrome P450 (CYP) enzyme 3A (CYP3A), with clinically significant effects (Bailey et al. 1994), as discussed in the next subsection (see "Metabolism").

Metabolites then enter the systemic circulation, and those that have been transformed to water-soluble compounds ("conjugated") may be excreted directly by the kidney. Parenteral drug administration (im or iv) eliminates first-pass metabolism, so the bioavailability of parenteral drugs is closer to 100%, and the intramuscular or intravenous dose required may be correspondingly smaller than the oral dose. It should be noted that the relatively small muscle mass of the average elderly patient makes intramuscular dosing painful and renders absorption erratic. For these reasons, the intramuscular route of drug administration is the least desirable for geriatric patients.

Drugs in the systemic circulation are distributed to target organs (such as the brain), back to the liver, or to peripheral storage sites such as fat or muscle. Distribution to peripheral sites is significantly affected by aging, as fat stores increase and lean body mass decreases. These changes in the aging individual result in a larger volume of distribution for lipophilic (fat-soluble) drugs, including almost all psychotropic agents (Thompson et al. 1983a, 1983b). Since drug half-life is directly related to volume of distribution, this change has profound effects on geriatric prescribing (Greenblatt et al. 1986), as detailed later in this chapter (see "Drug Half-Life"). Other properties determining a drug's distribution include its affinity for different tissues and the extent of its plasma protein binding (von Moltke et al. 1995). As Figure 1–1 suggests, the various sites of distribution are actually in competition with the brain for the drug. The greater the uptake in peripheral sites (e.g., larger adipose stores taking up more lipophilic drug), the less drug there is in the systemic circulation and the less drug there is available to brain receptors. In fact, only a small proportion of most administered drugs ever reaches these target receptors (von Moltke et al. 1995).

In contrast to half-life, duration of drug action is inversely related to volume of distribution. Lipophilic drugs are more readily taken up by the larger volume of adipose tissue found in elderly persons, such that drug concentration in plasma falls more quickly below the minimum effective threshold (von Moltke et al. 1995). For lipophilic drugs such as diazepam, initial use in elderly patients is, in principle, characterized by brief duration of effect but long life in the system; with repeated dosing, the potential exists for considerable accumulation in the system (von Moltke et al. 1995).

For lithium and other hydrophilic (water-soluble) drugs, the volume of distribution actually decreases with aging, so that more drug is present in the systemic circulation and proportionately more drug reaches the brain (Salzman 1998). This is one reason that smaller doses of lithium are required for older patients, although the major reason relates to reduced renal clearance, as noted later in this chapter (see "Clearance").

Metabolism

Aging is associated with decreased hepatic blood flow and reduced hepatic metabolism of many medications (Thompson et al. 1983a, 1983b). Demethylation reactions converting tertiary to secondary amines (e.g., amitriptyline to nortriptyline) are less efficient in elderly patients, and this is associated with accumulation of more active tertiary compounds (Salzman 1998). More importantly, phase I oxidation reactions of several CYP enzymes involved in the metabolism of many psychotropic drugs are significantly affected by aging (Greenblatt et al. 1986).

Phase I Processes (Cytochrome P450 Metabolism)

Three CYP families are of particular interest in psychopharmacology: CYP1, CYP2, and CYP3 (Nemeroff et al. 1996). As shown in Table 1–1, each CYP enzyme has specific substrate drugs, enzyme inhibitors, and enzyme inducers (Richelson 1997). Some drugs (e.g., carbamazepine) appear on more than one list, as substrates, inhibitors, or inducers for one or more enzymes. For most drugs, substrates are oxidatively metabolized by CYP enzymes (in phase I processes) to inactive or less active metabolites. In the presence of enzyme inducers, the oxidation reaction is facilitated, and the active parent compound is metabolized more rapidly. In the presence of enzyme inhibitors, the proportion of active parent compound stays high relative to that of inactive metabolite. When more than one inhibitor is co-ingested, significant enzyme inhibition can result.

Genetic differences in the presence or activity of certain CYP enzymes also are seen and account for much of the observed interindividual variability in serum levels of certain psychotropic drugs found with the same administered dose. *Slow* (or "poor") *metabolizers,* having low or no activity of an enzyme, could be expected to have difficulty metabolizing and excreting substrates for that enzyme, resulting in high levels of active drug. *Extensive metabolizers,* having higher levels and activity of the enzyme, could be expected to metabolize and excrete those substrates readily, at times resulting in low levels of active drug (Richelson

Table 1–1. Substrates, inhibitors, and inducers of known cytochrome P450 enzymes

1A2	2C19	2C9	2D6	3A
		Substrates		
caffeine	amitriptyline	celecoxib	amitriptyline	alprazolam
clozapine	citalopram	diclofenac	amphetamine	amitriptyline
cyclobenzaprine	clomipramine	flurbiprofen	clomipramine	amlodipine
fluvoxamine	cyclophosphamide	fluvastatin	codeine	atorvastatin
haloperidol	diazepam	glipizide	desipramine	buspirone
mexiletine	imipramine	ibuprofen	dextromethorphan	CALCIUM CHANNEL BLOCKERS
naproxen	lansoprazole	irbesartan	donepezil	carbamazepine
pentazocine	nelfinavir	losartan	flecainide	cerivastatin
riluzole	omeprazole	naproxen	haloperidol	chlorpheniramine
tacrine	pantoprazole	phenytoin	imipramine	clarithromycin
theophylline	phenytoin	piroxicam	lidocaine	cyclosporine
	topiramate	sulfamethoxazole	methadone	diazepam
		tamoxifen	metoprolol	diltiazem
		tolbutamide	mexiletine	erythromycin
		torsemide	mirtazapine	felodipine
		warfarin	nortriptyline	haloperidol
			ondansetron	indinavir

Table 1–1. Substrates, inhibitors, and inducers of known cytochrome P450 enzymes *(continued)*

1A2	2C19	2C9	2D6	3A
			oxycodone	lovastatin
			paroxetine	methadone
			propafenone	midazolam
			propranolol	nefazodone
			risperidone	nifedipine
			tamoxifen	nisoldipine
			thioridazine	pimozide
			timolol	quinidine
			tolterodine	quinine
			tramadol	ritonavir
			trazodone	saquinavir
			venlafaxine	sildenafil
				simvastatin
				tacrolimus
				tamoxifen
				trazodone
				triazolam
				verapamil
				vincristine

Table 1–1. Substrates, inhibitors, and inducers of known cytochrome P450 enzymes (*continued*)

1A2	2C19	2C9	2D6	3A
		Inhibitors		
cimetidine	cimetidine	amiodarone	amiodarone	amiodarone
fluoroquinolones	fluoxetine	fluconazole	chlorpheniramine	cimetidine
fluvoxamine	fluvoxamine	fluoxetine	cimetidine	clarithromycin
	ketoconazole	fluvastatin	clomipramine	erythromycin
	lansoprazole	fluvoxamine	fluoxetine	fluoxetine
	omeprazole	isoniazid	haloperidol	fluvoxamine
	paroxetine	metronidazole	methadone	grapefruit juice
	sertraline	paroxetine	indinavir	indinavir
	topiramate	zafirlukast	paroxetine	itraconazole
			perphenazine	ketoconazole
			quinidine	MACROLIDE ANTIBIOTICS
			ritonavir	nefazodone
			sertraline	nelfinavir
			terbinafine	ritonavir
				saquinavir
				troleandomycin

Table 1–1. Substrates, inhibitors, and inducers of known cytochrome P450 enzymes (*continued*)

1A2	2C19	2C9	2D6	3A
		Inducers		
carbamazepine	carbamazepine	chloral hydrate		carbamazepine
rifampin	phenobarbital	phenobarbital		phenobarbital
hydrocarbons from	rifampin	rifampin		phenytoin
smoking				rifabutin
				rifampin
				ritonavir
				St. John's-wort

Source. Adapted and prepared with consultation from David A. Flockhart, M.D., Ph.D. (2001).

1997). Available data regarding individual enzymes and ethnic differences in the proportion of individuals who are poor metabolizers are summarized below (Nemeroff et al. 1996; Richelson 1997). Laboratory methods to identify slow metabolizers by genotyping may soon be clinically available for the CYP2D6 and CYP2C19 enzymes.

CYP1A2. The CYP1A2 enzyme is involved in the metabolism of clozapine, tacrine, haloperidol, olanzapine, propranolol, fluvoxamine, and imipramine, in addition to important nonpsychotropic drugs, procarcinogens, and promutagens. In a minority of Caucasians, African Americans, and Asians, this enzyme is deficient or has low activity (slow metabolizers) (Richelson 1997). CYP1A2 activity declines with aging and is very significantly inhibited by the selective serotonin reuptake inhibitor (SSRI) fluvoxamine (Ereshefsky et al. 1996). Known inducers include carbamazepine, rifampin, and hydrocarbons inhaled in cigarette smoke.

CYP2C19. In 18%–23% of Asians, 3%–5% of Caucasians, and 2% of African Americans, the CYP2C19 enzyme is deficient or has low activity (Richelson 1997).

CYP2C9. The CYP2C9 enzyme is important in geriatrics because inhibition by fluoxetine or fluvoxamine (both significant inhibitors) can be associated with increased levels of important active drugs, such as *S*-warfarin, when these drugs are used in combination. Other substrates include nonsteroidal anti-inflammatory drugs, certain angiotensin II antagonists and oral hypoglycemic agents, sulfamethoxazole, and tamoxifen.

CYP2D6. CYP2D6 is a major enzyme that is involved in metabolism of many psychotropic drugs, including analgesics, antidepressants, antipsychotics, mood stabilizers, and β-blockers. For most drugs, oxidative metabolism by CYP2D6 yields less active metabolites; the exceptions include analgesics such as codeine and tramadol, which are administered as pro-drugs and must be metabolized to have the desired pharmacodynamic effect (Poulsen et al. 1996). In 3%–10% of Caucasians and as many as 2% of African Americans and Asians, the CYP2D6 enzyme is deficient or has low activity (Richelson 1997). Psychotropic inhibitors of this enzyme include paroxetine, fluoxetine, sertraline, and fluvoxamine (strength of inhibition: paroxetine > fluoxetine >> sertraline > fluvoxamine). Inducers include carbamazepine and phenytoin. Available data suggest that CYP2D6 activity does not decline with normal aging (Ereshefsky et al. 1996), although mutations giving rise to the slow metabolizer phenotype have been associated with Parkinson's disease (Smith et al. 1992) and dementia with Lewy bodies.

CYP3A. Members of the CYP3A subfamily are the most abundant of the CYP enzymes and are important in the metabolism of a large and diverse group of drugs, both psychotropic and nonpsychotropic. These enzymes are expressed in both the intestinal wall and the liver. Psychotropic substrates include antidepressants, antipsychotics, and sedative-hypnotics. Significant inhibitors include antiretroviral agents, antifungal agents, certain antibiotics, and grapefruit juice. Among psychotropic agents, inhibitors include nefazodone, fluvoxamine, and, to a lesser extent, fluoxetine. Certain of the antihistamine substrates for this enzyme (including terfenadine and astemizole) and the gastric motility drug cisapride are highly cardiotoxic at high serum levels, causing torsades de pointes tachycardia when their metabolism by CYP3A4 is inhibited; all three drugs have now been withdrawn from the U.S. market. Inducers of CYP3A4 include carbamazepine, rifampin, phenytoin, St.-John's-wort, phenobarbital, steroids such as dexamethasone, chronic ethanol consumption, and hydrocarbons inhaled in cigarette smoke. Clearance of drugs metabolized primarily by CYP3A appears to decrease with aging (Pollock 1998).

Phase II Processes

In contrast to the phase I metabolic processes, phase II processes of conjugation (also known as *glucuronidation*), acetylation, and methylation are unaffected by normal aging (Greenblatt et al. 1986; Hammerlein et al. 1998), although they may be affected by malnutrition and extreme old age (Pollock 1998). Medications metabolized primarily through conjugation, such as lorazepam and oxazepam among benzodiazepines, are thus theoretically preferred agents in the elderly population.

Protein Binding

Serum albumin levels are often in the low or low-normal range in elderly patients. For protein-bound drugs, this lower albumin level affects the free fraction (percent bound vs. unbound) but does not affect free drug concentration, as shown in Figure 1–2. Decreased protein binding does not affect the amount of "active" drug (Greenblatt et al. 1982a); unbound drug is also available for distribution, metabolism, and excretion (Greenblatt et al. 1986). Change in protein binding does, however, affect interpretation of total drug concentrations. In general, where the free fraction of a drug is high because of lowered albumin levels, the measured concentration of the drug will underestimate the amount of drug acting on the target organ. This is because the laboratory measurement is of total drug concentration rather than free drug concentration, unless the latter is specifically reported as such (Greenblatt et al. 1982a). In other words, when albumin levels are low, it is of potential concern that the patient could develop toxic symptoms at apparently "therapeutic" drug levels. Aside from this, altered protein binding is not generally an overriding clinical concern in the elderly population.

Clearance

Clearance is the volume of blood per unit of time from which a drug is removed from the systemic circulation by hepatic metabolism and renal excretion, measured in units of cc/minute. Clearance is the most significant physiological determinant of steady-state plasma concentration (von Moltke et al. 1995) and is inversely related to that quantity, as follows:

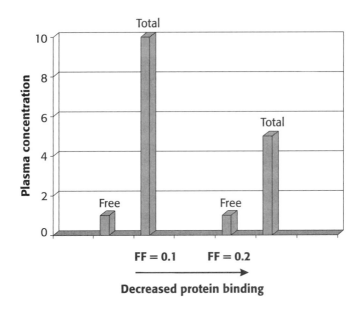

Figure 1–2. Effect of changes in protein binding on free fraction, total concentration, and free drug concentration.
Note that free drug concentration is not affected.
Source. Reprinted from von Moltke LL, Greenblatt DJ, Harmatz JS, et al.: "Psychotropic Drug Metabolism in Old Age: Principles and Problems of Assessment," in *Psychopharmacology: The Fourth Generation of Progress.* Edited by Bloom FE, Kupfer DJ. New York, Raven, 1995, pp. 1461–1469. Copyright 1995, Lippincott Williams & Wilkins. Used with permission.

concentration at steady state = dosing rate/clearance

Aging is associated with reduced clearance of many drugs because of declines in glomerular filtration rate, hepatic blood flow, and hepatic metabolism, among other factors (Greenblatt et al. 1982b). Reduced clearance results in increased steady-state concentration, with enhanced therapeutic effects as well as toxicity. Reduced clearance can be offset by a decrease in dosing rate, in which smaller doses and/or longer intervals are used such that the total dose per unit time is lower (Greenblatt et al. 1982b). Reduced clearance is a major physiological reason for the "start low and go slow" maxim in geriatric psychopharmacology. For drugs cleared partly or entirely by renal excretion of intact drug, clearance declines with age in proportion to the decline in glomerular filtration rate (GFR) (Greenblatt et al. 1982b). This applies to lithium as well as hydroxylated metabolites of various drugs, some of which are pharmacologically active, such as hydroxy-nortriptyline, hydroxy-bupropion, hydroxy-venlafaxine, and hydroxy-risperidone (Pollock 1998). A mean 35% reduction in GFR in elderly patients compared with younger patients has been reported (Rowe et al. 1976). This finding is not universal, however; as many as one-third of individuals show no decline in GFR with aging (Rowe et al. 1976). Because of this heterogeneity, dosing adjustments for reduced GFR are based on the individual patient's creatinine clearance. Ideally, this clearance is measured by a timed urine collection. When a timed urine collection is not feasible, creatinine clearance (CC, in mL/min) can be roughly calculated as follows:

$$CC = [(140 - age) \times weight\ (kg)]/72 \times serum\ creatinine\ level\ (mg/dL)$$

For *females,* the resulting value is multiplied by a correction factor of 0.85.

The "Drug Summary" sections of this handbook note available information on dosage adjustments required for patients with reduced creatinine clearance.

Drug Half-Life

Drug half-life is related to clearance as follows:

$$half\text{-}life = (0.693 \times volume\ of\ distribution)/clearance$$

Note that half-life is dependent on both volume of distribution and clearance, either one of which could be significantly affected by aging (von Moltke et al. 1995). As a hybrid variable, half-life is less useful than clearance itself in pharmacokinetic research. It is discussed here because it has clinical utility in calculating the time to steady state and the time to washout of a drug. Steady state is reached in four to five half-lives for a given drug. During titration, time to steady state determines how soon the clinician can increase or decrease the dose. On discontinuation of a drug, it takes four to five half-lives for the drug to wash out. Since clearance is reduced in the elderly, the half-life of many psychotropic drugs is increased. From the equation above, it can also be seen that half-life for lipophilic drugs would be further increased because of an increased volume of distribution with aging.

As noted in the drug summary sections of this handbook, half-lives vary considerably among drugs. In general, drugs with short half-lives can be associated with between-dose withdrawal symptoms, and use of these agents can be problematic if doses are missed. On the other hand, and much more important for elderly patients, drugs with long half-lives can accumulate over time, and this accumulation can lead to toxic effects. Such accumulation could occur, for example, with amitriptyline, chlordiazepoxide, or diazepam when used in elderly patients.

Pharmacodynamics and Aging

Compared with pharmacokinetics, the pharmacodynamic changes of aging—the effects of aging on the body's response to drugs—have been less well investigated. Increased pharmacodynamic sensitivity to drugs with aging has been postulated but not conclusively demonstrated. In general, pharmacodynamic response is a function of neuronal receptor number and affinity, signal transduction, cellular response, and homeostatic regulation (Tumer et al. 1992). Reduced density of muscarinic, μ opioid, and dopamine$_2$ (D$_2$) receptors has been noted as a concomitant of aging (Hammerlein et al. 1998; Pollock 1998). The ability to up-regulate or down-regulate postsynaptic receptors may also decrease with aging (Salzman 1998). Most enzyme activities are reduced with aging, except for monoamine oxidase B activity, which is increased. The functional results of these changes are likely to be significant but at this time are poorly characterized.

The Practice of Geriatric Psychopharmacology

Considering the interplay of physical disease and psychiatric dysfunction in elderly patients, as well as the effects of nonpsychotropic medications on cognitive, emotional, and motor functions, it is particularly important that a medical history and examination be conducted before a psychotropic agent is prescribed in this population. Table 1–2 lists recommended routine screening procedures for this purpose (Thompson et al. 1983a, 1983b). Evaluation of cognitive function is crucial and should precede any effort to obtain informed consent for treatment, since substituted judgment may be required. Whenever possible, nonpharmacological measures such as supportive or educative psychotherapy and environmental modification should be used, and other somatic treatments, such as ECT, should be considered, so that polypharmacy is minimized.

Maximizing Therapeutic Effects

In geriatric psychopharmacology, as in general psychopharmacology, a major reason for treatment nonresponse is incorrect diagnosis. In geriatrics, however, the risk of incorrect diagnosis is increased by the presence of comorbid physical conditions and the use of other prescribed medications. Partial treatment also confounds diagnosis. In addition to taking a careful longitudinal history and corroborating that history (e.g., by speaking with family members), it is important to obtain a medication-free baseline whenever possible. The patient should be detoxified from alcohol and other nonprescribed drugs. If diagnostic uncertainty remains (as it often does), diagnostic hypotheses can be formulated and tested one at a time, with use of indicated treatments.

The categorical approach of DSM to psychiatric diagnosis has, for the most part, been applied successfully to geriatrics, but

Table 1–2. Recommended routine screening procedures for psychotropic use in elderly patients

History

Is a medical illness causing the "psychiatric" symptoms?

Is a drug the patient is currently taking causing the psychiatric symptoms?

Has the patient had these or other psychiatric symptoms in the past?

If so, what was the diagnosis and what medication, if any, was therapeutically effective? What side effects, if any, developed?

Physical examination

Is there evidence of neurological, renal, hepatic, or other medical disease that would further increase the patient's risk for side effects?

Establish baseline function: orthostatic vital signs.

Mental status

Is there a psychiatric illness of recent onset?

Is there evidence of dementia or delirium?

Laboratory studies

Is there evidence of decreased hepatic synthesizing function (i.e., decreased serum albumin) or decreased renal function (i.e., decreased creatinine clearance)?

Is there evidence from laboratory evaluation that a medical illness is causing the "psychiatric" symptoms?

Establish baseline function: CBC with platelets, electrolytes, TSH, cholesterol, triglycerides, ECG.

Drug interactions

What adverse drug interactions might develop if the psychotropic drug were added to medications the patient is currently taking?

Note. CBC = complete blood cell count; ECG = electrocardiogram; TSH = thyroid-stimulating hormone.
Source. Adapted with permission from Thompson TL, Moran MG, Nies AS: "Psychotropic Drug Use in the Elderly, Part 1." *New England Journal of Medicine* 308: 134–138, 1983a. Copyright 1983, Massachusetts Medical Society. Adapted 2001. All rights reserved.

it is often true that elderly patients present with a forme fruste of a disease. For example, patients with dementia often present with symptoms of major depression that do not meet the full criteria for a major depressive episode. Whether all such patients should be treated for depression is the subject of some debate.

Setting up a clear treatment plan can help resolve some of these uncertainties. First, target symptoms are identified. Whenever possible, objective ratings of effect are used, with use of standardized scales with published normative data. An initial dose and titration schedule are selected, as are the frequency of monitoring, target dose or target serum level of medication, and expected stop date. For reasons noted previously, medications are administered to elderly patients in smaller initial doses, with smaller dosing increments, on a more slowly titrating schedule than for younger patients. For drugs prescribed "as needed" (prn), clear guidance regarding target symptoms must be provided, and in many cases administration should be supervised or monitored by someone other than the patient.

Choice of drug is influenced by several factors, including comorbid medical or neurological diagnoses, hypothesized neurotransmitter deficits, expected side-effect profile, and prior positive response to a drug. Interactions with existing medications must be considered. As part of routine screening (discussed earlier), evidence of hepatic dysfunction, renal dysfunction, or a blood dyscrasia (e.g., leukopenia) is sought. Creatinine clearance is measured or calculated according to the formula described earlier.

A second important reason for treatment nonresponse is inadequacy of the drug trial. An *adequate* drug trial is defined as a sufficient amount of drug taken for a sufficient period of time. What constitutes sufficient time varies widely among drugs and classes. For pharmacokinetic reasons such as increased half-life of drugs (discussed earlier), sufficient time periods to observe responses in elderly patients are often much longer than those for younger patients. For many drugs in current use, sufficient amount can be confirmed by serum drug levels. In obtaining a drug level, optimal sampling time is the period just before a regular dose is administered ("trough level"), after a steady state at that dose has been achieved.

The value of drug level monitoring for adequacy of a drug trial is limited when the "therapeutic range" of the drug has not been established or when the drug's active metabolites are not assayed. Aside from confirming adequacy, however, drug levels are sometimes obtained to confirm suspected noncompliance (looking for a negligible detectable level) or toxicity (looking for a level an order of magnitude or more above the laboratory reference value). Theoretically, the level of any drug could be determined for these latter two purposes, limited only by the laboratory's ingenuity in generating reference values. When drug level is being considered as an explanation for clinical toxicity in geriatric patients, however, it is worth remembering that, in some cases, these patients can develop drug toxicity even at apparently "therapeutic" levels.

A basic rule in geriatric psychopharmacology is to "do one thing at a time." This applies particularly to nonurgent situations; in these cases, monotherapy is used as far as possible before changes or additions are made. In more urgent situations, such as admission of a delirious patient who is taking multiple psychotropic medications or treatment of a depressed patient with psychotic features, it is often true that several drugs are withheld or started simultaneously.

The treatment plan set up initially can provide needed inertia to maintain the course of a treatment trial despite the small setbacks that invariably occur. During the response waiting period, periodic determinations of partial versus no response are made in order to decide whether the trial should be continued. For example, it would be unwise to maintain a patient with major depression on sertraline for 12 weeks if no response was seen by 6 weeks at a dose of 100–150 mg daily.

Improving Compliance

Medication noncompliance is a problem that may be seriously underestimated by clinicians who prescribe medications for geriatric patients. The risk of noncompliance increases dramatically with number of prescribed medications, number of doses per day, and increasing cognitive and physical disability (Corlett 1996; Ostrom et al. 1985). Factors contributing to noncompliance in elderly patients include lack of information about how to take medication, lack of understanding about the importance of medications in managing disease symptoms, irrational fears about side effects, actual experience of side effects (particularly unexpected ones), forgetfulness, and physical incapacity (Corlett 1996).

In improving compliance, collaboration between the doctor and elderly patient as well as the caregiver is critical (Morrow et al. 1996). It is often a good idea to ask the patient or caregiver to repeat oral instructions to ascertain that they have been understood. It is always necessary as well to provide written information and instructions (Newell et al. 1999).

Simplifying the treatment plan has perhaps the greatest effect on compliance. Whenever possible, use once-daily dosing at bedtime. For medications that must be taken more often, specify actual times the drugs are to be taken that the patient finds acceptable. Try to avoid varying schedules such as every-other-day regimens. Memory aids such as pillboxes used to organize medications to be taken at particular times are well accepted by elderly patients and are essential for those with more complicated regimens. Calendar-style written medication schedules are also helpful. Cuing devices such as wristwatch or pillbox alarms that remind patients of medication times are rated highly by some patients.

Physical incapacities are particularly important to note in elderly patients who self-administer medications (Thwaites 1999). For those with disabling conditions such as arthritis, nonchildproof caps may be required. For those with visual deficits, large-print labels may be needed. For those who have trouble swallowing pills, consideration can be given to use of available liquid preparations or sprinkles.

Minimizing Adverse Effects

For the pharmacokinetic and pharmacodynamic reasons noted earlier in this chapter, effective doses of medications for geriatric patients are often much lower than those for younger patients— on the order of one-third to one-half the "usual" dose. Keeping medication at the lowest effective dose is the single most important step in minimizing side effects for geriatric patients.

Another variable that can be manipulated to minimize adverse effects is that of between-dose fluctuation in drug level. Drug A given 10 mg once daily has a higher peak and lower trough level than the same drug given 5 mg twice daily, despite yielding the same average steady-state concentration. Since peak levels can be associated with symptoms of toxicity, dividing the dose often has the effect of reducing toxic effects. The trade-off in doing so is that the potential for noncompliance probably increases.

As noted earlier, monodrug therapy is preferred to polydrug therapy in treating conditions responsive to one drug. Effective treatment of many geriatric patients, however, requires informed polypharmacy. For this reason, it is essential that geriatric psychopharmacologists become knowledgeable about drug interactions in addition to adverse drug effects. Interacting drugs should be avoided if possible, but if it is not possible to do so, the drugs should be administered as far apart in time as feasible. For medications with particularly dangerous potential interactions, such as monoamine oxidase inhibitors, it is recommended that patients wear identification bracelets and/or carry cards warning against the dangers of administering drugs such as meperidine (Demerol) or pressor amines (Jenike 1989).

It is often true that bad outcomes with medication can be minimized if developing side effects are detected early. For this reason, it is critically important that patients and their families and caregivers are fully educated as to signs of potentially serious reactions as well as expectable nuisance side effects. In addition, in this population, there should be a low threshold for obtaining tests such as electrocardiograms to monitor cardiac side effects.

Containing Costs

Medication cost is cited as the reason for noncompliance by a significant number of elderly patients (Col et al. 1990), particularly those with restrictive drug plans who have limited, fixed incomes. Creative solutions—for example, weekly dosing of medications such as the long-acting SSRI antidepressant fluoxetine or use of a pill cutter to generate donepezil 5-mg doses from 10-mg tablets—must be tailored to the individual patient. Informed prescribing of generic drugs may introduce huge cost savings to the patient, but newer drugs with more benign side-effect profiles may have much higher patient acceptance and compliance rates. For reasons such as these, it is critical that prescribing clinicians be fully acquainted with the facts about psychotropic medications derived from systematic, controlled studies rather than adhering to advertising propaganda or bowing to ill-conceived regulatory measures.

Summary Guidelines:
The Practice of Geriatric Psychopharmacology

- Clarify diagnosis.

- Obtain a drug-free baseline, if possible.

- Identify target symptoms.

- Use objective ratings of effect.

- Use doses and titration schedules recommended for geriatrics.

- Make only one medication change at a time, if possible.

- Use monotherapy as far as possible.

- Simplify instructions to the patient.

- Give instructions in writing.

- Use pillboxes and other compliance aids.

- Monitor closely for changes in vital signs, bowel and bladder function, and vision or for development of abnormal limb or mouth movements.

- Ask explicitly about relevant side effects.

- Reassess the need for the drug at regular intervals.

- Obtain drug levels when indicated.

- Document adequacy of all drug trials.

Chapter Summary

- With aging, there tends to be an increase in fat stores and a decrease in lean body mass, resulting in a larger volume of distribution for lipophilic (fat-soluble) drugs, including almost all psychotropic agents.

- For lipophilic drugs such as diazepam, use in elderly patients is characterized by brief duration of effect on initial dosing but long life in the system; with repeated dosing, the potential exists for considerable accumulation in the system.

- Aging is associated with significant decreases in the rate and extent of metabolic processes of oxidation and demethylation (but not of synthetic processes such as glucuronidation).

- Aging is associated with reduced clearance of many drugs because of declines in glomerular filtration rate and hepatic blood flow, among other factors.

- Reduced drug clearance results in increased steady-state drug concentration.

- Since clearance is reduced in elderly persons, the half-lives of many psychotropic drugs are increased.

- Drugs with long half-lives can accumulate over time, and this accumulation can lead to toxic effects.

- Reduced clearance in elderly patients can be offset by use of smaller doses and/or longer dosing intervals, resulting in less drug administered per unit time.

- Altered protein binding with aging rarely has important clinical effects, although it can affect interpretation of drug levels.

References

Bailey DG, Arnold JMO, Spence JD: Grapefruit juice and drugs: how significant is the interaction? Clin Pharmacokinet 26:91–98, 1994

Col N, Fanale JE, Kronholm P: The role of medication noncompliance and adverse drug reactions in hospitalizations of the elderly. Arch Intern Med 150:841–845, 1990

Corlett AJ: Aids to compliance with medication. BMJ 313:926–929, 1996

Ereshefsky L, Riesenman C, Lam YW: Serotonin selective reuptake inhibitor drug interactions and the cytochrome P450 system. J Clin Psychiatry 57 (8, suppl):17–25, 1996

Greenblatt DJ, Sellers EM, Koch-Weser J: Importance of protein binding for the interpretation of serum or plasma drug concentrations. J Clin Pharmacol 22:259–263, 1982a

Greenblatt DJ, Sellers EM, Shader RI: Drug disposition in old age. N Engl J Med 306:1081–1088, 1982b

Greenblatt DJ, Abernethy DR, Shader RI: Pharmacokinetic aspects of drug therapy in the elderly. Ther Drug Monit 8:249–255, 1986

Hammerlein A, Derendorf H, Lowenthal DT: Pharmacokinetic and pharmacodynamic changes in the elderly. Clin Pharmacokinet 35:49–64, 1998

Jenike MA: Geriatric Psychiatry and Psychopharmacology: A Clinical Approach. St Louis, MO, Mosby Year Book, 1989

Morrow DG, Leirer VO, Andrassy JM, et al: Medication instruction design: younger and older adult schemas for taking medication. Human Factors 38:556–573, 1996

Nemeroff CB, DeVane CL, Pollock BG: Newer antidepressants and the cytochrome P450 system. Am J Psychiatry 153:311–320, 1996

Newell SA, Bowman JA, Cockburn JD: A critical review of interventions to increase compliance with medication-taking, obtaining medication refills, and appointment-keeping in the treatment of cardiovascular disease. Prev Med 29:535–548, 1999

Ostrom JR, Hammarlund ER, Christensen DB, et al: Medication usage in an elderly population. Med Care 23:157–164, 1985

Pollock BG: Psychotropic drugs and the aging patient. Geriatrics 53 (suppl 1):S20–S24, 1998

Poulsen L, Arendt-Nielsen L, Brosen K, et al: The hypoalgesic effect of tramadol in relation to CYP2D6. Clin Pharmacol Ther 60:636–644, 1996

Richelson E: Pharmacokinetic drug interactions of new antidepressants: a review of the effects on the metabolism of other drugs. Mayo Clin Proc 72:835–847, 1997

Rowe JW, Andres R, Tobin JD: Age-adjusted standards for creatinine clearance. Ann Intern Med 84:567–569, 1976

Salzman C: Clinical Geriatric Psychopharmacology, 3rd Edition. Baltimore, MD, Williams & Wilkins, 1998

Smith CAD, Gough AC, Leigh PN, et al: Debrisoquine hydroxylase gene polymorphism and susceptibility to Parkinson's disease. Lancet 339: 1375–1377, 1992

Thompson TL, Moran MG, Nies AS: Psychotropic drug use in the elderly, Part 1. N Engl J Med 308:134–138, 1983a

Thompson TL, Moran MG, Nies AS: Psychotropic drug use in the elderly, Part 2. N Engl J Med 308:194–199, 1983b

Thwaites JH: Practical aspects of drug treatment in elderly patients with mobility problems. Drugs Aging 14:105–114, 1999

Tumer N, Scarpace PJ, Lowenthal DT: Geriatric pharmacology: basic and clinical considerations. Annu Rev Pharmacol Toxicol 32:271–302, 1992

von Moltke LL, Greenblatt DJ, Harmatz JS, et al: Psychotropic drug metabolism in old age: principles and problems of assessment, in Psychopharmacology: The Fourth Generation of Progress. Edited by Bloom FE, Kupfer DJ. New York, Raven, 1995, pp 1461–1469

PART 1

Major Psychotropic Drug Classes

2

Antipsychotics

Patterns of antipsychotic medication use in elderly patients have changed considerably over the past decade. Partly in response to restrictions introduced by the Nursing Home Reform Amendments of the Omnibus Budget Reconciliation Act (OBRA) of 1987, antipsychotic use in institutional settings has decreased. These medications are now used for a narrower range of indications, and lower doses are used along with slower dose titration. For pharmacokinetic and pharmacodynamic reasons discussed in this chapter, there has been a move away from prn (as needed) use. There has been increasing recognition that antipsychotics should not be prescribed chronically for many elders and that periodic reassessment of need is critical. More recently, there has been increased use of newer "atypical" agents, in view of initial reports of their demonstrated superiority to reference "typical" agents, efficacy in both positive and negative symptoms, mood-stabilizing and antidepressant effects, lower relapse rates when used chronically, lower incidence of associated extrapyramidal symptoms

(EPS) and tardive dyskinesia, and the suggestion of a possible association with improvement in cognitive function (Pickar 1995). In fact, most of these claims have yet to be validated for the geriatric population, and although the claims may be valid for clozapine, they may not necessarily be valid for other atypical agents.

Pharmacokinetics

In general, antipsychotics are well absorbed. Absorption may be affected by antacids and histamine$_1$ (H$_1$) receptor blockers such as cimetidine that change gastric pH (Salzman 1998). Bioavailability of most low-potency antipsychotics (chlorpromazine, thioridazine, mesoridazine, clozapine, and quetiapine) is variable, so dosing ranges are wide, and no single "correct" dosage is associated with optimal response. Dosage ranges for most higher-potency agents (haloperidol, risperidone, and olanzapine) are narrower, and titration is therefore more routine. For agents with few active metabolites (e.g., clozapine), serum levels can be used as an approximate gauge of appropriate dosing range for a particular patient.

Antipsychotics are highly lipid soluble. In the average elderly patient, these drugs have a large volume of distribution and slow elimination and achieve high concentrations in the brain. The large volume of distribution also limits the duration of action of a single dose of antipsychotic. Antipsychotics are highly protein bound, mainly to albumin. As noted in Chapter 1, albumin concentration declines with aging, disease, and malnutrition (Salzman 1998). Changes in serum protein concentrations are of concern because they can affect interpretation of laboratory tests that measure serum drug levels, as discussed in Chapter 1 (see "Protein Binding").

Antipsychotics are metabolized primarily in the liver, first undergoing oxidation by enzymes of the cytochrome P450 (CYP) system, then undergoing glucuronidation before being excreted in the urine. Some drugs (e.g., clozapine) undergo demethylation, a type of oxidation reaction that becomes less efficient with aging, resulting in longer times to steady state and to elimination. As noted in Chapter 1, the activities of certain CYP enzymes such as CYP1A2 and CYP3A4 decline with aging, and clearance of substrates such as clozapine is thus decreased (Ereshefsky 1996). In contrast, activity of CYP2D6 is unaffected by aging alone (Pollock and Mulsant 1995) but may be affected by cigarette smoking and CYP2D6 genotype (Pan et al. 1999). Antipsychotics metabolized by each of these enzymes are included in Table 1–1 in Chapter 1.

Clearance of an antipsychotic medication depends on the age of the patient as well as the class of drug (Ereshefsky 1996). The same antipsychotic dose administered to a younger patient and an elderly patient may yield a serum concentration of drug in the older patient that is twice that in the younger patient (Salzman et al. 1995). This is one reason for the "start low and go slow" adage in prescribing drugs to geriatric patients. In general, atypical antipsychotics are associated with smaller clearance decrements with aging than are typical agents (Ereshefsky 1996), so, in general, doses of these newer drugs for elderly patients are more similar to those for younger patients. Moreover, a gender difference may prove to be clinically important; the atypical agents have been found experimentally to be cleared more rapidly in men than in women (Ereshefsky 1996).

Antipsychotic medications are released slowly from lipid storage sites, so when toxic effects develop, they can last for weeks (Salzman 1998). Moreover, measurable antipsychotic drug metabolites may persist in urine as long as 3 months after discontinuation of these drugs (Ereshefsky 1996).

Pharmacodynamics and Mechanism of Action

At the drug-receptor interface, the level of receptor occupancy is an important determinant of therapeutic response as well as of the likelihood of developing side effects. For typical antipsychotics, therapeutic response is associated with a dopamine$_2$ (D$_2$) receptor occupancy threshold of 60%–70% (Heinz et al. 1996). D$_2$ receptor occupancy of 80% or more is associated with extrapyramidal effects, and occupancy as low as 55%–65% is associated with akathisia (Farde et al. 1992). Recent studies using functional neuroimaging techniques have repeatedly demonstrated that low doses of haloperidol are associated with adequate receptor occupancy rates, such that neither outcome nor response time differs from that seen with high doses; for example, in patients treated with haloperidol at a dose of 2 mg daily for 2 weeks, receptor occupancy was shown to be on the order of 70% (Kapur et al. 1996).

Clinically effective doses of clozapine, in contrast to typical agents, are associated with a wide D$_2$ receptor occupancy range between individuals (Heinz et al. 1996; Nordstrom et al. 1995). Moreover, a greater than 80% serotonin$_2$ (5-HT$_2$) receptor occupancy rate has been found for clozapine serum concentrations associated with only 20% D$_2$ occupancy (Nordstrom et al. 1995). Risperidone, olanzapine, quetiapine, and ziprasidone also demonstrate much greater 5-HT$_2$ than D$_2$ affinity. One mechanism thought to underlie atypicality is potent 5-HT$_2$ antagonism coupled with relatively weak D$_2$ antagonism, leading to good efficacy and low potential for extrapyramidal effects (Pickar 1995). Risperidone differs from the other atypical medications in that it shows greater D$_2$ receptor affinity at higher doses; in fact, extrapyramidal effects are seen at doses above 4 mg daily (Kopala et al. 1997).

Typical antipsychotics, in general, have significant effects at dopamine D$_2$ receptors (antipsychotic and motor effects), histamine H$_1$ receptors (sedation and weight gain), α_1-adrenergic receptors (blood pressure effects), and muscarinic M$_1$ receptors (anticholinergic effects). Side-effect profiles of individual agents differ because relative affinities for each of these receptor populations differ. Specific drugs are selected on the basis of side effects as well as the patient's history of response. In the treatment of elderly patients, agents with high affinity for α_1 and M$_1$ receptors are best avoided because of problems with hypotension and anticholinergic side effects, as discussed later in this chapter. Age-related pharmacodynamic changes also occur. With some antipsychotics, therapeutic effects are achieved and toxic effects are seen at lower serum drug levels in older compared with younger patients. With haloperidol, for example, serum levels associated with therapeutic improvement in older schizophrenic patients (0–10.4 ng/mL), and especially older patients with dementia (0.32–1.44 ng/mL) (Lacro et al. 1996), were significantly lower than serum levels associated with therapeutic improvement in younger patients (2–15 ng/mL) (Van Putten et al. 1992).

Drug Interactions

Significant drug interactions involving antipsychotics are shown in Table 2–1. In general, antipsychotic agents appear to have little potential to interfere with the metabolism of other drugs through CYP enzymes, but other drugs may significantly inhibit their metabolism. Perphenazine, being a potent CYP2D6 inhibitor, is an exception to this rule.

A potentially serious interaction of clozapine and benzodiazepines involves cardiovascular and respiratory depression and has been associated with sudden death. Benzodiazepines are best discontinued before clozapine is initiated in elderly patients and added to an existing clozapine regimen only after clozapine titration is complete.

Indications

Antipsychotic medications are appropriately used in the management of various disorders associated with psychotic symptoms such as delusions, ideas of reference, hallucinations, disordered thought, and loss of reality testing. Psychotic disorders that affect the elderly population are listed in Table 2–2.

Table 2–1.   Antipsychotic drug interactions

Antipsychotic	Interacting drug	Potential interaction
All classes	Antacids (e.g., Maalox)	Impaired absorption
	β-Blockers	Increased levels of both
	Ethanol; other CNS depressants	Additive CNS depression
All antipsychotics except clozapine (possibly also olanzapine and quetiapine)	Levodopa	Decreased antiparkinsonian effect because of dopamine receptor blockade
Low-potency antipsychotics (typical and atypical)	Anticholinergic drugs	Additive anticholinergic effects
Typical antipsychotics	Lithium	Neurotoxicity; increased extrapyramidal effects
Clozapine	Benzodiazepines	Syncope and respiratory arrest
	Carbamazepine	Increased risk of agranulocytosis; ataxia
	CYP1A2, CYP2D6, and CYP3A4 inhibitors	Increased clozapine level
	CYP1A2 and CYP3A4 inducers	Decreased clozapine level

Table 2–1. Antipsychotic drug interactions *(continued)*

Antipsychotic	Interacting drug	Potential interaction
Olanzapine	CYP1A2 and CYP2D6 inhibitors	Increased olanzapine level
	CYP1A2 inducers	Decreased olanzapine level
Pimozide	CYP3A4 inhibitors	Increased pimozide level
	CYP3A4 inducers	Decreased pimozide level
Quetiapine	CYP3A4 inhibitors	Increased quetiapine level
	CYP3A4 inducers	Decreased quetiapine level
Risperidone	CYP2D6 inhibitors	Increased risperidone level

Source. Adapted from Pies 1998.

Table 2–2.   Psychotic disorders affecting the elderly

Delirium

Dementia with psychotic symptoms[a]

Depression with psychotic symptoms

Mania

Schizophrenia (including brief reactive psychosis and schizophreniform disorder)

Schizoaffective disorder

Delusional disorder

Secondary psychotic states (e.g., alcohol/drug intoxication or withdrawal, hyperthyroidism, cerebrovascular disease)

[a]In patients with dementia with Lewy bodies, use of antipsychotics other than clozapine (and possibly other atypical agents) may be associated with acute exacerbation of motor symptoms, delirium, and episodes of unresponsiveness.

The use of typical antipsychotic medications to treat nonpsychotic behavioral disturbances in the context of dementia in elderly patients is controversial. Specific behavioral problems for which antipsychotics have been tried include "agitation," wandering, irritability, repetitive vocalization, belligerence, insomnia, and aggression. On the one hand, considerable anecdotal experience and several controlled studies have demonstrated that typical antipsychotics have at best only modest efficacy in treating nonpsychotic disruptive behaviors, and this efficacy is largely attributable to their sedative effects (Coccaro et al. 1990; Schneider et al. 1990). Moreover, since tolerance develops to sedative effects, doses are escalated to maintain control of symptoms, with concomitant increased risk of side effects. On the other hand, these agents continue to be widely used for treatment of these behaviors, and they do have a long track record of efficacy, albeit a modest one. Unlike typical agents, atypical antipsychotics have mood-stabilizing properties that make them more likely to be efficacious in treating nonpsychotic "agitation" in dementia. A randomized, controlled trial of risperidone among elderly patients with dementia showed that a dose of 1 mg daily was optimal in controlling aggressive behavior while minimizing extrapyramidal effects (Katz et al. 1999). Other medications used in the treatment of disruptive behavior in the context of dementia are discussed in Chapter 8.

Efficacy

With treatment, symptoms of schizophrenia typically remit in a particular order: acute agitation first; then hallucinations, delusions, and thought disorder; and then, much later, functional improvement with improvement in negative symptoms. Whether this order of symptom remission also applies to other psychotic disorders such as psychotic depression is not clear. Rate of response is said to mirror rate of onset, such that more acute syndromes resolve more quickly. Our experience with the atypical agents suggests that risperidone has a faster onset of action than other atypical antipsychotics.

Clozapine, as the prototypical atypical antipsychotic, has set a new standard of efficacy, ameliorating not only positive symptoms but also negative symptoms, abnormal movements, and certain cognitive impairments (Jann 1991; Jibson and Tandon 1998; Pickar 1995). Clozapine has been shown to be superior to chlorpromazine in long-term treatment and in cases of treatment resistance. Olanzapine and risperidone have been shown in preliminary studies to be more effective in general than haloperidol, as gauged by improvement in scores on the Brief Psychiatric Rating Scale and the Positive and Negative Syndromes Scale (Marder et al. 1997). Risperidone has been found to be equivalent in efficacy to clozapine in a nongeriatric sample of patients with treatment-resistant schizophrenia (Bondolfi et al. 1998).

Clinical Use

Choice of Antipsychotic

Antipsychotic formulations and strengths are listed in Table 2–3. The specific choice of an antipsychotic depends on several factors:

Table 2–3. Antipsychotic formulations and strengths

Generic name	Trade name	Relative potency	Tablets (mg)	Capsules (mg)	SR forms (mg)	Liquid concentrate	Liquid suspension or elixir	Syrup	Injectable form
Typical antipsychotics									
chlorpromazine[a]	Thorazine	100	10, 25, 50, 100, 200		30, 75, 150, 200, 300	30 mg/mL, 100 mg/mL		10 mg/ 5 mL	10 mg/mL, 25 mg/mL
droperidol	Inapsine	1							2.5 mg/mL
fluphenazine	Prolixin	2	1, 2.5, 5, 10			5 mg/mL	0.5 mg/mL, 2.5 mg/5 mL		2.5 mg/mL
fluphenazine decanoate	Prolixin Decanoate								25 mg/mL
haloperidol	Haldol	2	0.5, 1, 2, 5, 10, 20			2 mg/mL			5 mg/mL
haloperidol decanoate	Haldol Decanoate								50 mg/mL, 100 mg/ mL

Table 2–3. Antipsychotic formulations and strengths (*continued*)

						Available formulations			
							Liquid		
Generic name	Trade name	Relative potency	Tablets (mg)	Capsules (mg)	SR forms (mg)	Liquid concentrate	suspension or elixir	Syrup	Injectable form
loxapine	Loxitane	10		5, 10, 25, 50		25 mg/mL			50 mg/mL
mesoridazine	Serentil	50	10, 25, 50, 100			25 mg/mL			25 mg/mL
molindone	Moban	10	5, 10, 25, 50, 100			20 mg/mL			
perphenazine	Trilafon	8	2, 4, 8, 16			16 mg/5 mL			5 mg/mL
pimozide	Orap	1	1, 2						
thioridazine	Mellaril	95	10, 15, 25, 50, 100, 150, 200			30 mg/mL, 100 mg/mL	5 mg/mL, 20 mg/mL		
thiothixene	Navane	5		1, 2, 5, 10, 20		5 mg/mL			2 mg/mL, 5 mg/mL
trifluoperazine	Stelazine	5	1, 2, 5, 10			10 mg/mL			2 mg/mL

Table 2–3.   Antipsychotic formulations and strengths (*continued*)

Generic name	Trade name	Relative potency	Tablets (mg)	Capsules (mg)	SR forms (mg)	Liquid concentrate	Liquid suspension or elixir	Syrup	Injectable form
Atypical antipsychotics									
clozapine	Clozaril	100	25, 100						
olanzapine	Zyprexa	5	2.5, 5, 7.5, 10, 15						
	Zyprexa Zydis	5	5, 10, 15, 20						
quetiapine	Seroquel	100	25, 100, 200						
risperidone	Risperdal	1–2	0.25, 0.5, 1, 2, 3, 4			1 mg/mL			
ziprasidone	Geodon			20, 40, 60, 80					

aAlso available in suppository form (25 and 100 mg).

how acutely a response is needed, whether the patient has a medical condition limiting the use of a particular agent, whether the patient's illness has demonstrated treatment refractoriness, whether primarily positive or positive and negative symptoms are targeted, and whether chronic therapy is anticipated. In addition, prior response to a particular agent is noted, and potential compliance problems are considered in cases in which depot antipsychotics may be used.

The drug of choice for emergency sedation of the psychotic elderly patient in settings such as the intensive care unit is the butyrophenone antipsychotic haloperidol, administered intravenously. This medication has a rapid onset of action and, compared with other available drugs, has little autonomic and cardiovascular effect, although prolongation of the corrected QT interval (QT_c) on the electrocardiogram (ECG) has been noted. Droperidol, which has also been recommended in this context, has more of an effect on the QT_c interval than haloperidol (Reilly et al. 2000). More detailed information on the dosage and administration of these medications can be found later in this chapter (see "Treatment of Selected Syndromes and Disorders With Antipsychotics" and "Specific Drugs" sections).

For less emergent situations when intravenous access is not available, haloperidol can be administered intramuscularly or an oral liquid formulation can be used. In general, atypical antipsychotics are not useful for emergency sedation because of their slow onset of action and, until recently, the unavailability of parenteral formulations. Possible exceptions to this include liquid risperidone and intramuscular and sublingual olanzapine. Clinical experience in the geriatric population at this point is insufficient to recommend these options.

In nonemergency situations, atypical antipsychotics are becoming the treatments of choice for elderly patients because of their efficacy as well as superior side-effect profiles. Atypical agents must be used with caution in the geriatric population because of associated orthostatic hypotension, sedation, impaired glucose tolerance and emergence of diabetes mellitus, and other drug-specific side effects such as significant anticholinergic effects with clozapine and possibly olanzapine. With regard to clozapine in particular, overshadowing these other concerns is the risk of agranulocytosis. Agranulocytosis can occur even with scrupulous white blood cell monitoring and can, in rare cases, be fatal. For this reason, despite its proven superiority, clozapine is still reserved for patients who do not respond to or do not tolerate other antipsychotic medications; it is also used for the specific purpose of treating tardive dyskinesia or other movement disorders in the context of psychotic illness (Small et al. 1987). Other specific recommendations for antipsychotic use in selected patient populations are shown in Table 2–4.

Table 2–4. Antipsychotic agents: specific recommendations for selected patient groups

Medical condition	Recommendation
Cardiovascular	
Recent myocardial infarction	Haloperidol usually safe
Chronic congestive heart failure	Haloperidol usually safe
Arrhythmia/QT_c prolongation	Avoid pimozide, thioridazine, mesoridazine
Orthostatic hypotension	Avoid low-potency agents, risperidone
Diabetes (type 1 or 2)	Avoid clozapine and olanzapine
Glaucoma (closed-angle)	Avoid highly anticholinergic agents (thioridazine, clozapine)
Hepatic insufficiency	Decrease dosage of any antipsychotic, including atypical agents
Neurological	
Delirium	Avoid highly anticholinergic agents; use haloperidol, droperidol
Dementia (dementia of the Alzheimer's type, vascular dementia)	Avoid highly anticholinergic agents; use haloperidol, risperidone, quetiapine

Table 2–4. Antipsychotic agents: specific recommendations for selected patient groups *(continued)*

Medical condition	Recommendation
Neurological *(continued)*	
Dementia with Lewy bodies	Avoid antipsychotics if possible; consider low-dose clozapine, quetiapine, olanzapine, ziprasidone
Parkinson's disease or drug-induced parkinsonism	Avoid high-potency agents; consider low-dose clozapine, quetiapine, olanzapine, ziprasidone
Seizures	Consider haloperidol or molindone; if clozapine is used, co-administer anticonvulsant (valproate)
Other	
Tardive dyskinesia	Use clozapine, olanzapine, quetiapine, ziprasidone
Obesity	Consider molindone
Prostatic hypertrophy	Avoid highly anticholinergic agents
Renal insufficiency	Antipsychotic dosage adjustment generally not required
Suicidality	Avoid thioridazine, mesoridazine, pimozide

As noted earlier, clinical experience with atypical antipsychotic agents to date suggests that at least certain atypical agents do not work as quickly as typical agents in acutely psychotic patients; it may take 3 weeks to several months to observe meaningful clinical effects in elderly patients. For this reason, typical agents are often used with the acutely psychotic elder to "lead in" to atypical use, with overlap and then discontinuation of the typical medication (Stahl 1999). In our experience, elderly patients without significant medical comorbidity can tolerate initiation of both agents simultaneously.

Although it is true that atypical agents cost more than typical agents, medication cost is actually only a small fraction of the total cost of patient care. A number of published studies have now clearly demonstrated cost savings in overall patient care with clozapine versus haloperidol and olanzapine versus haloperidol. These savings are attributed to decreased rates of hospitalization and decreased use of residential care with the newer agents.

Alternative Formulations

As shown in Table 2–3, most typical antipsychotics are available in several formulations. In terms of speed with which the medication enters the systemic circulation, intravenous formulations are the fastest, followed by short-acting intramuscular, oral liquid, oral capsule, oral tablet, and long-acting (depot) intramuscular. The time to onset of action for oral liquids is approximately the same as that for intramuscularly administered drugs (Ereshefsky 1996). Some side effects (e.g., hypotension) may occur because of too-rapid onset of action; for this reason, oral liquid formulations may be less desirable than oral capsules or tablets for many geriatric patients.

There is no consensus regarding the appropriate use and dosing of decanoate antipsychotics in elderly patients. These agents are convenient and ensure compliance in patients for whom this is an otherwise insurmountable problem, and at least haloperidol decanoate may be associated with a decreased incidence of extrapyramidal effects because of slow release. On the other hand, decanoate antipsychotics are painful when injected and may be erratically absorbed in patients with small muscle mass. In general, they have been understudied in the elderly population. In addition, with fluphenazine decanoate, a significant fraction of the injected dose is released within hours, introducing a greater risk of extrapyramidal effects. Although some recommend against the use of decanoate medications in elders (Salzman 1998), we have found them to be effective and well tolerated in a subset of elderly patients with chronic psychosis and persistent compliance problems.

The equivalent geriatric decanoate dose of a stable oral dose of haloperidol is calculated by multiplying the daily oral dose (mg) by a factor of 10 and administering this dose intramuscularly every 4 weeks. A daily oral dose of 2 mg, for example, could be substituted by 20 mg of haloperidol decanoate given every 4 weeks. Fluphenazine decanoate is usually initiated in geriatric patients at a dose of 6.25 mg (0.25 cc), which is added to the patient's oral regimen. A second dose of 6.25 mg is then given after 2–4 weeks, after which the oral medication is tapered slowly and discontinued. The effective dose (in mg) and dosing interval for fluphenazine decanoate are then determined empirically; intervals range from 2 weeks to 2 months.

Baseline Laboratory Studies

Before treatment with an antipsychotic medication is initiated, the elderly patient should have a white blood cell count (WBC), liver function panel (aspartate transaminase [AST], alanine transaminase [ALT], alkaline phosphatase, and bilirubin), and an ECG (Salzman 1998). For patients being considered for treatment with clozapine or olanzapine, baseline fasting blood sugar and serum triglyceride levels should be obtained (Gaulin et al. 1999; Osser et al. 1999).

Dose and Dose Titration

A general rule for antipsychotic dosing in the elderly patient is that the total daily dose (target dose) is ideally not more than twice the "relative potency" value (shown in Table 2–3), even for acutely psychotic patients. For example, haloperidol is prescribed at dosages of 4 mg daily or less, and olanzapine is prescribed at dosages of 10 mg daily or less, in elderly patients. One exception to this rule is droperidol, which is sometimes used to quell psychotic agitation at relatively higher doses, used with careful monitoring of QT_c interval, blood pressure, and respiratory rate, as discussed later in this chapter (see "Cardiac Conduction Changes"). For all antipsychotics, therapy is initiated at the lowest feasible dosage, and some patients never require more than this minimum. Others do require upward dosage titration, depending on factors such as age (young-old vs. old-old), sex, creatinine clearance, hepatic function, and diagnosis. In general, elderly patients with schizophrenia require higher total daily doses, and those with dementia-related psychotic symptoms require lower doses, of antipsychotics (Lacro et al. 1996).

As a rule, antipsychotics are administered to elderly patients initially in divided doses (twice daily to three times daily). For clozapine, risperidone, quetiapine, and low-potency typical agents, continued divided dosing (usually twice daily) is recommended to minimize problems from side effects such as orthostatic hypotension (Ereshefsky 1996). For olanzapine and high-potency typical antipsychotics, a switch to a single bedtime dose can be made when the targeted total daily dose is reached (Ereshefsky 1996).

Antipsychotic medications are titrated as rapidly as tolerated to target doses presumed to be therapeutic, as detailed in the specific drug summary at the end of this chapter. In practice, initial titration usually proceeds at a rate of one to two dose increases per week. For medications with a wide dosing range (e.g., quetiapine), increases above the initial target dose are made after steady state is attained, to avoid "overshooting" the minimal therapeutic dosage for the individual patient.

PRN Use of Antipsychotics

When antipsychotic medications are used to control psychosis, standing rather than prn doses are used because consistent levels of drug at the receptor site are required for antipsychotic effect. Drugs with fast onset of action, such as risperidone, and many typical antipsychotics can be used prn, in situations such as the following: the prn dose is used 1) to supplement a small standing dose, with the intention of "adding" the total amount (in mg) ingested and subsequently adjusting the standing dose upward; 2) to minimize the amount of drug given, when the intention is to lower the dose; or 3) to manage unexpected behaviors that cannot be managed with other agents. In the last-mentioned case, limits as to how many prn doses can be given apply to patients in long-term care facilities. When antipsychotic medications are used prn, the effect of an individual dose is probably more related to general sedation than to specific antipsychotic effects.

Increasingly, benzodiazepines are coprescribed for psychotic patients requiring prn medication, particularly with the advent of atypical antipsychotics, most of which are not used prn. As noted in Chapter 5 ("Anxiolytic and Sedative-Hypnotic Medications"), however, benzodiazepines are problematic for many elderly patients because of side effects of sedation, cognitive impairment, and gait instability. In addition, the combination of benzodiazepines with clozapine can be dangerous in this population, as noted earlier. In view of these observations, careful consideration should be given to other agents such as trazodone for prn use in elderly patients taking antipsychotics. Although sedating antihistamines such as hydroxyzine (Vistaril) or diphenhydramine (Benadryl) may be safe for occasional one-time use for this purpose, repeated dosing of these medications is associated with serious anticholinergic side effects (including cognitive impairment) in elderly patients.

Monitoring Treatment

In addition to scales used to measure improvement in targeted symptoms, other parameters are monitored to ensure patient safety. Vital signs, including temperature and orthostatic blood pressure and pulse, are taken at least daily during dose titration for inpatients, and orthostatic vital signs are taken at each visit during dose titration for outpatients. Weight is monitored in all antipsychotic-treated patients, particularly those taking the atypical agents clozapine and olanzapine. Assessment for abnormal movements is performed at least monthly during dosage titration. During maintenance treatment, it is a reasonable practice to complete a scale for the assessment of abnormal movements, such as the Abnormal Involuntary Movement Scale (AIMS), every 3–6 months.

For phenothiazines other than clozapine, a WBC should be repeated within the first 2 months of treatment, or sooner if infection develops. For all antipsychotic-treated elderly patients, clinical monitoring for evidence of hepatic dysfunction (e.g., malaise, nausea, jaundice) is crucial; in addition, it is a reasonable but by no means universal practice to check liver function tests every 3–6 months. Clozapine treatment requires more intensive hematological surveillance (see Table 2–5 and guidelines in the specific drug summary on clozapine at the end of this chapter).

Other reasonable recommendations for patients treated with clozapine or olanzapine include fasting blood sugar determination every 6 months and serum triglyceride level determination every 12 months.

Serum Antipsychotic Levels

For any antipsychotic, extreme values reported on serum level measurement may be helpful: a zero level could confirm suspected noncompliance or possibly suggest that a patient might be an ultra-rapid metabolizer; a very high level could confirm suspected toxicity. Most commercial laboratories perform these measurements. For purposes of therapeutic-level monitoring, only drugs with few active metabolites are usefully assayed, and not all of these drugs have been adequately studied. Among antipsychotics, only clozapine, haloperidol, fluphenazine, thiothixene, and perphenazine have established therapeutic ranges, and only haloperidol has a therapeutic range established specifically for elderly patients. For haloperidol decanoate, the same therapeutic range as for the short-acting drug is used, as long as the sample is drawn after steady state has been attained.

Managing Treatment Resistance

As noted in Chapter 1 ("Introduction to Geriatric Psychopharmacology"), apparent treatment resistance can be a function of wrong diagnosis, noncompliance, or inadequacy of a drug trial.

Table 2–5. Leukopenia, granulocytopenia, and agranulocytosis: definitions and suggested clinical management

Problem phase	WBC or absolute neutrophil count (per mm³)	Clinical findings	Treatment plan
Mild leukopenia Mild granulocyto- penia	WBC: 3,000–3,500 ANC: 1,000–1,500	Monitor closely for clinical symptoms, such as lethargy, fever, sore throat, and weakness.	1. Monitor patient closely. 2. Institute twice-weekly WBC tests with differentials. 3. Clozapine (Clozaril) therapy may continue. 4. Treat infections appropriately.
Moderate leukopenia Moderate granulo- cytopenia	WBC: 2,000–3,000 ANC: 1,000–1,500	Monitor closely for clinical symptoms, such as lethargy, fever, sore throat, and weakness.	1. Discontinue clozapine at once and notify CNR. 2. Institute WBC tests with differentials every day until WBC ≥ 3,000/mm³, then twice weekly until WBC ≥ 3,500/mm³. 3. Treat infections appropriately. 4. Clozapine therapy may be reinstituted (with twice-weekly monitoring) when WBC ≥ 3,000/mm³ and ANC ≥ 1,500/mm³. 5. Once WBC ≥ 3,500/mm³, must follow weekly for 6 months without any leukopenia, then biweekly WBC monitoring may be instituted.

Table 2–5. Leukopenia, granulocytopenia, and agranulocytosis: definitions and suggested clinical management (*continued*)

Problem phase	WBC or absolute neutrophil count (per mm³)	Clinical findings	Treatment plan
Severe leukopenia Severe granulocyto-penia	WBC: <2,000 ANC: 500–1,000	Monitor closely for clinical symptoms, such as lethargy, fever, sore throat, and weakness.	1. Discontinue clozapine at once and notify CNR. 2. Consult with a hematologist for current treatment options. 3. Treat infections aggressively. 4. Monitor patient daily until WBC ≥ 3,500/mm³ and ANC ≥ 1,500/mm³ (usually about 2 weeks). 5. Clozapine must *not* be restarted. 6. Perform WBC tests for at least 4 weeks after discontinuation of clozapine.

Table 2–5. Leukopenia, granulocytopenia, and agranulocytosis: definitions and suggested clinical management (*continued*)

Problem phase	WBC or absolute neutrophil count (per mm^3)	Clinical findings	Treatment plan
Agranulocytosis	ANC: <500	Evidence of a local infection (sore throat; skin, nail, or tooth abscess) or systemic infection (fever, lethargy, weakness, malaise) represents a medical emergency.	1. Discontinue clozapine at once and notify CNR. 2. Consult with a hematologist to determine appropriate treatment regimen. 3. Treat infections aggressively. 4. Consider admission for symptomatic agranulocytosis. 5. Consider treating patient with a G-CSF/GM-CSF drug until ANC > 1,000/mm^3. 6. Monitor patient daily until WBC ≥ 3,500/mm^3 and ANC ≥ 1,500/mm^3. 7. Clozapine must *not* be restarted. 8. Perform WBC tests for at least 4 weeks after discontinuation of clozapine.

Note. ANC = absolute neutrophil count; CNR = Clozaril National Registry; G-CSF = granulocyte colony-stimulating factor; GM-CSF = granulocyte-macrophage colony-stimulating factor; WBC = white blood cell count.

Initial management follows a logical sequence of confirming the diagnosis, ascertaining compliance, and adjusting the medication dose. Dosage adjustments can be made on the basis of a drug level or the presence or absence of important side effects, such as EPS in the case of antipsychotics. The patient with a poor therapeutic response to an antipsychotic in the presence of EPS may benefit more from a dosage decrease than a dosage increase.

True treatment resistance, when the patient has failed two adequate antipsychotic trials, may be more prevalent among elderly patients than among younger patients. In general, patients with illnesses that are truly "treatment resistant" should first be switched to an atypical agent other than clozapine, and an adequate dosage of that agent should be maintained for 6–12 weeks (Marder 1996). If there is a response, the trial should be maintained up to 16 weeks. If there is no response to the first atypical medication tried, a trial of another nonclozapine atypical medication should be considered. Again, this trial should be maintained for 6–12 weeks, with an extension up to 16 weeks for a partial response.

If there is still an inadequate response, a trial of clozapine should be considered. This trial should be continued, if possible, for a period of 6–12 months. Alternatively, consideration should be given to adding a typical antipsychotic to the atypical agent, either in an oral formulation or a long-acting intramuscular formulation. In addition, adjunctive therapies such as mood stabilizers could be used to augment a partial response (Marder 1996), as described in Chapter 4 ("Mood Stabilizers").

Patients with dementia that is resistant to antipsychotic medications may be treated using the same general algorithm, but they may show intolerance to high doses of antipsychotics.

Switching Antipsychotics

Increasingly, elderly patients currently undergoing treatment with typical antipsychotic agents are being switched to atypical agents because of better efficacy for negative symptoms and lesser risk of tardive dyskinesia. In addition, clozapine-treated patients may opt to switch to another atypical agent such as risperidone to lessen the risk of agranulocytosis and avoid required blood draws.

In switching from one antipsychotic to another, it is generally safer to taper and discontinue one agent before starting the second. When this is not feasible because of the severity of psychotic symptoms, the second drug can be added to the first, which can then be tapered and discontinued (a strategy known as "cross tapering"). When antipsychotics are co-administered, careful attention should be paid to cardiac conduction and other potential adverse effects. Abrupt (one-step) antipsychotic switching is rarely necessary but, when attempted, is most safely accomplished in an inpatient setting, where the patient can be monitored closely.

In the course of cross tapering to switch from a typical antipsychotic to an atypical antipsychotic, a therapeutic response is sometimes seen that is followed by clinical worsening as the cross tapering proceeds. In this situation, it is difficult to know whether the problem is the decreasing level of the typical agent, the increasing level of the atypical agent, or some interaction. If it is clinically reasonable to do so, it is best to complete the cross tapering to give the second medication an adequate trial as monotherapy. Then the typical agent can be added back, if needed. A substantial minority of patients treated with an atypical antipsychotic apparently require a conventional antipsychotic to "top off" its effects, at least periodically (Stahl 1999). There are no published studies looking at these combinations in elderly patients, so there is little to guide clinical practice in this area.

Adjunctive Treatments

In the context of short-term antipsychotic treatment for acute psychosis in the elderly, co-administration of a benzodiazepine such as lorazepam (Ativan) can reduce the dose of antipsychotic needed. As noted earlier, however, these medications are not without adverse effects in elderly patients, and they are relatively contraindicated for patients taking clozapine. For the "agitated" psychotic patient, trazodone or gabapentin is another good option, and for the more severely psychotic and medically ill patient, electroconvulsive therapy (ECT) may be the best alternative.

In the treatment of chronic psychotic disorders, other interventions assume greater importance: milieu therapy, social and functional skills training, coping skills, and education. Other long-term medication adjuncts include trazodone, lithium, valproate, and other newer anticonvulsants, antidepressants, calcium channel blockers, β-blockers, and psychostimulants (Pies and Dewan 2001).

Discontinuation of Antipsychotics

Elders with schizophrenia are best maintained long term on a stable low dose of antipsychotic, preferably an atypical agent. For those without schizophrenia, periodic attempts to reduce the dosage of antipsychotics are recommended, and even mandated for patients in long-term care facilities. To minimize withdrawal symptoms, dosage reduction should proceed slowly. In our experience, conventional antipsychotics given at the recommended geriatric (low) dosages should be tapered over 2 weeks, at minimum. Clozapine withdrawal is complicated by the drug's anticholinergic and anti-adrenergic activity and by the potential for rebound psychosis, such that the taper is best performed over a minimum of 4 weeks in elderly patients. An only slightly less protracted withdrawal period may apply to thioridazine because of its anticholinergic properties.

Antipsychotic Overdose in Elderly Patients

Many antipsychotic medications are nonlethal when taken alone in overdose. Exceptions include highly anticholinergic agents as well as agents associated with significant prolongation of the QT_c interval at high doses, including droperidol, haloperidol, thioridazine, mesoridazine, and fluphenazine. Antipsychotic drugs are not removed by dialysis. Activated charcoal can decrease absorption of clozapine and other antipsychotics if given within 1 hour of ingestion. In monitored settings such as the emergency room, anticholinergic (M_1 receptor) effects can be reversed with physostigmine 1–2 mg iv or im (Schneider 1993).

Side Effects

In general, high-potency antipsychotics carry a high risk of inducing extrapyramidal effects and a low risk of seizures, whereas low-potency antipsychotics carry the risks of hypotension, sedation, peripheral autonomic effects, anticholinergic effects, and greater risk of seizures. Typical antipsychotics carry a much greater risk of tardive dyskinesia than do atypical agents. Atypical antipsychotics more closely resemble the low-potency typical agents in presenting a low risk of extrapyramidal effects, the exception being risperidone at doses of 4 mg daily or greater (Kopala et al. 1997). Table 2–6 shows the relative severity of selected side effects for various typical and atypical compounds.

Many geriatric psychopharmacologists avoid the use of low-potency agents in elderly patients because cardiac effects, particularly orthostatic hypotension, are more dangerous in this population than are extrapyramidal effects. What this predicts about the future use of individual atypical agents is not yet clear, although the trend clearly favors the use of low doses of atypical agents in geriatric patients. In each case, however, a risk-benefit assessment must be made before proceeding with treatment.

It is important to note that the rate of titration greatly influences the incidence of side effects—hence the recommendation to "start low and go slow" in older patients. Other factors include the rate of absorption and the frequency of dosing. For elderly patients, it is advisable to give small doses, divide doses (at least

Table 2–6.   Relative severity of side effects of antipsychotic drugs

Generic name	Trade name	Side effects[a]			
		Sedation	Extrapyramidal (dopamine receptor) effects	Anticholinergic (M_1 receptor) effects	Orthostasis (α_1-adrenergic receptor)
Typical antipsychotics					
chlorpromazine	Thorazine	+++	+	++ to +++	+++
droperidol	Inapsine	+++	0 to +	0 to +	+++
fluphenazine	Prolixin	+	+++	+	+
haloperidol	Haldol	+	+++	+/–	+
loxapine	Loxitane	++	++	+	++
mesoridazine	Serentil	+++	+	++	++
molindone	Moban	+	++	+	+
perphenazine	Trilafon	+	++	+	++
pimozide	Orap	+	+++	+	+
thioridazine	Mellaril	+++	+	+++	+++
thiothixene	Navane	+	+++	+	+
trifluoperazine	Stelazine	+	+++	+	+

Table 2–6. Relative severity of side effects of antipsychotic drugs (*continued*)

Generic name	Trade name	Sedation	Side effects[a]			
			Extrapyramidal (dopamine receptor) effects	Anticholinergic (M$_1$ receptor) effects	Orthostasis (α_1-adrenergic receptor)
Atypical antipsychotics						
clozapine	Clozaril	+++	+/−	+++	+++
olanzapine	Zyprexa	++	+	+	+
quetiapine	Seroquel	++	+/−	+	++
risperidone	Risperdal	+	++	+	++ to +++
ziprasidone	Geodon	++	+	−	++

[a]+++ = substantial; ++ = moderate; + = mild; +/− = minimal; 0 = none.
Source. Adapted from Pies 1998.

initially), titrate slowly, and avoid oral liquid and short-acting parenteral formulations unless specifically indicated.

Anticholinergic Effects

Peripheral effects of cholinergic receptor blockade include dry mouth, blurred vision, exacerbation of glaucoma, constipation, urinary retention, and tachycardia, all of which are potentially serious in elderly patients. Central effects of cholinergic receptor blockade include drowsiness, irritability, disorientation, impaired memory and other cognitive dysfunction, assaultiveness, and delirium. Patients with dementia characterized by cholinergic hypofunction are likely to be particularly affected. When these symptoms are mistaken for escalating psychosis, the dosage of antipsychotic may be increased, resulting in worsening dysfunction.

Relative anticholinergic effects of various antipsychotic agents are listed in Table 2–6. Among typical agents, droperidol is the least anticholinergic, and thioridazine and its metabolite mesoridazine are the most anticholinergic. Among atypical agents, risperidone and quetiapine are the least anticholinergic, and clozapine is the most anticholinergic.

Cardiovascular Effects

Orthostatic Hypotension

Significant orthostatic hypotension, defined as a drop in systolic blood pressure of more than 20 mm Hg on assuming a sitting or standing position, is associated with α_1-adrenergic receptor antagonism. Relative orthostatic effects of various antipsychotic medications are shown in Table 2–6. Orthostasis is more common in elderly patients, in patients with reduced cardiac output, and in patients taking other α_1-adrenergic receptor blocking medications. The importance of this problem in older patients cannot be overstated. Orthostatic hypotension is associated with falls, myocardial infarction, stroke, and lesser degrees of ischemic brain injury. In most cases, orthostasis develops early in the course of antipsychotic treatment. Since orthostasis is highly dependent on speed of absorption and peak plasma level, it may occur more frequently with parenterally administered or oral liquid formulations.

For patients with baseline orthostasis, antipsychotic medications with low affinity for the α_1 receptor, such as haloperidol, fluphenazine, and olanzapine, are preferred. Standard care for the patient with orthostasis is discussed in Chapter 3 in the context of antidepressants (see "System-Specific Side Effects").

Cardiac Conduction Changes

For all patients with preexisting conduction abnormalities, including anything more than a first-degree atrioventricular block, antipsychotic medication should be used with caution. Droperidol, thioridazine, mesoridazine, perphenazine, and high-dose haloperidol and fluphenazine should be avoided (Reilly et al. 2000). ECG and serum levels of electrolytes (especially potassium) should be monitored regularly. Plasma levels of antipsychotics may be useful in this context but are not as sensitive as the ECG itself in demonstrating cardiotoxicity.

In any patient, high-dose haloperidol or droperidol administered intravenously can be associated with prolongation of the QT_c and, in some cases, torsades de pointes tachycardia. If the baseline QT_c is prolonged, these drugs should be used with caution (Di Salvo and O'Gara 1995; Frye et al. 1995). Prolongation of the QT_c beyond 25% of baseline or to greater than 450 ms may predict the development of torsades and should prompt immediate discontinuation of intravenous haloperidol or droperidol (Di Salvo and O'Gara 1995). The U.S. Food and Drug Administration required labeling changes in 2000 to warn users about significant QT_c prolongation with thioridazine and mesoridazine, also associated with torsades de pointes tachycardia.

Venous Thromboembolism

Rarely, clozapine use is associated with pulmonary embolism and venous thrombosis (Hagg et al. 2000). It may be that this side effect is not dose dependent and that it is more common in men. If venous thromboembolism is suspected, clozapine should be discontinued.

Dermatological Effects

An allergic reaction to antipsychotic medication is usually seen as a pruritic, maculopapular rash affecting the face, neck, upper thorax, and extremities. The rash is seen most often within weeks of initiating therapy but can occur with dose increases. It resolves with discontinuation of the offending agent. If antipsychotic therapy is resumed, a drug from another class should be selected.

Endocrinological Effects

Diabetes Mellitus

Both clozapine and olanzapine are associated with impaired glucose tolerance and the development of diabetes mellitus (Henderson et al. 2000; Wirshing et al. 1998), which is at least partly independent of weight gain (Henderson et al. 2000). In patients with preexisting type 1 diabetes, these agents can introduce severe glucose dysregulation. These drugs should be used with caution in patients at risk for diabetes mellitus by virtue of a positive family history, obesity, or sedentary lifestyle. In elderly patients prescribed clozapine or olanzapine, fasting blood sugar should be checked periodically, as noted earlier. If diabetes does develop, it can usually be controlled with diet, exercise, and oral hypoglycemic agents. Severe glucose dysregulation may necessitate a switch to a different antipsychotic.

Hyperprolactinemia

Typical antipsychotics and risperidone may be associated with increased prolactin secretion, with symptoms of gynecomastia, galactorrhea, and impotence in men. In elderly patients, prolactin elevations may be problematic in patients with prolactin-secreting pituitary tumors and possibly in patients with breast cancer.

Atypical agents other than risperidone do not routinely result in significant elevation in levels of prolactin (Casey 1997).

SIADH

A syndrome of inappropriate antidiuretic hormone secretion (SIADH) can occur with typical as well as atypical antipsychotic treatment, especially in debilitated patients. The resulting hyponatremia may be associated with delirium, disorientation, or memory impairment. SIADH is distinguished from polydipsia (i.e., excessive water intake) by urine osmolality: relatively high urine osmolality is found with SIADH, whereas very low osmolality is found with polydipsia and water intoxication.

Gastrointestinal Effects

Antiemetic Effects

Most typical antipsychotics have antiemetic effects at low doses mediated by an action or actions on the chemoreceptor trigger zone. Typical antipsychotics with these effects include droperidol and all phenothiazines except thioridazine (Theoharides 1996).

Sialorrhea

In some patients, clozapine treatment is complicated by a condition of copiously increased saliva known as *sialorrhea*. Several studies have demonstrated that patients with sialorrhea do not, in fact, have increased saliva flow, but that clozapine interferes with the swallowing reflex, resulting in increased salivary pooling (Pearlman 1994; Rabinowitz et al. 1996). Impaired swallowing combined with sedation puts the patient at risk of aspiration. This problem might not be unique to clozapine; in the experience of the authors, it can be found with risperidone as well. None of the existing treatments is satisfactory for elderly patients; although anticholinergic medications such as trihexyphenidyl (Artane) can decrease saliva flow below baseline, these medications have other undesirable effects in elders. In addition, stimulating the swallowing reflex by chewing gum also has limits in patients with any degree of dysphagia.

Genitourinary Effects

Antipsychotic blockade of α_1-adrenergic receptors can be associated with failure to ejaculate and impotence in treated men (Theoharides 1996). Antipsychotic drugs with high anticholinergic activity can precipitate urinary retention, particularly in male patients with benign prostatic hypertrophy. Urinary incontinence may be a side effect of clozapine or olanzapine therapy, possibly also a function of anti-adrenergic effects. Incontinence has been treated with the adrenergic agonist ephedrine at a dosage of 25 mg po qd or bid. Other agents that have been used in younger patients include oxybutynin and intranasal desmopressin.

Hematological Effects

Decline in WBCs can be seen with typical antipsychotics, particularly low-potency phenothiazines. Agranulocytosis (absolute neutrophil count < $500/mm^3$) is a potentially life-threatening condition associated with clozapine therapy and, much more rarely, with other phenothiazines (chlorpromazine, fluphenazine, perphenazine, thioridazine, and trifluoperazine). The atypical agents risperidone, olanzapine, and quetiapine do not significantly increase agranulocytosis risk (Casey 1997). The risk of agranulocytosis with clozapine and other medications is highest in the first few months of treatment, but it can occur at any time and is not a dose-dependent problem; the overall risk is about 0.5%.

Weekly WBCs are required for the first 6 months of clozapine treatment and for a minimum of 4 weeks after clozapine discontinuation. If cell counts remain acceptable during the first 6 months of treatment (WBC at least $3,000/mm^3$ and absolute neutrophil count at least $1,500/mm^3$), WBC checks can be done every other week thereafter. Other drugs with the potential for bone marrow suppression, including amoxicillin, carbamazepine, captopril, sulfonamides, and PTU, should be avoided in combination with clozapine (McEvoy et al. 2000). Specific recommendations for management of leukopenia and agranulocytosis are shown in Table 2–5.

Hepatic Effects

Increases in serum transaminase levels (AST and ALT) of 1.5–2 times normal levels are common in the first few weeks of treatment with typical as well as atypical antipsychotics (Casey 1997; Fuller et al. 1996). The usual clinical course is a return to normal values (Casey 1997). Higher increases in transaminase levels (3 times normal levels or higher), elevation of alkaline phosphatase levels, or elevation of bilirubin levels should be cause for stopping the implicated medication. In addition, the patient should be monitored clinically for jaundice, malaise, and anorexia. Patients with a history of obstructive jaundice or preexisting liver disease should not be treated with phenothiazine antipsychotics (Salzman 1998).

Musculoskeletal System Effects

Treatment with atypical antipsychotics and haloperidol has been associated with a variable elevation in serum creatine kinase (CK) level (MM form) in the absence of obvious musculoskeletal pathology in about 10% of patients (Meltzer et al. 1996). In a minority of these patients, the elevation is extreme, in the range seen with rhabdomyolysis, although no evidence has been found of consequent impairment of renal function. It has been hypothesized that the increased CK activity might reflect changes in cell membrane permeability that particularly affect skeletal muscle in susceptible individuals (Meltzer et al. 1996). Whatever the cause, this effect has to be taken into account whenever CK is used to diagnose disorders such as acute myocardial infarction or neuroleptic malignant syndrome (NMS).

Neuropsychiatric Effects

Cognitive Impairment

Typical antipsychotics are reputed to be associated with some degree of cognitive impairment, as determined by decrease in

Mini-Mental State Exam (MMSE) score with treatment. In contrast, patients treated with risperidone have been found to have improvement over time on measures of alertness and attention (Lussier and Stip 1998) and in MMSE score (Jeste et al. 1996). In a study of olanzapine versus haloperidol, impaired cognitive efficiency persisted past the first day only in haloperidol-treated patients (Tollefson et al. 1997). Although atypical agents in general appear to be superior to typical agents in preserving cognitive function, the relative superiority of individual atypical agents is not yet established.

Extrapyramidal Symptoms

Acute extrapyramidal effects of typical oral antipsychotics, including akathisia and parkinsonism, may occur in the majority of elderly patients. These motor effects greatly influence the quality of life for the treated elder; can significantly affect functional ability, including walking and eating; and increase the incidence of adverse events such as falls. Despite these effects, routine prophylaxis with antiparkinsonian drugs is not recommended for elders, even in the initial phases of treatment, since almost all such drugs have anticholinergic effects that are seriously problematic in most older people. When antipsychotic-treated elders develop EPS, attempts are made to discontinue or lower the dosage of medication or to add or switch to an atypical agent. If the offending antipsychotic is discontinued, the EPS should resolve within about 2 months, but in some cases signs and symptoms persist for a year or more (Eimer 1992). If additional treatment of parkinsonism is required, amantadine can be used; this agent is a dopamine reuptake blocker and dopamine$_2$ (D$_2$) receptor agonist that is well tolerated at low doses (e.g., 12.5–50 mg bid).

　　Parenteral, as opposed to oral, administration of haloperidol and droperidol is associated with a greatly reduced incidence of EPS. Also, in general, atypical agents are associated with rates of EPS lower than those seen with typical agents (see Table 2–6). Clozapine is not associated with parkinsonism at any dose and has a low prevalence of associated akathisia (Chengappa et al.

1994). Quetiapine is similar to clozapine in its profile of extrapyramidal effects. Olanzapine added to a typical antipsychotic has been found to improve EPS in elderly patients (Sajatovic et al. 1998). Although doses of olanzapine greater than about 35 mg daily can cause EPS in nonelderly patients, this dosage is far above the geriatric dose ceiling. Ziprasidone's potential to cause EPS appears equivalent to that of olanzapine. Risperidone is poised between the typical and atypical agents in its extrapyramidal profile; at daily doses above 4 mg in elders, it may have effects as pronounced as the typical antipsychotics, whereas at low daily doses (1 mg or less), it has little extrapyramidal effect, except perhaps akathisia. In our experience, dysphagia is another manifestation of EPS with risperidone and can be problematic even at low doses among patients with cranial nerve dysfunction (e.g., those with vascular dementia).

Neuroleptic Malignant Syndrome

The central features of NMS include high fever, muscle rigidity, fluctuating consciousness, and autonomic instability. Laboratory abnormalities frequently include elevations in CK, WBC, and liver function tests. The syndrome occurs most often with antipsychotic treatment but can also occur with dopamine agonist withdrawal (e.g., with levodopa or pramipexole), lithium treatment, and possibly selective serotonin reuptake inhibitor treatment. In practice, this syndrome is uncommon in elderly patients, but its incidence may be increased by neurological disease or debilitation or by a rapid rate of initial antipsychotic titration. The risk of NMS is believed to be lower with atypical antipsychotic agents, although there have been case reports of the syndrome's developing in patients treated with all marketed atypical agents. Use of serum CK levels to guide diagnosis is confounded by the association of CK level elevation with atypical antipsychotic treatment in the absence of other signs or symptoms of NMS, as discussed earlier (see "Musculoskeletal System Effects").

Neuroleptic malignant syndrome represents a medical emergency that is managed in a monitored setting with aggressive hydration and treatment of comorbid medical illness. Specific treatment of NMS is described in our discussion of the treatment of movement disorders (see Chapter 7: "Treatment of Movement Disorders").

Seizures

Low-potency typical antipsychotic agents and clozapine are associated with an increased risk of seizures (McEvoy et al. 2000). For any antipsychotic, there is an increased incidence of seizures whenever there is a history of past seizure or structural brain disease. The correlation of clozapine and seizures is dose dependent; in patients of mixed age, the rate is 1% at dosages of less than 300 mg daily (Casey 1997). Tonic-clonic seizures may be preceded by myoclonus or drop attacks. In addition, epileptiform activity on the electroencephalogram may predict later development of seizures. Patients with any of these presaging events, or those who develop clinical seizures, should be treated with dose reduction and more gradual titration or with addition of an anticonvulsant such as valproic acid, or possibly with gabapentin.

Tardive Dyskinesia

Tardive dyskinesia (TD) is a syndrome of abnormal involuntary movements associated with antipsychotic medication treatment. The syndrome occurs more frequently among elderly patients, and its incidence is related to duration of antipsychotic use. Clinical characteristics and treatment of TD are discussed in the chapter on movement disorders (see Chapter 7: "Treatment of Movement Disorders").

Ocular Effects

Three types of ocular effects of antipsychotic treatment may be seen: pigmentation, pigmentary retinopathy, and lens opacification (i.e., cataracts). Pigmentation of the conjunctiva, cornea, lens, or retina is usually a benign side effect of low-potency phenothiazine antipsychotics. Pigmentary retinopathy is a serious condition that can result in irreversible visual impairment associated with use of thioridazine at high doses (greater than 800 mg daily in patients of mixed age) and perhaps mesoridazine. Elderly patients who must be treated with thioridazine should have regular ophthalmological examinations. Lens opacification (i.e., cataracts) is a potential side effect of the atypical agent quetiapine (Seroquel) and can occur as well with other phenothiazines. Although a recent survey suggested that the incidence of cataracts with quetiapine treatment is low, systematic surveillance for the development of cataracts among treated patients was poor. Until more information is available, it is recommended that careful ophthalmological examination with a slit lamp be performed within the first few weeks of initiation of quetiapine therapy in elderly psychotic patients and at 6-month intervals thereafter.

Sedation

Histamine H_1 receptor binding underlies sedation and weight gain, both of which are commonly seen in antipsychotic-treated patients. Table 2–6 shows relative sedative effects of various typical and atypical antipsychotic agents. Sedation in elderly patients is associated with decreased oral intake, increased risk of falls, and increased risk of aspiration. Tolerance to sedation from antipsychotic medication often develops within a few days to several weeks. For certain patients, particularly those taking a combination of medications, sedation persists. When these patients require treatment over an extended period, high-potency (less sedating) antipsychotic drugs are preferred.

Weight Gain

All currently marketed antipsychotics (except perhaps molindone) are associated with weight gain, which may be significant (Richelson 1996). Although the mechanisms of this drug effect are not well understood, it is thought to relate both to histamine H_1 receptor binding and to hypothalamic dysregulation. In our experience, clozapine and olanzapine are associated with the most weight gain, and haloperidol and risperidone are associated with the least. Weight gain is more likely to occur in elderly patients with diabetes or those with restricted activity. Weight gain can significantly complicate the care and treatment of patients with diabetes, hypertension, or hypercholesterolemia. Co-administration of the histamine$_2$ (H_2) receptor antagonist nizatidine (Axid) 150 mg po bid (the same dosage used for acute treatment of peptic ulcer or maintenance treatment of gastro-esophageal reflux disease) was found in one case to control olanzapine-associated weight gain (Sacchetti et al. 2000); the clinical utility of this observation has yet to be determined for elderly patients. The antipsychotic ziprasidone carries a lower risk of weight gain compared with other atypical antipsychotics.

Clozapine, olanzapine, and perhaps quetiapine are also associated with significant elevations in serum triglyceride (but not cholesterol) levels. Treatment options include switching to an antipsychotic that is less associated with weight gain, such as a typical agent, or adding a lipid-lowering drug.

Treatment of Selected Syndromes and Disorders With Antipsychotics

Delirium

Definitive treatment of the cause of delirium (e.g., correction of hyponatremia) always takes precedence over symptomatic treatment. Symptomatic treatment is not always required, but when it is (e.g., for control of agitation and psychosis), high-potency antipsychotics are used. Although some patients are effectively treated with an oral formulation, patients posing a danger to themselves or others are best treated with a parenteral formulation. For reasons noted earlier, the intravenous route is preferred. Haloperidol remains the drug of choice for treating agitation (with or without psychosis) in elderly patients with delirium. It should be used according to the following guidelines: 0.5–2.0 mg bolus iv (or im), with the dose repeated or doubled every 30 minutes until the patient is calm (Jacobson 1997; Jacobson and

Schreibman 1997). Most patients respond to one or two doses. When doses escalate into the range of 5 to 10 mg, consideration should be given to adjunctive use of a benzodiazepine such as lorazepam 0.5–1.0 mg. As an alternative, an infusion of haloperidol may be used, with the haloperidol started at 1 mg/hour and the dosage titrated to effect. Ceiling rates of 15–25 mg/hour of haloperidol have been documented in younger patients (Fish 1991). As noted in the earlier discussion of cardiac conduction effects of parenteral haloperidol, QT_c duration must be monitored.

If no further antipsychotic medication is administered, agitation will reemerge 6–12 hours after behavioral control has been achieved. For this reason, haloperidol should be continued and tapered over several days, with exact dosing guided by frequent clinical assessment. In general, one-half the dose effective in controlling agitation is given on day two in divided doses, and the medication is tapered over three to five days (Fish 1991).

Risperidone and olanzapine are in use at some centers for the treatment of delirium (Sipahimalani and Masand 1998), although controlled studies of these applications are lacking in geriatric patients. A published case series of risperidone treatment that included four geriatric patients with delirium had mixed results; only two of the geriatric patients showed improvement (Sipahimalani et al. 1997). In our experience, the need for slow initial titration of risperidone in elders and the latency to effect for olanzapine are both limiting for treatment of delirium. Another alternative to haloperidol is droperidol, which is preferred to haloperidol by some clinicians because it is more sedating, has a faster onset of action and more rapid clearance, and has fewer extrapyramidal effects. Although bolus injection of droperidol has been associated with hypotension, continuous infusion of droperidol 1–20 mg/hour has been shown to provide excellent behavioral control without hypotension (Frye et al. 1995). A recent study showed that treatment with droperidol confers a significantly greater risk of QT_c prolongation compared with haloperidol, however, so this medication should now be considered a distant second choice (Reilly et al. 2000).

According to anecdotal reports, the acetylcholinesterase inhibitor donepezil is being used with some success for symptomatic treatment of delirium in hospital settings. Our experience is that donepezil 5 mg po qd can be effective and well tolerated but may not be as immediately effective as haloperidol. For critically ill patients whose movements pose a medical hazard, such as those on ventilators or intra-aortic balloon pumps, and terminally ill cancer patients, more aggressive treatment of agitation may be needed. Adams (1984) proposed a highly effective regimen that is a combination of haloperidol, lorazepam, and hydromorphone.

Delusional Disorder

The same treatment principles apply to delusional disorder as to schizophrenia (discussed later in this section), except that delusional disorders may be much less responsive to treatment, and there is usually less need to control acute agitation. Chronic therapy may be indicated, and for this purpose the lowest effective dose and preferential use of atypical antipsychotics are recommended.

Dementia With Psychotic Symptoms

Alzheimer's disease, vascular dementia, dementia with Lewy bodies, and other etiologies of dementia are frequently associated with psychotic symptoms at some stage of the illness (Tariot 1996). In dementia with Lewy bodies, psychotic symptoms in the form of visual hallucinations are in fact a central feature of the psychopathology. In other dementias, nonspecific features such as "sundowning," or nighttime agitation, may occur. In view of the potentially serious consequences of administering typical antipsychotics to patients with dementia with Lewy bodies, the differential diagnosis of dementia in elderly patients is critical (Ballard et al. 1998; McKeith et al. 1995). For patients with dementia with Lewy bodies, clozapine is the only antipsychotic that has consistently been shown to improve symptoms without (in most cases) worsening motor function. Sensitivity to extrapyramidal effects of low-dose risperidone in patients with Lewy body dementia has been reported (McKeith et al. 1995). Other, newer atypical agents may be useful in this context but have been inadequately studied for this indication.

For patients with non–Lewy body dementia, typical or atypical agents can be used. These medications are best prescribed at very low doses on a standing rather than prn basis. For sundowning, the antipsychotic can be given 1–2 hours before the time of usual behavioral disturbance to take advantage of sedative effects. A randomized, controlled trial of haloperidol for psychosis and disruptive behavior in Alzheimer's disease demonstrated that doses of 2–3 mg daily provide the best balance of efficacy and side effects, with doses below 1 mg daily being no more effective than placebo (Devanand et al. 1998). A randomized, controlled trial of risperidone in a large cohort of elderly patients with dementia (dementia of the Alzheimer's type, vascular dementia, or mixed) demonstrated that an optimal dose of risperidone 1 mg daily was effective in reducing behavioral pathology (Katz et al. 1999; Kumar and Brecher 1999). Quetiapine may also be effective for this indication (McManus et al. 1999). Ziprasidone has been understudied in this population.

Depression With Psychotic Symptoms

The treatment of choice for elderly patients with major depression with psychotic features is ECT, which induces rapid remission. Alternatively, an antipsychotic such as olanzapine or risperidone can be started in combination with an antidepressant such as venlafaxine or citalopram. Medications in general have a longer latency to effect than ECT. When a course of ECT is completed, the antidepressant effect must be maintained, either with further ECT or with antidepressant medication.

Mania

Acute manic episodes in elderly patients are often associated with significant thought disorganization in addition to the positive psychotic symptoms of delusions and hallucinations. These symptoms are effectively treated with administration of an antipsychotic such as olanzapine with the mood stabilizer, along with prn use of a benzodiazepine, usually lorazepam or oxazepam. If risperidone is used in this context, the starting dose should be low (0.25 mg qd or bid) to avoid undesirable activating effects. When the acute manic episode has resolved to the point that the psychotic symptoms have subsided, the antipsychotic may be tapered and withdrawn. Increasingly, however, bipolar patients receive maintenance therapy with atypical antipsychotics for their mood-stabilizing effects.

Parkinson's Disease With Psychosis

Parkinson's disease is a degenerative disease that significantly affects motor function but can also be associated with psychotic symptoms. In addition, drugs such as levodopa used to treat patients with Parkinson's disease may secondarily give rise to psychosis. In both clinical situations, low-dose atypical antipsychotics may be useful. As noted earlier, the atypical antipsychotics show greater affinity for serotonin receptors than for dopamine receptors, and at clinically effective doses these agents could be expected to interfere less with prodopaminergic effects of Parkinson's disease drugs. Although the logistics of co-administration of these classes of drugs are not well worked out, it makes sense to separate their administration by giving the atypical antipsychotic at bedtime and the last dose of levodopa at dinnertime.

Of the atypical antipsychotics, clozapine is the most effective for this indication, possibly followed by quetiapine, but mixed results have been obtained with olanzapine and risperidone. Low-dose thioridazine may also be used but is no longer a drug of first choice. The dosage of clozapine used for this indication ranges from 6.25 mg every other day to 150 mg daily, with most patients treated effectively with 50 mg daily or less. The dosage of quetiapine is usually in the range of 12.5 to 150 mg daily, with most patients treated with 100 mg daily or less.

Personality Disorders

When antipsychotics are used in the treatment of personality disorders, specific target symptoms (e.g., paranoid ideation) are identified, and treatment is time-limited. For example, an elderly patient with borderline personality disorder with a current exacerbation involving fears of poisoning may be effectively treated with haloperidol 0.25 mg po bid for 2 weeks. In addition, mood-stabilizing atypical antipsychotics such as olanzapine may prove to be useful for longer-term treatment of psychotic symptoms in patients with personality disorders.

Schizoaffective Disorder

The same treatment principles apply to schizoaffective disorder as to schizophrenia (see below), except that true schizoaffective disorder often necessitates combined therapy with a mood stabilizer or antidepressant, or ECT. Atypical antipsychotic monotherapy is an emerging treatment alternative that is particularly attractive for elderly patients with schizoaffective disorder, although it is possibly more effective for those with the bipolar subtype than for those with the depressed subtype. In our experience to date, the atypical antipsychotic of first choice is olanzapine, which is started at 2.5 mg qhs and titrated to a usual target dose of 10 mg qhs. Risperidone is also effective but can be activating for some patients, particularly during initial titration; it may be best used in combination with a mood stabilizer. Insufficient data are available to recommend quetiapine for this indication. Clozapine is highly effective and would be the drug of choice if not for its adverse effects.

Schizophrenia

In the treatment of acute psychosis in elderly patients, it is important to avoid using excessively large doses of medication. Both clinical and in vivo receptor-binding studies have shown that for most patients, there is no advantage in using any more than haloperidol 4 mg (total daily dose) or its equivalent in terms of either rapidity or completeness of response. For controlling aggression and other excessive motor behaviors, a benzodiazepine can be co-prescribed.

For maintenance treatment of schizophrenia in elderly patients, the patient should be reassessed at least every 3–6 months. At these intervals, attempts should be made to reduce the dosage of antipsychotic and to maintain the patient at the lowest effective dosage. Increasingly, these interval assessments are used to begin a crossover from a typical to an atypical agent for maintenance treatment.

Secondary Psychotic Syndromes

Symptoms of delusions, hallucinations, or thought disorganization can occur as secondary symptoms in the context of various medical disorders, including cerebrovascular disease and hyperthyroidism. These symptoms can occur with or without changes in level of consciousness and sensorium characteristic of delirium. Treatment first involves optimization of therapy directed at the underlying medical condition. An atypical antipsychotic at a low dosage (e.g., risperidone 0.25 mg bid) may be started concurrently and the dosage titrated to effect. The antipsychotic is tapered and withdrawn, if possible, when the medical condition has been stabilized.

Substance Intoxication and Withdrawal

Delusions or hallucinations can occur in the context of alcohol and other drug intoxication or withdrawal. In most cases, these psychotic symptoms either resolve with the intoxication or withdrawal syndrome itself or are responsive to benzodiazepine therapy. In some cases, however, persistent alcoholic hallucinosis can be seen. In persistent cases, patients are treated with low doses of atypical antipsychotics (e.g., olanzapine 5 mg po qhs) to avoid inducing akathisia, since this condition can increase alcohol craving. Most cases of persistent hallucinosis prove to be relatively refractory to treatment.

As noted in the chapter on the treatment of substance-related disorders (see Chapter 6: "Treatment of Substance-Related Disorders"), the mainstay of treatment for delirium tremens is benzodiazepine therapy. Antipsychotics have a role in severe cases in which benzodiazepines are not sufficient to contain symptoms. In those cases, there is usually an intercurrent medical or psychiatric illness that is complicating withdrawal.

Chapter Summary

- The same antipsychotic dose administered to a younger patient and an elderly patient may yield a serum concentration of drug in the older patient that is twice that in the younger patient.

- With some agents, therapeutic effects are achieved and toxic effects are seen at lower serum drug concentrations in older compared with younger patients.

- A general rule for antipsychotic dosing in the elderly patient is that the total daily dose (target dose) is ideally not more than twice the "relative potency" value (see Table 2–3).

- Antipsychotic medications are used on a standing rather than a prn basis because consistent levels of drug at the receptor site are required for antipsychotic effect.

- In treating elderly patients, give small doses, divide doses (at least initially), and titrate the dosage slowly.

- In general, elders with schizophrenia require higher doses of antipsychotics than elders with dementia.

- Some patients treated with an atypical antipsychotic require a second (typical) antipsychotic to "top off" its effect, at least periodically.

- Conventional high-potency antipsychotics (e.g., haloperidol) are the drugs of choice for emergency sedation of delirious, medically ill patients.

- Atypical antipsychotics are the drugs of choice for long-term treatment of psychotic illness such as schizophrenia in elderly patients.

- Low-potency typical antipsychotics are in general best avoided in elderly patients because of the risk of hypotension, sedation, and anticholinergic effects.

References

Adams F: Neuropsychiatric evaluation and treatment of delirium in the critically ill cancer patient. Cancer Bull 36:156–160, 1984

Ballard C, Grace J, McKeith I, et al: Neuroleptic sensitivity in dementia with Lewy bodies and Alzheimer's disease. Lancet 351:1032–1033, 1998

Bondolfi G, Dufour H, Patris M, et al: Risperidone versus clozapine in treatment-resistant chronic schizophrenia: a randomised double-blind study. Am J Psychiatry 155:499–504, 1998

Casey DE: The relationship of pharmacology to side effects. J Clin Psychiatry 58 (10, suppl):55–62, 1997

Chengappa KNR, Shelton MD, Baker RW, et al: The prevalence of akathisia in patients receiving stable doses of clozapine. J Clin Psychiatry 55:142–145, 1994

Coccaro EF, Kramer E, Zemishlany Z, et al: Pharmacologic treatment of noncognitive behavioral disturbances in elderly demented patients. Am J Psychiatry 147:1640–1645, 1990

Devanand DP, Marder K, Michaels KS, et al: A randomized, placebo-controlled dose-comparison trial of haloperidol for psychosis and disruptive behaviors in Alzheimer's disease. Am J Psychiatry 155:1512–1520, 1998

Di Salvo TG, O'Gara PT: Torsades de pointes caused by high-dose intravenous haloperidol in cardiac patients. Clin Cardiol 18:285–290, 1995

Eimer M: Considerations in the pharmacologic management of dementia-related behavioral symptoms. Consult Pharm 7:921–933, 1992

Ereshefsky L: Pharmacokinetics and drug interactions: update for new antipsychotics. J Clin Psychiatry 57 (11, suppl):12–25, 1996

Farde L, Nordstrom AL, Wiesel FA, et al: PET-analysis of central D_1- and D_2-dopamine receptor occupancy in patients treated with classical neuroleptics and clozapine: relation to extrapyramidal side effects. Arch Gen Psychiatry 49:538–544, 1992

Fish DN: Treatment of delirium in the critically ill patient. Clin Pharm 10:456–466, 1991

Frye MA, Coudreaut MF, Hakeman SM, et al: Continuous droperidol infusion for management of agitated delirium in an intensive care unit. Psychosomatics 36:301–305, 1995

Fuller MA, Simon MR, Freedman L: Risperidone-associated hepatotoxicity. J Clin Psychopharmacol 16:84–85, 1996

Gaulin BD, Markowitz JS, Caley CF, et al: Clozapine-associated elevation in serum triglycerides. Am J Psychiatry 156:1270–1272, 1999

Hagg S, Spigset O, Soderstrom TG: Association of venous thromboembolism and clozapine. Lancet 355:1155–1156, 2000

Heinz A, Knable MB, Weinberger DR: Dopamine D_2 receptor imaging and neuroleptic drug response. J Clin Psychiatry 57 (11, suppl):84–88, 1996

Henderson DC, Cagliero E, Gray C, et al: Clozapine, diabetes mellitus, weight gain, and lipid abnormalities: a five-year naturalistic study. Am J Psychiatry 157:975–981, 2000

Jacobson SA: Delirium in the elderly. Psychiatr Clin North Am 20:91–110, 1997

Jacobson S, Schreibman B: Behavioral and pharmacologic treatment of delirium. Am Fam Physician 56:2005–2012, 1997

Jann MW: Clozapine. Pharmacotherapy 11:179–195, 1991

Jeste DV, Eastham JH, Lacro JP, et al: Management of late-life psychosis. J Clin Psychiatry 57 (3, suppl):39–45, 1996

Jibson MD, Tandon R: New atypical antipsychotic medications. J Psychiatr Res 32:215–228, 1998

Kapur S, Remington G, Jones C, et al: High levels of dopamine D_2 receptor occupancy with low dose haloperidol treatment: a PET study. Am J Psychiatry 153:948–950, 1996

Katz IR, Jeste DV, Mintzer JE, et al: Comparison of risperidone and placebo for psychosis and behavioral disturbances associated with dementia: a randomized, double-blind trial. J Clin Psychiatry 60:107–115, 1999

Kopala LC, Good KP, Honer WG: Extrapyramidal signs and clinical symptoms in first-episode schizophrenia: response to low-dose risperidone. J Clin Psychopharmacol 17:308–313, 1997

Kumar V, Brecher M: Psychopharmacology of atypical antipsychotics and clinical outcomes in elderly patients. J Clin Psychiatry 60 (suppl 13): 5–9, 1999

Lacro JP, Kuczenski R, Roznoski M, et al: Serum haloperidol levels in older psychotic patients. Am J Geriatr Psychiatry 4:229–236, 1996

Lussier I, Stip E: The effect of risperidone on cognitive and psychopathological manifestations of schizophrenia. CNS Spectrums 3:55–69, 1998

Marder SR: Management of treatment-resistant patients with schizophrenia. J Clin Psychiatry 57 (11, suppl):26–30, 1996

Marder SR, Davis JM, Chouinard G: The effects of risperidone on the five dimensions of schizophrenia derived by factor analysis: combined results of the North American trials. J Clin Psychiatry 58:538–546, 1997

McEvoy GK, Litvak K, Welsh OH, et al: AHFS Drug Information. Bethesda, American Society of Health-System Pharmacists, 2000

McKeith IG, Ballard CG, Harrison RW: Neuroleptic sensitivity to risperidone in Lewy body dementia (letter; comment). Lancet 346:699, 1995

McManus DQ, Arvanitis LA, Kowalcyk BB: Quetiapine, a novel antipsychotic: experience in elderly patients with psychotic disorders. J Clin Psychiatry 60:292–298, 1999

Meltzer HY, Cola PA, Parsa M: Marked elevations of serum creatine kinase activity associated with antipsychotic drug treatment. Neuropsychopharmacology 15:395–405, 1996

Nordstrom AL, Farde L, Nyberg S, et al: D_1, D_2, and 5-HT_2 receptor occupancy in relation to clozapine serum concentration: a PET study of schizophrenic patients. Am J Psychiatry 152:1444–1449, 1995

Osser DN, Najarian DM, Dufresne RL: Olanzapine increases weight and serum triglyceride levels. J Clin Psychiatry 60:767–770, 1999

Pan L, Vander Stichele R, Rosseel MT, et al: Effects of smoking, CYP2D6 genotype, and concomitant drug intake on the steady state plasma concentrations of haloperidol and reduced haloperidol in schizophrenic inpatients. Ther Drug Monit 21:489–497, 1999

Pearlman C: Clozapine, nocturnal sialorrhea, and choking (letter). J Clin Psychopharmacol 14:283, 1994

Pickar D: Prospects for pharmacotherapy of schizophrenia. Lancet 345: 557–562, 1995

Pies RW: Handbook of Essential Psychopharmacology. Washington, DC, American Psychiatric Press, 1998

Pies RW, Dewan M: The difficult to treat patient with schizophrenia, in The Difficult-to-Treat Psychiatric Patient. Edited by Dewan M, Pies R. Washington, DC, American Psychiatric Publishing, 2001, pp

Pollock BG, Mulsant BH: Antipsychotics in older patients. A safety perspective. Drugs Aging 6:312–323, 1995

Rabinowitz T, Frankenburg FR, Centorrino F, et al: The effect of clozapine on saliva flow rate: a pilot study. Biol Psychiatry 40:1132–1134, 1996

Reilly JG, Ayis SA, Ferrier IN, et al: QTc-interval abnormalities and psychotropic drug therapy in psychiatric patients. Lancet 355:1048–1052, 2000

Richelson E: Preclinical pharmacology of neuroleptics: focus on new generation compounds. J Clin Psychiatry 57 (11, suppl):4–11, 1996

Sacchetti E, Guarneri L, Bravi D: H_2 antagonist nizatidine may control olanzapine-associated weight gain in schizophrenic patients. Biol Psychiatry 48:167–168, 2000

Sajatovic M, Perez D, Brescan D, et al: Olanzapine therapy in elderly patients with schizophrenia. Psychopharmacol Bull 34:819–823, 1998

Salzman C: Clinical Geriatric Psychopharmacology, 3rd Edition. Baltimore, MD, Williams & Wilkins, 1998

Salzman C, Satlin A, Burrows AB: Geriatric psychopharmacology, in The American Psychiatric Press Textbook of Psychopharmacology, 2nd Edition, Edited by Schatzberg AF, Nemeroff CB. Washington, DC, American Psychiatric Press, 1998, pp 961–970

Schneider LS: Efficacy of treatment for geropsychiatric patients with severe mental illness. Psychopharmacol Bull 29:501–524, 1993

Schneider LS, Pollock VE, Lyness SA: A metaanalysis of controlled trials of neuroleptic treatment in dementia. J Am Geriatr Soc 38:553–563, 1990

Sipahimalani A, Masand PS: Olanzapine in the treatment of delirium. Psychosomatics 39:422–430, 1998

Sipahimalani S, Sime RM, Masand PS: Treatment of delirium with risperidone. International Journal of Geriatric Psychopharmacology 1:24–26, 1997

Small JG, Milstein V, Marhenke JD, et al: Treatment outcome with clozapine in tardive dyskinesia, neuroleptic sensitivity, and treatment-resistant psychosis. J Clin Psychiatry 48:263–267, 1987

Stahl SM: Antipsychotic polypharmacy, Part 1: therapeutic option or dirty little secret? J Clin Psychiatry 60:425–426, 1999

Tariot PN: Treatment strategies for agitation and psychosis in dementia. J Clin Psychiatry 57 (suppl 14):21–29, 1996

Theoharides TC: Essentials of Pharmacology, 2nd Edition. Boston, MA, Little, Brown, 1996

Tollefson GD, Beasley CM, Tran PV, et al: Olanzapine versus haloperidol in the treatment of schizophrenia and schizoaffective and schizophreniform disorders: results of an international collaborative trial. Am J Psychiatry 154:457–465, 1997

Van Putten T, Marder SR, Mintz J, et al: Haloperidol plasma levels and clinical response: a therapeutic window relationship. Am J Psychiatry 149:500–505, 1992

Wirshing DA, Spellberg BJ, Erhart SM, et al: Novel antipsychotics and new onset diabetes. Biol Psychiatry 44:778–783, 1998

Generic name	clozapine
Trade name	Clozaril
Class	Dibenzodiazepine
Half-life	12 hours (range 4–66 hours)
Mechanism	Blockade of serotonin, dopamine, α-adrenergic, and acetylcholine receptors
Available formulation	Tablets: 25, 100 mg (both scored)
Starting dose	6.25–12.5 mg qd
Titration	Increase by 6.25–12.5 mg every 7 days, as tolerated (may be added to a high-potency typical antipsychotic that is tapered when clozapine dose is at target or at 100 mg daily)
Typical daily dose	Schizophrenia: 100 mg bid for acute treatment; lower dose for maintenance. Psychosis in Parkinson's disease: 6.25–50 mg
Dosage range	6.25–400 mg daily (divided doses)
Therapeutic serum level	Parent compound: 200–350 ng/mL (for schizophrenia; not established for Parkinson's disease)

Comments: The new gold standard of efficacy. Particularly useful for patients with Parkinson's disease and related disorders (including dementia with Lewy bodies) or TD. Lowest doses (e.g., 6.25 mg, prepared by pharmacy) used for very elderly and patients with dementia. Divided doses are recommended. Not used prn. Like olanzapine, clozapine has a more prolonged latency to response compared with other agents; latencies of 6 weeks to several months are not uncommon in elderly patients. Response may not plateau for 12 months, especially for negative symptoms. *Drug interactions:* Potential interaction with benzodiazepines associated with sudden death; add benzodiazepines only after clozapine titration is complete. Other drug interactions mediated by cytochrome P450 1A2, 2D6, and 3A4 enzymes. *Adverse effects* (include): agranulocytosis, NMS, deep venous thrombosis and pulmonary embolism, impaired glucose tolerance, increased serum CK levels, increased serum triglyceride levels, seizures, tachycardia, confusion, sedation, dizziness, and salivary pooling. See Table 2–5 for guidelines on management of leukopenia. Routine WBC monitoring weekly for 6 months, then every other week if WBC and absolute neutrophil count values have been acceptable. Serum lipid assay (triglycerides) checked yearly. To discontinue (for reasons other than leukopenia), decrease dose gradually over 4–6 weeks and continue WBC monitoring for 4 weeks after discontinuation. For missed doses or if patient discontinues on own more than 48 hours, drug must be retitrated, starting with lowest dose.

Generic name	droperidol
Trade name	Inapsine
Class	Butyrophenone
Half-life	2.3 hours
Mechanism of action	Blockade of dopamine and α-adrenergic receptors
Available formulation	Injectable: 2.5 mg/mL
Starting dose	1–3 mg iv or im
Titration	Repeat if needed at same or doubled dose after 30–60 minutes
Typical daily dose	Up to 5 mg
Dosage range	1–10 mg daily
Therapeutic serum level	Not established

Comments: Used as a second-line agent for emergency sedation of the psychotic elderly patient. Has antiemetic effects. Available for parenteral use only. Onset in 3–10 minutes; peak effect in 30 minutes. Usual duration of action 2–4 hours but may extend to 12 hours. More sedating than haloperidol and confers a greater risk of prolonging QT_c compared with haloperidol but is associated with lower risk of EPS. *Adverse effects* (include): hypotension, respiratory depression, and NMS.

Generic name	fluphenazine
Trade name	Prolixin, Permitil
Class	Phenothiazine
Half-life	Oral form (HCl): 33 hours Decanoate form: approximately 7–10 days
Mechanism of action	Blockade of dopamine, α-adrenergic, and anticholinergic receptors
Available formulations	Oral forms: Tablets: 1, 2.5, 5, 10 mg Liquid concentrate: 5 mg/mL Liquid suspension: 0.5 mg/mL, 2.5 mg/5 mL Injectable: 2.5 mg/mL Decanoate (im) form: 25 mg/mL
Starting dose	Oral: 0.25–0.5 qd or bid Decanoate: 6.25 mg (dementia: 1.25 mg)
Titration	Oral: increase by 0.25–0.5 mg at 4- to 7-day intervals, as tolerated
Typical dose	Oral: 1 mg bid Decanoate: 12.5 mg every 2–4 weeks (dementia: 3.75 mg every 2–4 weeks)
Dosage range	Oral: 0.25–4 mg daily (divided doses) Decanoate: 6.25–100 mg/month
Therapeutic serum level	0.2–2 ng/mL (unselected ages)

Comments: High-potency conventional antipsychotic; a phenothiazine derivative. Effect profile similar to that of haloperidol. Liquid form not compatible with liquids containing caffeine, tannin (tea), or pectinates (apple juice). With oral or intramuscular HCl formulation, onset of sedative action within 1 hour and biological effect persisting 24 hours; once-daily dosing is feasible after initial titration. Decanoate peaks in

8–36 hrs, with second peak in 1–2 weeks. Decanoate can be given in small doses every 2–3 weeks. Steady state may take longer than the 3–4 months observed in younger populations. Extensively metabolized in the liver; substrate and inhibitor of CYP2D6. *Adverse effects* (include): cardiovascular (e.g., orthostasis, dysrhythmias), extrapyramidal effects, TD, NMS, seizures, anticholinergic effects (e.g., dry mouth, constipation, urinary retention, blurred vision), sexual dysfunction, weight gain, agranulocytosis, and other hematological abnormalities.

Generic name	haloperidol
Trade name	Haldol
Class	Butyrophenone
Half-life	20 hours
Mechanism of action	Blockade of dopamine receptors
Available formulations	Short-acting forms: Tablets: 0.2, 1, 2, 5, 10, 20 mg Liquid concentrate: 2 mg/mL Injectable: 5 mg/mL Decanoate form: 50 mg/mL, 100 mg/mL
Starting dose	0.25–0.5 mg qd or bid
Titration	Increase by 0.25–0.5 mg at 4- to 7-day intervals, as tolerated
Typical dose	Short-acting: 1 mg bid Decanoate: 25 mg/month
Dosage range	0.25–4 mg daily Depot: 25–100 mg/month
Therapeutic serum level	0.32–10.4 ng/mL (for elderly patients; lower end of range for patients with dementia, higher end for patients with schizophrenia)

Comments: A drug of choice in elderly patients requiring rapid treatment of psychotic symptoms and for agitation in delirium. Onset of effect with intramuscular administration in 30–60 minutes, with substantial improvement in 2–3 hours. Faster onset with intravenous administration. 60% bioavailability with oral administration because of first-pass metabolism. Biological effect persists 24 hours; once-daily dosing is feasible after initial titration. Decanoate time to peak 3–9 days, half-life 3 weeks, dosing interval 1 month. Metabolized in liver; substrate mainly of CYP3A4. Asians show lower dose:concentration ratios compared with Caucasians. Minimal hypotensive and anticholinergic effects. *Adverse effects* (include): extrapyramidal syndromes, TD, and NMS.

Generic name	loxapine
Trade name	Loxitane
Class	Dibenzoxazepine
Half-life	Biphasic: 5 hours/12–19 hours
Mechanism of action	Blockade of dopamine, adrenergic, and anticholinergic receptors.
Available formulations	Capsules: 5, 10, 25, 50 mg Liquid concentrate: 25 mg/mL Injectable: 50 mg/mL
Starting dose	5–10 mg qd or bid
Titration	Increase by 5–10 mg (qd or bid) at 4- to 7-day intervals, as tolerated
Typical daily dose	40 mg (divided bid to qid)
Dosage range	10–80 mg daily
Therapeutic serum level	Not established

Comments: Not a drug of choice in elderly patients. Rapidly and completely absorbed. Onset of sedative effect in 20–30 minutes; peak sedative effect in 1.5–3 hours; duration of sedation 12 hours. Extensive first-pass metabolism. Extensive hepatic metabolism, to active metabolites. Excreted in urine and feces. *Drug interactions:* epinephrine (inhibits vasopressor effect), other CNS depressants, other anticholinergic agents. *Adverse effects:* drowsiness, extrapyramidal effects (may be worse with intramuscular dosing than with oral dosing), TD, NMS, seizures, agranulocytosis, leukopenia, hypotension (especially orthostatic), tachycardia, dysrhythmias, ECG changes, syncope, dizziness, fatigue, dry mouth, constipation, urinary retention, blurred vision, retinal pigmentation, renal failure, hepatotoxicity, cholestatic jaundice, weight gain, ocular pigmentation, and rhabdomyolysis.

Generic name	molindone
Trade name	Moban
Class	Dihydroindolone
Half-life	20–40 hours
Mechanism of action	Blockade of dopamine, adrenergic, and anticholinergic receptors
Available formulations	Capsules: 5, 10, 25 mg Tablets: 5, 10, 25, 50, 100 mg Liquid concentrate: 20 mg/mL
Starting dose	5 mg bid
Titration	Increase by 5–10 mg at 4- to 7-day intervals, as tolerated
Typical daily dose	20 mg
Dosage range	10–100 mg daily
Therapeutic serum level	Not established

Comments: Not a drug of choice in elderly patients. The only antipsychotic not associated with weight gain. Rapidly absorbed; peak levels in 90 minutes. Duration of action 36 hours or more. Metabolized in the liver; substrate of CYP2D6 enzyme; excreted in urine and feces. *Drug interactions:* Metabolism inhibited by SSRIs and quinidine. Additive effect with other CNS depressants. May block effect of guanethidine; may cause neurotoxicity with lithium. *Adverse effects:* drowsiness, frequent extrapyramidal effects, TD, NMS, seizures, dry mouth, constipation, urinary retention, blurred vision, retinal pigmentation, weight gain, hypotension, tachycardia, dysrhythmias, photosensitivity, hyperpigmentation, agranulocytosis, and leukopenia.

Generic name	olanzapine
Trade name	Zyprexa, Zyprexa ZYDIS
Class	Thienobenzodiazepine
Half-life	30 hours (range 21–54 hours)
Mechanism of action	Blockade of serotonin, dopamine, muscarinic, histamine, and adrenergic receptors
Available formulations	Tablets: 2.5, 5, 7.5, 10, 15 mg Orally disintegrating tablets: 5, 10, 15, 20 mg
Starting dose	2.5 mg qd (hs)
Titration	Increase by 2.5 mg after 3–4 days
Typical daily dose	5–10 mg qd (hs)
Dosage range	2.5–15 mg daily
Therapeutic serum level	>9 ng/mL (not well established)

Comments: May be a drug of choice in elderly patients. Chemical analog of clozapine, without significant hematological effects. Like clozapine, olanzapine has more prolonged latency to response compared with other agents; latency of 6 weeks to several months not uncommon in elderly patients. Some patients who do not respond to or cannot tolerate clozapine do respond to olanzapine. Higher target dose may be required when making a change from clozapine to olanzapine. ZYDIS preparation dissolves rapidly in saliva and can be swallowed with or without liquid. Olanzapine peaks at 5–8 hours; not used prn. Substrate of CYP1A2 and 2D6. Clearance reduced in elderly and in women; increased in smokers. *Adverse effects* (include): orthostatic hypotension, sedation, weight gain, loss of glycemic control, elevated serum triglyceride levels, anticholinergic effects (e.g., constipation), nausea, dizziness (not orthostatic), tremor, insomnia, overactivation, akathisia, TD, and NMS.

Generic name	perphenazine
Trade name	Trilafon
Class	Piperazine
Half-life	20–40 hours
Mechanism of action	Blockade of dopamine, adrenergic, and anticholinergic receptors
Available formulations	Tablets: 2, 4, 8, 16 mg Liquid concentrate: 16 mg/5 mL Injectable: 5 mg/mL
Starting dose	2–4 mg qd or bid
Titration	Increase by 2–4 mg at 4- to 7-day intervals, as tolerated
Typical daily dose	8 mg
Dosage range	2–32 mg daily
Therapeutic serum level	0.8–2.4 ng/mL (unselected ages)

Comments: Not a drug of choice in elderly patients. Peak levels in 4–8 hrs; effects persist for 24 hours. Well absorbed. Extensive first-pass metabolism. Extensive metab-olism in liver; substrate and inhibitor of CYP2D6. Excreted in urine and bile. *Drug interactions:* see Table 1–1 in Chapter 1 for other CYP2D6 inhibitors and substrates. Additive effects with other CNS depressants and anticholinergics, and decreased effectiveness of certain antihypertensives. *Adverse effects:* sedation, anticholinergic effects > EPS; ECG changes, hypotension (especially orthostatic), tachycardia, dysrhythmias, rest-lessness, anxiety, TD, NMS, seizures, hyperpigmentation, rash, dry mouth, constipation, urinary retention, blurred vision, weight gain, sexual dysfunction, agranulocytosis, leukopenia, cholestatic jaundice, retinal pigmenta-tion, and decreased visual acuity.

Generic name	quetiapine
Trade name	Seroquel
Class	Dibenzothiazepine
Half-life	6 hours
Mechanism of action	Blockade of serotonin, dopamine, histamine, and α_1- and α_2-adrenergic receptors
Available formulation	Tablets: 25, 100, 200, 300 mg
Starting dose	25 mg qd (qhs)
Titration	Increase by 25 mg every 2–4 days, as tolerated
Typical daily dose	50–100 mg bid
Dosage range	50–400 mg (divided bid or tid)
Therapeutic serum level	Not established

Comments: May be a drug of choice in elderly patients. Chemical analog of clozapine and olanzapine. Should be given consistently in relation to meals. Peak plasma concentration in 1–2 hours. Steady state achieved within 2 days. Metabolized in liver to inactive metabolites. Substrate of CYP3A4. *Adverse effects* (include): Sedation, orthostatic hypotension, dizziness, agitation, insomnia, headache, and NMS. Lens changes, possibly associated with cataracts, may be associated with chronic use; manufacturer recommends slit-lamp examination on initiation of treatment and every 6 months thereafter.

Generic name	risperidone
Trade name	Risperdal
Class	Benzisoxazole
Half-life	24 hours (risperidone + 9-hydroxy metabolite)
Mechanism of action	Blockade of serotonin and dopamine receptors
Available formulations	Tablets: 0.25, 0.5, 1, 2, 3, 4 mg Liquid concentrate: 1 mg/mL
Starting dose	0.5 mg qhs or 0.25 mg bid
Titration	Increase slowly by 0.25–0.5 mg at 7-day intervals, as tolerated
Typical daily dose	0.5 mg bid
Dosage range	0.25–3 mg daily (divided bid)
Therapeutic serum level	Not established

Comments: A drug of choice in elderly patients, provided low starting doses and slow titration are used to avoid hypotension and activation/ akathisia. Effective within the first week for acute psychotic symptoms. Initial titration requires close monitoring for hypotension. Peak plasma concentrations in 1 hour. Metabolized extensively via the CYP2D6 enzyme system; has active metabolites. Decreased clearance in renal and hepatic disease. Liquid concentrate compatible with coffee, water, orange juice, and lowfat milk; not compatible with tea or cola. Not recommended by manufacturer for prn use. *Adverse effects* (include): hypotension (especially orthostasis), tachycardia, dysrhythmias, ECG changes, syncope, sedation, headache, dizziness, restlessness, akathisia, anxiety, extrapyramidal effects, TD, and NMS (rare).

Generic name	thioridazine
Trade name	Mellaril
Class	Phenothiazine
Half-life	21–25 hours
Mechanism of action	Blockade of dopamine, adrenergic, and anticholinergic receptors
Available formulations	Tablets: 10, 15, 25, 50, 100, 150, 200 mg Liquid concentrate: 30 mg/mL, 100 mg/mL Liquid suspension: 25 mg/5 mL, 100 mg/ 5 mL
Starting dose	10–25 mg qd or bid
Titration	Increase by 10–25 mg at 4- to 7-day intervals, as tolerated
Typical daily dose	75 mg
Dosage range	10–200 mg (OBRA 1987 maximum = 75 mg)
Therapeutic serum level	1.0–1.5 µg/mL

Comments: Recommended now only as a second- or third-line agent for patients whose illness is refractory to treatment with other drugs. Formerly widely used for treatment of psychosis in patients with Parkinson's disease and in psychotic elderly patients requiring sedation. The FDA required labeling changes in July of 2000 to warn users about significant QT_c prolongation associated with torsades de pointes tachycardia. *Drug interactions:* Contraindicated for use with fluvoxamine, propranolol, pindolol, and any inhibitor of CYP2D6 (e.g., fluoxetine, paroxetine; see Table 1–1 in Chapter 1). Other significant drug interactions with guanethidine, meperidine, norepinephrine, and epinephrine. Primarily metabolized to mesoridazine. Liquid form should be diluted only in acidified tap water, distilled water, or fruit juice such as orange or grape. *Adverse effects:* Highly sedating, with marked anticholinergic effects (e.g., constipation, urinary retention, visual blurring). Dosages higher than 75 mg daily associated with cognitive impairment in elderly patients. Other adverse effects include NMS, orthostatic hypotension, agranulocytosis, and retinitis pigmentosa (at very high dosages). OBRA = Omnibus Budget Reconciliation Act of 1987.

Generic name	ziprasidone
Trade name	Geodon
Class	Benzisothiazolyl piperazine
Half-life	7 hours
Mechanism of action	Blockade of serotonin, dopamine, α_1-adrenergic, and histamine receptors; serotonin and norepinephrine reuptake inhibition
Available formulation	Capsules: 20, 40, 60, 80 mg
Starting dose	20 mg bid with food
Titration	Increase as tolerated at intervals of 3 days (or more)
Typical daily dose	80 mg (divided bid)
Dosage range	40–160 mg daily (divided bid)
Therapeutic serum level	Not established

Comments: Newly marketed atypical antipsychotic with little reported experience in the geriatric population. Although less associated with weight gain than are other atypical agents, cardiovascular effects are likely to make this a second-line drug in elderly patients. Well absorbed orally, with peak concentrations in 6–8 hours. Fatty food increases absorption. Nearly entirely (99%) protein bound. Metabolized in the liver by aldehyde oxidase and CYP3A4. Excreted in urine and feces. *Drug interactions:* avoid use with other drugs that act to prolong the QT_c interval; avoid use with significant CYP3A4 inhibitors; risk of significant hypotension with antihypertensive agents; may antagonize the effects of dopamine agonists. *Adverse effects:* QT_c interval prolongation, orthostatic hypotension, somnolence, EPS, transient prolactin level elevation, nausea, and rash. Baseline ECG and follow-up ECG recommended to determine QT_c effects.

3

Antidepressants

In current practice, medications labeled as "antidepressants" are used for a variety of indications beyond major depression, as listed in Table 3–1. The class of serotonin selective reuptake inhibitor (SSRI) antidepressants, in particular, has expanded the utility of antidepressant medications to include treatment of various anxiety disorders in elderly patients. SSRIs are viewed by many clinicians as the agents of first choice for treatment of geriatric depression, although electroconvulsive therapy (ECT) and several of the newer antidepressant agents are also useful as first-line therapies. Tricyclic antidepressants (TCAs) have assumed a more limited role despite demonstrated efficacy, mainly because of cardiovascular side effects. St.-John's-wort has a wider acceptance than its efficacy and safety probably merit, but it may be useful for a subgroup of depressed elders. Monoamine oxidase inhibitors (MAOIs) available in the United States are used as third-line agents, mainly in treatment-refractory cases.

Table 3–1.   Indications for antidepressant medication

Established indications

Unipolar major depression

Bipolar depression

Atypical depression

Melancholic depression

Psychotic depression

Secondary depression[a]

Dysthymic disorder

Bulimia

Complicated bereavement

Insomnia

Pain syndromes (neuropathic pain, atypical chest pain, etc.)

Panic disorder

Obsessive-compulsive disorder

Generalized anxiety disorder

Posttraumatic stress disorder

Possible/investigational uses

Aggression in dementia

Social phobia

Chronic fatigue syndrome/fibromyalgia

Emotional lability in personality disorders

Alcohol craving

Cocaine craving

Neurotic skin excoriation

Irritable bowel syndrome

[a]Depression in the context of medical disease affecting brain function, such as cancer, cardiovascular disease, dementia, diabetes, Parkinson's disease, and stroke.

Pharmacokinetics

Antidepressant formulations and strengths are listed in Table 3–2. With the exception of fluoxetine, paroxetine, nefazodone, and high-dose venlafaxine, antidepressants have linear kinetics, meaning that each dose increase yields a proportionate serum level increase. In general, antidepressants are rapidly and completely absorbed in the small intestine, but bioavailability is decreased secondary to first-pass metabolism. Food can significantly delay absorption of many antidepressants, but this delay probably has little clinical relevance.

Most antidepressants are highly lipophilic. As noted in Chapter 1, increased fat stores in elderly patients are associated with an increased volume of distribution for lipophilic drugs, with consequent lengthening of half-lives. Most antidepressants are also highly tissue- and protein-bound; one exception is venlafaxine. Antidepressants undergo different degrees of first-pass metabolism, yielding a range of bioavailability values. Cytochrome P450 (CYP) enzymes in the intestinal mucosa and liver catalyze oxidation reactions (demethylation and hydroxylation) involved in the primary metabolic pathway for antidepressants.

Whether the ratio of dose to concentration changes with normal aging depends largely on age-related changes in clearance for a particular drug. For example, aging is associated with decreased clearance of tertiary TCAs (e.g., imipramine and amitriptyline), and reduced doses of these medications are indicated in elders. On the other hand, aging is not associated with reduced clearance of desipramine, and full antidepressant doses and drug levels for desipramine are required in treating depression in elders (Nelson et al. 1995). Clearance of bupropion, nefazodone, and trazodone is decreased with aging, although variably.

Decreased renal function significantly affects clearance of water-soluble antidepressant metabolites. For drugs such as TCAs, such metabolite accumulation is clinically significant. For example, the concentration of a metabolite of nortriptyline (E10 hydroxy-nortriptyline) increases with decreased glomerular fil-

Table 3–2.   Selected antidepressant formulations and strengths

Generic name	Trade name	Tablets (mg)	Capsules (mg)	SR forms (mg)	Liquid (concentrate, suspension, or elixir)	Injectable form
Tricyclic antidepressants						
desipramine	Norpramin	10, 25, 50, 75, 100, 150	25, 50			
nortriptyline	Pamelor		10, 25, 50, 75		10 mg/5 mL	
Selective serotonin reuptake inhibitors						
citalopram	Celexa	20, 40			10 mg/5 mL	
fluoxetine	Prozac	10	10, 20, 40	90[a]	20 mg/5 mL	
paroxetine	Paxil	10, 20, 30, 40			10 mg/5 mL	
sertraline	Zoloft	25, 50, 100				
Psychostimulants						
dextroamphetamine	Dexedrine	5, 10		5, 10, 15		
methylphenidate	Ritalin	5, 10, 20		10, 20		

Table 3–2. Selected antidepressant formulations and strengths *(continued)*

Generic name	Trade name	Tablets (mg)	Capsules (mg)	SR forms (mg)	Liquid (concentrate, suspension, or elixir)	Injectable form
Novel antidepressants						
bupropion	Wellbutrin	75, 100		100, 150		
	Wellbutrin SR					
	Zyban					
mirtazapine	Remeron	15, 30, 45				
	Remeron SolTab	15, 30, 45				
nefazodone	Serzone	50, 100, 150, 200, 250				
trazodone	Desyrel	50, 100, 150, 300				
venlafaxine	Effexor	25, 37.5, 50, 75, 100		37.5, 75, 150		

^aProzac weekly.

tration rate, whereas the clearance of the parent compound is unaffected (Young et al. 1987). The metabolite is associated with prolonged cardiac conduction, is negatively correlated with clinical improvement, and is half as potent as the parent compound in noradrenergic uptake effects (Pollock et al. 1992; Schneider et al. 1990). An analogous situation applies to desipramine (Kitanaka et al. 1982) and probably to other TCAs. Serum drug levels do not routinely take metabolite levels into account, although assay for metabolite levels can be specifically ordered. Although desmethylvenlafaxine is also renally excreted, evidence to date suggests that the clinical significance of accumulation of this metabolite for normally aging patients is probably minimal (McEvoy et al. 2000).

Pharmacodynamics and Mechanism of Action

TCAs have broad-ranging receptor binding and reuptake inhibitory effects, including the following: serotonin, norepinephrine, and, to a lesser extent, dopamine reuptake inhibition; muscarinic, histamine, and α_1-adrenergic receptor binding; and ATPase inhibition, which results in stabilization of excitable cell membranes and slowing of cardiac conduction, a quinidine-like effect (McEvoy et al. 2000).

SSRI antidepressants act primarily to reduce serotonin reuptake and thereby enhance serotonergic neurotransmission. At higher doses (e.g., >60 mg fluoxetine), SSRIs also have limited reuptake effects on norepinephrine and dopamine (Tulloch and Johnson 1992), with sertraline having the greatest dopamine reuptake blocking effects. Paroxetine has weak affinity for muscarinic receptors; otherwise, the SSRIs have negligible receptor binding effects. SSRIs have been found experimentally to have a flat dose-response curve, such that the clinical practice of escalation to high doses is not warranted in many cases. In practice, however, some individual patients do require higher or lower doses than others, in part because of the wide variation among individuals in plasma levels attained at a given dose. In addition, for treatment of conditions such as obsessive-compulsive disorder (OCD), higher SSRI doses are routinely used.

Newer antidepressants have various receptor binding and inhibitory effects. Bupropion has a unique profile, with complex noradrenergic effects, dopamine inhibition at higher doses, and no serotonergic effects (McEvoy et al. 2000). Mirtazapine is the first of the so-called noradrenergic and specific serotonergic antagonists (NASSAs) with pre- and postsynaptic α_2-adrenergic receptor blocking effects, postsynaptic serotonin$_2$ (5-HT$_2$) antagonist affects, serotonin$_3$ (5-HT$_3$) antagonist effects, serotonin$_1$ (5-HT$_1$) agonist effects, and moderate histaminergic (H$_1$) affinity (Fawcett and Barkin 1998).

Nefazodone is a potent 5-HT$_2$ antagonist with the long-term effect of decreasing the number of cortical 5-HT$_2$ receptor binding sites; it is also a weak 5-HT$_2$ and norepinephrine reuptake inhibitor (McEvoy et al. 2000). m-Chlorophenylpiperazine (m-CPP), a minor metabolite of nefazodone, is an agonist at 5-HT$_{1A}$ and 5-HT$_{1C}$ sites and an antagonist at 5-HT$_2$ and 5-HT$_3$ sites. It is speculated that 5-HT$_2$ antagonism might limit the anxiogenic effects of serotonin reuptake inhibition, so that nefazodone may be more anxiolytic than SSRIs. Trazodone is a weak serotonin reuptake inhibitor and has differential serotonin agonist/antagonist effects, depending on dose (McEvoy et al. 2000). Venlafaxine is a serotonin and norepinephrine reuptake inhibitor and is a dopamine reuptake inhibitor at high dosages (>350 mg/day). Reboxetine is a selective norepinephrine reuptake inhibitor not yet marketed in the United States. The antidepressant mechanism of St.-John's-wort is not entirely clear but may involve serotonin reuptake inhibition and MAO inhibition (LaFrance et al. 2000).

Drug Interactions

With the possible exceptions of venlafaxine, mirtazapine, citalopram, and sertraline, inhibitory CYP interactions may be very significant for antidepressants. In general, SSRIs act as CYP enzyme inhibitors and are associated with elevated serum levels of the various substrates listed in Table 1–1 in Chapter 1; TCAs are themselves substrates but do not act as potent inhibitors (Greenblatt et al. 1998). Paroxetine and fluoxetine are very potent inhibitors of the CYP2D6 enzyme, while sertraline and citalopram are weaker inhibitors of this enzyme. Fluvoxamine is a very strong inhibitor of CYP1A2, with substrates including mexiletine and theophylline, as shown in Chapter 1 (Table 1–1); it also strongly inhibits CYP2C19 and moderately inhibits CYP2C9 and CYP3A. Drug interaction through enzyme inhibition is a major reason that fluvoxamine is not a first-line drug in treating elderly patients. Certain TCAs, SSRIs, and atypical antidepressants are substrates for CYP3A4, of which nefazodone is a potent inhibitor. Selected antidepressant drug interactions are listed in Table 3–3.

In general, a listed CYP interaction between a substrate and an inhibitor does not prohibit the co-prescription of those medications. An interaction simply means that when a substrate is prescribed in the presence of an inhibitor, the level of that substrate could become elevated. Accordingly, caution is used when substrates with narrow therapeutic indices are prescribed, and CYP inhibition is considered whenever adverse events occur during pharmacotherapy.

In contrast, CYP and other enzyme induction may be highly problematic. For example, St.-John's-wort is a CYP3A4 inducer, and this medication in cyclosporine-treated heart transplant patients may have been the cause of subtherapeutic cyclosporine levels and transplant rejection in several patients (Ruschitzka et al. 2000). In patients on antiretroviral agents such as indinavir, co-administration of St.-John's-wort has also been associated with subtherapeutic drug levels that could lead to loss of efficacy (Piscitelli et al. 2000).

Efficacy

The majority of depressed elderly patients eventually respond to aggressive treatment of their depression (Flint and Rifat 1996), al-

Table 3–3.   Antidepressant drug interactions

Antidepressant	Interacting drug	Potential interaction
MAOI	bupropion	Seizures
	buspirone	Hypertension
	guanadrel	Hypertension
	insulin and other hypoglycemic agents	Severe hypoglycemia
	levodopa	Hypertension with nonselective MAOIs; if you must use a nonselective MAOI with levodopa, be sure the levodopa is administered in combination with carbidopa (Sinemet)
	meperidine and its congeners; sympathomimetic agents	DO NOT COPRESCRIBE; risk of hypertensive crisis
	reserpine	Precipitation of mania
	SSRI	Avoid coprescribing; risk of serotonin syndrome
	succinylcholine	With phenelzine, prolonged neuromuscular blockade and apnea
	tolcapone	Toxicity
	tramadol	Toxicity
	triptans (except naratriptan)	Toxicity

Table 3–3. Antidepressant drug interactions *(continued)*

Antidepressant	Interacting drug	Potential interaction
mirtazapine	benzodiazepines, ethanol	Additive CNS depression; impaired cognitive and motor function
	MAOI	Cardiovascular, neurological toxicity
nefazodone	CYP3A substrates (e.g., alprazolam, cyclosporine, haloperidol, simvastatin)	Increased substrate levels via CYP3A inhibition
	digoxin	Possible digoxin toxicity
SSRI (see also individual agents)	MAOI; dextromethorphan and its congeners	Avoid coprescribing; risk of serotonin syndrome
fluoxetine paroxetine	CYP2D6 substrates (e.g., TCAs, flecainide, mexiletine, metoprolol)	Increased substrate levels via CYP2D6 inhibition
fluvoxamine	CYP1A2 substrates (e.g., propranolol, theophylline)	Increased substrate levels via CYP1A2 inhibition
	CYP2C19 substrates	Increased substrate levels via CYP2C19 inhibition
TCA	antihypertensive agents	Antihypertensive effects blocked for clonidine, guanethidine, guanfacine, guanadrel
	carbamazepine	Toxicity

Table 3–3. Antidepressant drug interactions *(continued)*

Antidepressant	Interacting drug	Potential interaction
TCA *(continued)*	CYP2D6 inhibitors (e.g., quinidine, SSRIs)	Increased TCA level and potential toxicity
	CYP3A4 inhibitors (e.g., ketoconazole, grapefruit juice)	Increased TCA level and potential toxicity
	CYP3A4 and CYP2D6 inducers	Decreased TCA level
	MAOI	Serotonin syndrome
	quinidine	Toxicity
	sympathomimetic agents	Hypertension
	thioridazine and other conventional antipsychotics	Increased level of TCA and/or antipsychotic
trazodone	buspirone, SSRIs	Serotonin syndrome; trazodone toxicity with fluoxetine
venlafaxine	MAOI	Cardiovascular, neurological toxicity

Note. CNS = central nervous system; CYP = cytochrome P450; SSRI = selective serotonin reuptake inhibitor; TCA = tricyclic antidepressant.

[a]See Table 1–1 in Chapter 1 for a listing of selected CYP interactions.

Source. Adapted from Pies 1998.

though elderly patients may be slower to respond than younger patients. Predictors of nonresponse include severe depression, presence of a comorbid personality disorder or chronic physical illness, adverse life events, prior treatment failure, "near delusional" status, and age (Nelson et al. 1994). The elderly are at chronic risk of undertreatment because of low expectations regarding recovery and fears about aggressive pharmacotherapy as well as ECT (Heeren et al. 1997). In fact, partial recovery is often accepted as the endpoint in the treatment of many elderly depressed patients, resulting in a high prevalence of chronic (and apparently treatment-refractory) depression in this population.

As with nongeriatric patients, elders with certain syndromes require cotreatment of various kinds. Those with psychotic depression require an antipsychotic, those with bipolar depression may require a mood stabilizer (and may not be good candidates for antidepressants), those with chronic pain syndromes may require other analgesics, and those with OCD and other anxiety disorders may require behavior therapy or cognitive therapy. In most cases, these cotreatments serve to enhance the efficacy of the antidepressant.

Clinical Use

The range of indications for antidepressant medications has broadened over the years, in part because of the introduction of SSRIs and other novel antidepressants with demonstrated efficacy in treating anxiety. A list of current indications for antidepressants is shown in Table 3–1. Specific treatment for most listed indications is covered in a later section (see "Treatment of Selected Syndromes and Disorders With Antidepressants").

A conundrum in treating elderly patients is the determination of which symptoms are due to medical illness or coprescribed medications and which might be attributable to depression. The inclusive approach, in which all symptoms (including anorexia and fatigue) are counted toward a diagnosis of depression, results in increased sensitivity but decreased specificity in diagnosis. The presence of "psychological" symptoms can assist the diagnostic effort, since helplessness, hopelessness, loss of self-esteem, feelings of worthlessness, excessive guilt, and wishes to die are not normal concomitants of medical illness.

Choice of Antidepressant

The initial decision in treating depression in the geriatric patient involves a risk-benefit assessment of pharmacotherapy versus other treatments, including ECT, psychotherapy, bright light therapy, and exercise therapy. The severity of the depression dictates whether ECT or pharmacotherapy is used in preference to other modalities. ECT remains the treatment of choice for depressed elderly patients with psychotic symptoms. ECT is more effective than pharmacotherapy in treating severe depression and induces remission rapidly, but its reputed superior safety compared with antidepressants has yet to be demonstrated by controlled study. In addition, it may be more costly than pharmacotherapy, in part because it requires a longer hospital stay (Manly et al. 2000). As an alternative to ECT, repeated transcranial magnetic stimulation (rTMS) would theoretically be preferred because general anesthesia is not required. Preliminary reports suggest, however, that rTMS is less effective in older than in younger depressed patients, with cerebral atrophy possibly confounding current stimulation protocols.

Psychodynamic, interpersonal, and cognitive therapies are appropriate for high-functioning geriatric outpatients and do not entail significant physical side effects. Behavior therapy is appropriate for almost any institutionalized patient and is often applied in tandem with other modalities. Bright light therapy can also be used in conjunction with pharmacotherapy for depression. In the authors' experience, adjunctive bright light therapy can be useful in the early stages of treatment before pharmacotherapy becomes effective, particularly when depression has its onset when ambient light is waning (e.g., fall months in the northern hemisphere).

Regular aerobic exercise can supplement or even supplant antidepressant medication in the treatment of mild to moderate geriatric depression, but it has a slower onset of effect and so requires a high level of motivation (Blumenthal et al. 1999).

The first consideration in choosing an antidepressant medication for an elderly patient is that of *medical comorbidity*. Table 3–4 lists selected antidepressant recommendations for particular medical subpopulations. Ischemic heart disease is a relative contraindication for TCAs (Roose and Glassman 1994). Inability to comply with dietary and over-the-counter medication limitations is a constraint to the prescription of MAOIs. Medications required for other conditions also guide therapy, since potential drug interactions must be taken into account.

For severe unipolar major depression, nortriptyline, venlafaxine, or bupropion is considered first-line therapy by some clinicians (Roose et al. 1994). For bipolar depression, bupropion or a SSRI such as paroxetine or citalopram may be chosen because of reduced likelihood of inducing mania (Thase and Sachs 2000). For atypical depression or dysthymic disorder, an SSRI may be preferred because of a favorable risk-benefit ratio, although there is some evidence that SSRI therapy might not successfully maintain remission in patients with atypical symptoms (McGrath et al. 2000). For primary anxiety disorders or for depression associated with significant anxiety, an SSRI, mirtazapine, venlafaxine, or nefazodone may be preferred, since these agents may be more anxiolytic than other antidepressants. For persistent insomnia, trazodone is a drug of choice in the elderly.

Other factors in choosing an antidepressant include the specific profile of symptoms (e.g., fluoxetine, venlafaxine, or bupropion for retarded depression vs. mirtazapine for agitated depression) and history of specific antidepressant response as well as family history of response, since what was effective in the past or for genetic relatives is probably more likely to be effective again. In addition, patient preference (in terms of expected "nuisance" side effects, such as dry mouth or blurred vision vs. impotence or weight gain) and cost are taken into account.

Table 3–4. Antidepressant recommendations for special populations

Clinical problem	Recommendation	Rationale
Alzheimer's disease	Avoid TCAs.	Anticholinergic effects worsen cognition.
Cardiac conduction abnormality (bundle branch block or intraventricular conduction delay)	Avoid TCAs.	Any TCA could worsen conduction disturbance.
	Use SSRI, bupropion, venlafaxine, or nefazodone.	Do not prolong cardiac conduction; rarely associated with arrhythmias.
Ischemic heart disease	Avoid TCAs.	Presence of TCA heightens risk of arrhythmia when ischemia occurs.
Post–myocardial infarction	Avoid TCAs.	Increased risk of mortality with TCAs.
Congestive heart failure	Avoid TCAs.	Severe orthostatic blood pressure changes can occur.
Diabetes	Avoid TCAs.	TCAs often have hyperglycemic effects.
	Use SSRI, bupropion, or venlafaxine.	SSRIs may have hypoglycemic effects. Bupropion and venlafaxine have little effect on glucose levels.
Epilepsy	Avoid bupropion	Bupropion is associated with increased seizure risk.

Table 3–4.   Antidepressant recommendations for special populations (*continued*)

Clinical problem	Recommendation	Rationale
Glaucoma	Avoid TCAs.	Anticholinergic effects of TCAs can precipitate angle closure.
	Use SSRIs, bupropion, nefazodone, or trazodone.	These agents lack anticholinergic effects. Trazodone lowers intraocular pressure in open-angle glaucoma.
Hepatic disease	Avoid TCAs (especially tertiary amines).	TCAs have a narrow therapeutic index.
	Use short-half-life SSRIs; venlafaxine; or bupropion (if no history of seizure).	These agents have a wide therapeutic index; however, must use lower starting doses in hepatic disease.
Obesity	Avoid SSRIs, TCAs, and MAOIs.	These agents are associated with significant weight gain when used chronically.
	Use bupropion, venlafaxine, psychostimulant, or, possibly, nefazodone.	These agents are associated with less weight gain with chronic use.
Polypharmacy (patient taking multiple medications)	Use citalopram, sertraline, venlafaxine, or bupropion.	These drugs have fewer drug interactions.

Table 3–4. Antidepressant recommendations for special populations (*continued*)

Clinical problem	Recommendation	Rationale
Pulmonary disease: apnea, COPD	Use SSRIs or trazodone.	SSRIs improve respiratory function in some cases. Trazodone does not usually cause respiratory depression.
Renal disease	Use SSRIs.	Metabolite clearance is less of an issue than with TCAs.

Note. COPD = chronic obstructive pulmonary disease; MAOI = monoamine oxidase inhibitor; SSRI = selective serotonin reuptake inhibitor; TCA = tricyclic antidepressant.
Source. Adapted from Pies 1998.

Certain antidepressants are preferred for geriatric patients. In general, these drugs lack significant anticholinergic effects, are less likely than other drugs to cause orthostatic hypotension, are not associated with daytime oversedation, and, with the exception of nortriptyline, are rarely associated with cardiac dysrhythmia. Antidepressants generally preferred for elders include the SSRIs citalopram, fluoxetine, paroxetine, and sertraline; the heterocyclics bupropion, mirtazapine, venlafaxine, and, possibly, reboxetine; and the TCA nortriptyline. For any particular patient, however, any one of these drugs might have disadvantages, so therapy must be individualized. Reboxetine is a selective norepinephrine reuptake inhibitor not yet marketed in the United States.

Although TCAs have several disadvantages in the treatment of geriatric patients, their efficacy in depression has been clearly demonstrated. Nortriptyline is the agent most used and recommended; tertiary amines are avoided in this population because of sedative and anticholinergic effects. Nortriptyline has for some time been considered the gold standard of tricyclic treatment for elderly patients because of its potency, linear kinetics, plasma level guidelines, relatively low potential for inducing orthostasis, and limited anticholinergic effects. However, it is no safer than other TCAs with respect to cardiac conduction effects. Nortriptyline treatment in one geriatric cohort was associated with increased triglyceride and VLDL (very-low-density lipoprotein) levels, increased heart rate, modest changes in cardiac conduction, and significant reduction in creatinine clearance after 7 months (Pollock et al. 1994). Side effects such as increased heart rate and anticholinergic effects, however well tolerated, could have significant long-term impact on quality of life for the treated elder (Roose and Suthers 1998). In general, nortriptyline is well tolerated in medically stable patients without dementia but less well tolerated in very old, frail, medically ill patients such as stroke patients (Flint 1997).

In view of concerns about the safety of administering TCAs to elderly patients, most clinicians now consider SSRIs and selected atypical agents to be the first-line treatment for depression in this population. There is, however, a long-standing controversy over the question of whether SSRIs are, in fact, equal in efficacy to TCAs in the treatment of severely depressed or melancholic patients. In terms of efficacy per se, we still prefer nortriptyline to an SSRI for this population, but note that nortriptyline is frequently contraindicated in geriatric patients because of cardiac disease. For this reason, atypical agents such as bupropion, venlafaxine, or mirtazapine are increasingly selected as first-line agents. It is the experience of the authors that many severely depressed geriatric patients who are not effectively treated with SSRIs do respond well to treatment with one of these atypical agents.

Despite methodological problems, studies of SSRIs have demonstrated clear effectiveness in mild to moderate depression in outpatients, dysthymic disorder, secondary depression, and the full range of anxiety disorders listed in Table 3–1. Fluoxetine is activating for most patients and may be particularly useful for patients with hypersomnia and psychomotor retardation, provided they are not co-administered drugs metabolized via CYP2D6 or CYP3A4 enzymes. In addition, the long half-lives of fluoxetine and norfluoxetine may confer some advantage in poorly compliant patients, because missed doses are not so problematic and because weekly dosing schedules may be possible. Fluoxetine is now FDA approved for the treatment of geriatric depression. Sertraline has been touted as superior for patients requiring treatment with other medications because of reduced CYP2D6 interactions. Paroxetine may be less useful in elderly patients with cognitive impairment because it does have anticholinergic effects, however weak. Citalopram appears to lack significant inhibitory effects on CYP enzymes and is not significantly activating or anxiogenic, so it may prove to be the SSRI of first choice among elderly patients. Systematic comparative studies of SSRIs in the geriatric population will help resolve this issue.

Irreversible MAOIs are not considered first-line agents in treating elderly patients because of serious and persistent side effects, such as orthostasis, and the need for dietary and medication restrictions. Irreversible MAOIs selective for MAO-B, such as selegiline (Deprenyl, Eldepryl), could theoretically obviate the need for such restrictions, but in practice the dosages effective against depression for many patients are high enough that selectivity is lost. MAOIs are used as second- or third-line agents in patients with atypical depression, bipolar depression, panic disorder, or depression refractory to treatment with other medications. Patients prescribed MAOIs should also be prescribed pyridoxine (vitamin B_6) 10–50 mg daily. A new class of agents not yet available in the United States is that of the reversible inhibitors of monoamine oxidase (RIMAs), agents lacking many of the disadvantages noted above for irreversible MAOIs. Moclobemide is a RIMA selective for MAO-A that may be particularly useful in treating patients with depression in the context of dementia.

Psychostimulants have found a treatment niche in the population of depressed, apathetic, medically ill geriatric patients, including those with dementia. Response to either methylphenidate or dextroamphetamine is often rapid, with effects seen in less than 24 hours. Energy, alertness, attention, and motivation may improve, but it is unclear whether this represents a true antidepressant response (Salzman 1992). These medications are considered safer than TCAs in patients with medical illness. They can prove problematic in patients with significant anxiety, since restlessness can be a side effect. As a rule, tolerance is not observed, but these agents have not been studied systematically over the long term. The potential exists for acute worsening of depression on discontinuation of these agents. They are used by some clinicians as accelerators in patients who later continue to take another antidepressant. They may also be useful in countering apathy and sexual dysfunction in SSRI-treated patients.

Similar to the SSRIs, newer antidepressants confer the significant advantage of having little or no muscarinic effects and, with the exception of nefazodone, little α_1-adrenergic effect. Nefazodone may be useful for elderly patients with prominent anxiety or insomnia, provided the patient is able to tolerate the associated sedation and hypotension, and provided that small initial doses with slow titration are used. Venlafaxine should theoretically be useful in the seriously depressed elderly population, considering its broad pharmacodynamic effects, but our experience is that blood pressure elevations do occur in elders treated with this medication, even at doses less than 100 mg daily.

ECT has high short-term efficacy in the treatment of major depression among elderly patients, but it also has a high relapse rate; to maintain the antidepressant response, antidepressant medication or maintenance ECT is required. In anticipation of ECT, nonessential psychotropic medications (particularly benzo-diazepines and mood stabilizers) may be discontinued, although this is by no means a universal practice. ECT protocols used for geriatric patients generally involve treatments two to three times weekly, but otherwise, protocols differ among centers. Some use nondominant unilateral treatment and switch to bilateral treatment only for nonresponders, whereas others start with bilateral treatment. With the pulse widths now in use, bilateral treatment is more effective than unilateral but may be associated with more severe cognitive impairment. A useful rule of thumb is that the patient recovering from an ECT session should have orientation to time and place return within about 10 minutes. Periods of disorientation of 45 minutes or more may predict more persistent memory impairment.

Alternative Formulations

The lack of available alternative formulations of antidepressants makes dosing quite inflexible, and this can be a serious problem, particularly for severely depressed patients who are not competent to decide about medications but refuse to take them. Amitriptyline, imipramine, and doxepin are the only antidepressants available for parenteral use in the United States, and none is a drug of choice for elderly patients. Oral solutions of nortriptyline, fluoxetine, paroxetine, citalopram, and doxepin are available, and sometimes these are accepted in juice or water by a patient refusing to take pills. In extreme cases, court permission can be sought to place needed medications in food for patients deemed incompetent, but this strategy introduces the risk that the patient will begin refusing food or will miss doses because of unfinished meals. In addition, this can prove to be a difficult issue for staff, who may continue to believe they are violating the patient's rights despite court approval.

For patients unable to swallow, rectal doxepin or rectal amitriptyline (50 mg in cocoa butter twice daily) may be tolerated. As noted earlier, however, neither of these medications is a drug of choice in elderly patients. When lithium is used as adjunctive therapy, lithium citrate can be used for patients who cannot swallow pills or who suffer intolerable gastrointestinal side effects from standard lithium formulations.

Baseline Laboratory Studies and Clinical Evaluation

Before initiating antidepressant treatment, a careful history should be obtained and corroborated regarding alcohol and illicit drug use. Chronic alcohol overuse in particular is not uncommon in the current elderly cohort and can be associated with significant depressive signs and symptoms. Patients with this history should undergo detoxification for a minimum of 2 weeks and then be reassessed. In many cases, depression remits with simple abstinence. If antidepressants are used after reassessment, it is important that abstinence be maintained for the duration of treatment, since the combination of medication and alcohol can be hepatotoxic.

Other historical information of note relates to cardiac disease, hypertension, prostatic enlargement, narrow-angle glaucoma, history of seizures, history of orthostasis or falls, sexual dysfunction, and drug allergies. These factors help guide the choice of antidepressant. Side effects and warnings for specific medications and classes are described in later sections. For patients with anxiety spectrum illness, consumption of caffeine and nicotine is important to quantify. For all patients, nonpsychiatric prescription medications and over-the-counter medications should be noted.

Recent stressors may be identified in the process of history taking. It is a common mistake to assume that depression is a "natural reaction" to the stresses of aging, but this argument becomes untenable in view of the facts that the large majority of elders endure stressors without ever becoming depressed, that even milder depressions may remit with appropriate pharmacotherapy, and that the presence of a "precipitating stressor" predicts neither the course of depression nor the response to treatment. The presence of recent stressors, rather than arguing against pharmacotherapy in the seriously depressed patient, argues for cotreatment with medication and psychotherapy.

Physical examination includes, at minimum, orthostatic vital signs, basic cardiac and pulmonary examination, and neurological examination. Neurological examination is directed toward uncovering focal signs suggestive of stroke, since depression associated with stroke requires a somewhat more aggressive treatment algorithm. Mental status examination focuses on immediate assessment of suicide risk, presence of psychotic features (delusions or hallucinations), presence of mixed mood features (mania or hypomania and depression), and cognition. The last-mentioned is usefully assessed with the Mini-Mental State Exam (Folstein et al. 1975). Depression and anxiety rating scales are also useful, particularly in fully delineating signs and symptoms such as somatic complaints that might later be attributed to medication.

Laboratory studies are performed either to uncover a physical condition that may be associated with depression or anxiety symptoms (e.g., anemia, hypothyroidism), to identify factors that could complicate medication treatment (e.g., bundle branch block, chronic renal insufficiency), or to uncover factors that might interfere with treatment response such as low B_{12} or folate levels (Fava et al. 1997). Routine studies include the following:

ECG, complete blood count, serum electrolyte (including K^+, Ca^{++}, Na^+, and Mg^{++}) levels, serum creatinine level, liver function tests (including aspartate transaminase [AST], alanine transaminase [ALT], and lactate dehydrogenase), B_{12} level, folate level, and an ultra-sensitive thyroid-stimulating hormone level.

A number of studies have reported variable success in using other laboratory tests to confirm and monitor depression. These tests include the dexamethasone suppression test, thyrotropin-releasing hormone test, platelet monoamine oxidase activity, platelet imipramine binding, and α_2-adrenergic receptor binding. In general, these tests are considered too nonspecific to be recommended for routine use.

Dose and Dose Titration

Details of initiating and titrating antidepressants are contained in the specific drug summaries at the end of this chapter. In general, for treatment of depressive spectrum disorders, the same dosage that induced remission is used for continuation and maintenance phase treatment.

When TCAs are used, careful attention must be paid to changes in blood pressure and pulse and to reports of dizziness. For inpatients, dose increments are made approximately every 3 days, as tolerated; for outpatients, dose increments are made every 5–7 days. For nortriptyline, the target dose can be determined by administering a 25-mg test dose, obtaining a plasma level at 24 hours, and using a dosing nomogram (Schneider et al. 1987).

For SSRIs, doses are initiated in the elderly at one-half the usual dose and are increased to the minimum effective dose after 1–2 weeks. In our experience, the minimum effective dose in elders for fluoxetine, paroxetine, and citalopram is usually 10–20 mg, and the minimum effective dose for sertraline is 50–100 mg. The patient is maintained at this dose for a period of 3–4 weeks before any further increments are made, since increasing the dose sooner is associated with more severe side effects but not more rapid response (Flint 1994, 1997).

For treatment of anxiety spectrum disorders as well as other conditions such as insomnia and aggression in dementia, little information is available from systematic study to inform target dosing. In general, treatment is initiated at the lowest possible dose and the dosage is titrated slowly. Anecdotal experience suggests that elderly patients with anxiety disorders such as panic disorder may initially require doses so small as to be achievable only with liquid suspension formulations (e.g., citalopram 2 mg daily). To achieve full remission of panic symptoms, however, these same patients require usual "antidepressant" doses. Furthermore, some elderly patients with panic disorder or OCD may require fluoxetine up to 60 mg for symptom control.

Course of Antidepressant Response

In elderly patients, significant antidepressant response sometimes requires up to 12 weeks of treatment. Although time to effect varies a great deal between individuals, in general, a minimum of 6 weeks of antidepressant treatment should be undertaken in an elderly patient before any prediction about "nonresponse" is made for that trial. Early responses (within days) can represent placebo responses that are not sustained over time. True responses usually involve a lag time of at least several weeks, although rapid dose escalation as well as use of particular agents may be associated with true early responses in some patients. For example, fast titration of venlafaxine can elicit an early response but, unfortunately, can also be associated with intolerable gastrointestinal side effects.

Little is known about the course of response in elderly patients to antidepressant medication for anxiety spectrum disorders such as panic disorder and OCD. Considering that latencies to response in younger patients are longer for these disorders than for depressive disorders, it might be reasonable to expect that latencies in elders would be especially prolonged. Some clinicians advocate continuing antidepressant treatment for OCD for 12 weeks before making any predictions about nonresponse.

Monitoring Antidepressant Therapy

Initiation of tricyclic and MAOI antidepressant therapy in elderly patients is often best accomplished in the inpatient setting so that important parameters such as blood pressure, pulse, and ECG can be adequately monitored. Frequency of follow-up visits during the initial stages of outpatient treatment is determined by the individual situation, but follow-up typically occurs on a weekly basis. During continuation and maintenance treatment, the elderly outpatient who is doing well at a stable dose of antidepressant medication should be seen at least every 3–4 months.

During the acute phase of treatment, patients taking TCAs should have regular determinations of orthostatic blood pressure and pulse as well as a baseline ECG. At steady state, the TCA blood level and a follow-up ECG should be obtained. Patients taking venlafaxine should have regular determinations of blood pressure, particularly supine diastolic pressure. Patients taking SSRIs require pulse checks for bradycardia, serum sodium checks because of the risk of hyponatremia, and examination for (rare) extrapyramidal symptoms. For all patients, suicidal ideation must be monitored, in view of the particular risk for this problem in the elderly population. In addition, weight loss in the acute phase of treatment with fluoxetine should be monitored.

During continuation and maintenance therapy, a reasonable (but by no means universal) standard of monitoring is as follows: for patients taking a TCA, an ECG, orthostatic blood pressure and pulse, electrolytes, serum creatinine, and liver function tests every 6 months. The TCA level should be rechecked with any dosage change or when a new medication with potential CYP interaction has been added. For patients treated with an SSRI, pulse checks (and ECG, if there is any indication of bradycardia), electrolytes, and liver function tests every 6 months are appropriate. In the absence of data regarding cardiac effects of long-term treatment with newer "atypical" antidepressants, recommendations regarding monitoring for these agents are the same as those for TCAs. Weight should also be monitored for patients treated with mirtazapine or an SSRI. For patients treated with an MAOI, orthostatic blood pressure and pulse should be obtained at each visit. In addition, because of the risk of fulminant hepatic failure, patients treated with phenelzine should have liver function tests regularly, at least during the first 6 months of therapy.

As discussed in Chapter 1 ("Introduction to Geriatric Psychopharmacology"), a serum level of any antidepressant can be obtained to determine noncompliance or toxicity. With regard to therapeutic level monitoring, data are available for nortriptyline, desipramine, and imipramine. In elderly patients, nortriptyline has a therapeutic window in the range of 50 to 150 ng/mL. In a recent randomized trial of two fixed serum levels of nortriptyline (40–60 ng/mL vs 80–120 ng/mL) in an elderly cohort, the lower level was associated with more residual depressive symptoms, and the higher with more constipation, but there was no difference between groups in the frequency of relapse to major depression over a 3-year period (Reynolds et al. 1999). In patients with dementia and depression, therapeutic levels of nortriptyline are not established, but lower doses are used. In addition, as noted earlier, nortriptyline's active hydroxy metabolite is renally excreted, and in patients with reduced creatinine clearance, this metabolite level can be elevated even when the parent drug level is in the normal range (Schneider et al. 1990). Although this metabolite can be assayed in many laboratories by special order, it is more important to follow the ECG to determine whether changes in cardiac conduction are seen.

The therapeutic threshold for desipramine in elderly patients is a serum level in the range of 105 to 125 ng/mL (Alexopoulos 1996; Nelson et al. 1995). Imipramine is not recommended for use in elderly patients. Therapeutic ranges for SSRI antidepressants have not been established, and, in fact, there is a very large between-individual variation in level for a given dose because of large differences in absorption and metabolism.

One criterion used to gauge response to therapy in major depression is 50% or greater reduction in score on a scale such as the Hamilton Rating Scale for Depression (Ham-D). This reduction may be adequate for mildly depressed patients, but for those with high initial scores, the 50% score could still be in the range representing significant depression. In these cases, a remission criterion is more appropriate, defined as a score of less than or equal to 7 (for the 17-item version) or 8 (for the 21-item version) on the Ham-D. Presumably, these scores would correspond to a return to "normal" functioning for the individual patient.

Duration of Treatment

Three stages of depression treatment are recognized (Flint 1997). During the *acute phase,* remission is induced. Remission can be defined as a return to the patient's presymptomatic baseline or to a cut-off score on a scale such as the Ham-D. Typically, this phase lasts 6–12 weeks. During the *continuation phase,* remission is preserved. Continuation therapy for elders should last for a minimum of 6 months, with 2 years being optimal for those with particularly severe or frequent episodes (Flint 1994, 1997). After completing a full course of continuation therapy, the patient is said to have "recovered." At that point, *maintenance phase* therapy is considered for susceptible patients, and this therapy is continued indefinitely.

Candidates for maintenance therapy include the following: patients with a history of three or more episodes of major depression; those with two or more rapidly recurrent episodes, pre-existing dysthymic disorder, onset of depression after age 60 years, prolonged or severe individual episodes, or poor response to acute treatment; and those with coexisting anxiety disorders or substance abuse (Hirschfeld and Schatzberg 1994). For continuation as well as maintenance therapy, full acute doses of antidepressant medication are recommended, as is continuation of any adjunctive treatment such as lithium (Flint and Rifat 2000). As noted earlier, in maintenance therapy with nortriptyline, when serum levels are maintained between 80 and 120 ng/mL, fewer residual depressive symptoms are seen, but constipation occurs more frequently. If such side effects cannot be managed, maintenance of a serum level in the range of 40 to 60 ng/mL is equally effective in preventing recurrence of major depressive episodes (Reynolds et al. 1999).

Little is known about duration of treatment for anxiety disorders in elderly patients. At least a subset of patients with severe forms of panic disorder or OCD require indefinite treatment with antidepressant medication. Others may respond to cognitive-behavioral therapy (CBT) alone or can have antidepressants tapered off after a course of CBT.

Managing Treatment Resistance

Treatment resistance occurs when there has been no response to an adequate amount of medication administered for a sufficient length of time. Adequate amount is reliably determined only for medications with known therapeutic blood levels: nortriptyline, desipramine, and imipramine. In determining "adequacy" for all other antidepressants, it is important to note that the ratio of dose to concentration varies widely among individuals. For this reason, a significant proportion of patients with illnesses labeled as "treatment resistant" respond to a simple increase in dose. For example, a patient treated with an SSRI such as citalopram 20 mg daily who shows a partial response at 8 weeks may experience remission of symptoms with an increase in dose to 30 mg daily. Furthermore, time to remission varies a great deal among elderly individuals, so other patients respond simply to a continuation of medication; a partial responder at 4 weeks may experience remission of symptoms at 8 weeks at the same dose. Chronically dysthymic patients may require 10 or more weeks for a full response.

A substantial minority of elderly patients do not respond to an adequate initial trial of antidepressant. For these patients, combination therapy, augmentation, acceleration, switching drugs, bright light therapy, and ECT can be considered.

Effective drug combinations usually target more than one

neurotransmitter system. Currently, bupropion is used in combination with SSRIs with good effect, and reboxetine may be used similarly in the future to complement SSRIs. Side effects of the combination of SSRI and bupropion are reportedly just additive. Since bupropion is stimulating, it may be associated with improvement in any SSRI-associated apathy as well as sexual side effects. When the SSRIs fluoxetine or paroxetine are selected, however, a lower dose of bupropion should be used, since the hydroxy- metabolite of bupropion is metabolized by the CYP2D6 enzyme, which is inhibited by these drugs.

Combination therapy involving SSRIs and TCAs can be highly effective and fast acting. Caution is advised, however, since serum TCA concentrations can be significantly elevated when SSRIs that inhibit their metabolism via CYP enzymes (particularly fluoxetine, fluvoxamine, and paroxetine) are co-administered. This may be hazardous for patients with ischemic heart disease or preexisting cardiac conduction abnormalities. In general, when these combinations are used, half of the usual dose of TCA is prescribed, along with a minimal effective dose of SSRI. Serum concentrations of TCA are monitored, if available. Although some clinicians recommend discontinuing one agent at the time that remission is achieved, with continuation monotherapy (Nelson et al. 1995), this strategy carries the risk of relapse.

Augmentation is used in cases of partial response and can be pharmacological or nonpharmacological; only the former is discussed here. The advantage of augmentation therapy over switching is that it does not require tapering and discontinuation of any medication, so the response is theoretically more rapid. The disadvantage is that yet another medication is introduced, with the potential for drug interactions.

Agents used for antidepressant augmentation include lithium, triiodothyronine (T_3), and estrogen. Lithium could be used to augment the effects of any antidepressant, but most clinical experience at this point has been with TCAs and SSRIs. In our experience, lithium augmentation is often effective in elderly patients but is not necessarily benign; side effects include serotonin syndrome, neurotoxicity, hypothyroidism, and renal dysfunction. Augmentation is usually started after a partial response is observed in a minimum 8-week trial with an adequate dose of the antidepressant. If no response is seen, a switch is made instead. Lithium augmentation is initiated in the same way as for treatment of bipolar disorder (see Chapter 4: "Mood Stabilizers"), and the lithium is maintained at a serum level of about 0.4 mmol/L, although some patients may require higher levels (Nelson 1998; Rouillon and Gorwood 1998). Some patients respond within a few days of augmentation, most respond within the first 3 weeks, and some (23%) respond with a delay of 3–4 weeks (Stein and Bernadt 1993).

Response rates for T_3 augmentation may be as high as those for lithium. T_3 therapy begins at a dose of 25 μg/day, which is increased to 50 μg/day in 1–2 weeks if no initial response is seen. Treatment is continued for 3 weeks before determining nonresponse (Wager and Klein 1988), at which point T_3 should be discontinued. T_3 augmentation should not be used in patients with coronary artery disease, cardiac dysrhythmia, or heart failure. Although T_3 is usually preferred for augmentation in unipolar depression, thyroxine (T_4) may also be effective, but information from controlled studies of T_4 is lacking.

Estrogen has diverse pharmacodynamic effects on the serotonergic, noradrenergic, and dopaminergic neurotransmitter systems. Estrogen has been reported to have mood-elevating as well as cognition-enhancing effects. Although controlled studies to establish the efficacy of estrogen in the treatment of major depression have yet to be published, our experience is that it may be effective both for primary treatment of depression and for augmentation therapy for certain women in the peri- or postmenopausal period at a dose of 0.625 mg daily of conjugated estrogen (Premarin).

Other agents used to accelerate or augment antidepressant response include modafinil, pindolol, and methylphenidate. Modafinil is a psychostimulant recently marked for narcolepsy that has been found effective at a dose of 200 mg daily (morning) in several reported cases involving elders (Menza et al. 2000). Overall, pindolol's effectiveness as an adjunct in antidepressant therapy has proven to be disappointing. Methylphenidate is started at 2.5 mg in the morning, then the dosage is increased by 2.5–5 mg every 2–3 days as tolerated to a maximum of 20 mg daily, usually given in divided doses before noon. Unlike augmenting agents, accelerating agents are not continued for the duration of antidepressant therapy; they are tapered and discontinued 2–3 weeks after the antidepressant is at the target dose. In general, antidepressant-stimulant combinations are characterized by rapid effect, easy titration of the stimulant, and absence of dangerous side effects. Stimulants should not be used with MAOIs and can be associated with hypertension in combination with atypical agents such as bupropion or venlafaxine.

For patients with treatment-resistant conditions showing no response to an initial trial or for those who do not respond to combination therapy or augmentation, switching is indicated. In general, switches are made to a medication with a broader spectrum of action (e.g., venlafaxine or mirtazapine) or to a medication in another class. In the case of a first trial of an SSRI, a second SSRI may be tried next, since nonresponse to one SSRI does not predict nonresponse to another. In our view, a patient in whom two SSRI trials have failed usually should receive a trial of a broader-spectrum agent.

In switching antidepressants in an elderly patient, the first drug is withdrawn gradually (over 1–2 weeks) as the second drug is titrated. Too-rapid withdrawal of venlafaxine or of short half-life SSRIs can be associated with a withdrawal syndrome, as discussed in the next section ("Side Effects"). It is important to monitor the patient for side effects and drug interactions during the switch-over period. For a switch from an irreversible MAOI, it is necessary to stop the MAOI and wait at least 2 weeks before starting any other antidepressant (including another MAOI), and even this washout may not be long enough for some patients. For a switch from fluoxetine to an irreversible MAOI, it is necessary to wait 5–6 weeks.

Discontinuation of Antidepressants

Except in cases in which toxicity is suspected, antidepressant medications should be tapered rather than abruptly discontinued. For most agents, tapering involves a gradual dosage reduction over a period of 2–4 weeks. For fluoxetine, the decline of serum level of drug occurs so slowly that the medication can be stopped when a dose of 10–20 mg of fluoxetine is reached. A withdrawal syndrome is seen in the 24–48 hours after a patient treated for as little as 3–4 weeks with paroxetine, sertraline, or fluvoxamine has the dose abruptly discontinued or decreased; this syndrome is more likely with paroxetine than with sertraline. A similar syndrome can occur with TCAs. Symptoms include nausea, vomiting, fatigue, myalgia, vertigo, headache, and insomnia (Rosenbaum et al. 1998).

Antidepressant Overdose

Overdose with TCAs is serious and can be fatal. For elderly patients, even a few days' supply of a TCA taken at one time can be fatal. The degree of QRS widening (>100 ms) is a more reliable indicator of TCA toxicity than a drug level and is correlated with central nervous system as well as cardiovascular compromise (Frommer et al. 1987). As QRS lengthens, complete heart block or reentry arrhythmias can develop, either of which can result in death (Glassman and Preud'homme 1993). Although TCA overdose affects many organ systems, the cause of death is usually cardiovascular. Other complications of TCA overdose include coma, seizures, hypertension, and hypotension (Frommer et al. 1987).

Side Effects

Relative severities of major side effects of antidepressant medications are shown in Table 3–5. Side effects that are significant in elderly patients include the following:

- Orthostatic hypotension
- Cardiac conduction disturbance
- Bleeding
- Constipation
- Urinary retention
- Blurred vision
- Sedation
- Dizziness
- Delirium
- Cognitive impairment
- Hyponatremia (syndrome of inappropriate antidiuretic hormone [SIADH])
- Sexual dysfunction
- Weight changes

These problems are more likely to be experienced by patients who are medically ill.

Most side effects occur early, usually within the first week of treatment. For most side effects, tolerance does not develop. This means that no matter how low the initiating dose and how slow the titration, the problem will persist. Tolerance often does develop to sedation, dizziness, gastrointestinal distress, some forms of sexual dysfunction, and possibly some domains of cognitive impairment. Importantly, tolerance does *not* develop to orthostasis (Glassman and Preud'homme 1993), cardiac rhythm disturbances, or delirium; these problems will usually not go away with time.

Overview of Side Effects by Medication Class

Tricyclic Antidepressants

All TCAs affect cardiac conduction and are relatively contraindicated in patients with ischemic heart disease, preexisting bundle branch block, or intraventricular conduction delay (Roose and Glassman 1994). Even nortriptyline and desipramine and their hydroxy metabolites affect cardiac conduction in vulnerable

Table 3–5. Relative severity of side effects of selected antidepressant drugs

Generic name	Trade name	Side effects			
		Sedation	Hypotension	Anticholinergic effects	Cardiac conduction
Heterocyclic antidepressants					
amitriptyline	Elavil	++++	++++	++++	+++
clomipramine	Anafranil	+++	+++	+++	+++
desipramine	Norpramin	+	++	+	+++
doxepin	Sinequan	++++	+++	+++	++
imipramine	Tofranil	+++	++++	+++	+++
nortriptyline	Pamelor	++	+	+	++
Selective serotonin reuptake inhibitors					
citalopram	Celexa	0 to +	0	0	0 to +
fluoxetine	Prozac	0 to +	0	0	0 to +
fluvoxamine	Luvox	0 to +	0	0	0
paroxetine	Paxil	0 to +	0	0 to +	0 to +
sertraline	Zoloft	0 to +	0	0	0 to +

Table 3–5. Relative severity of side effects of selected antidepressant drugs (*continued*)

Generic name	Trade name	Side effects			
		Sedation	Hypotension	Anticholinergic effects	Cardiac conduction
Atypical/novel agents					
bupropion	Wellbutrin	0 to +	0	0	0 to +
mirtazapine	Remeron	+++	+	0 to +	0 to +
nefazodone	Serzone	+++	++	0 to +	0 to +
trazodone	Desyrel	++++	++	+ ?	+
venlafaxine	Effexor	0 to +	0	0 to +	0 to +

Note. ++++ = substantial; +++ = moderate; ++ = mild; + = minimal; 0 = none; ? = not well characterized or understood.
Source. Adapted from Pies 1998.

individuals (Dietch and Fine 1990). All TCAs, especially tertiary amines (amitriptyline, doxepin, and imipramine), also have significant peripheral and central anticholinergic, sedative, and hypotensive effects. Tertiary amines are no longer considered agents of choice in treating elderly patients, aside from limited application in cancer patients.

Selective Serotonin Reuptake Inhibitors

With more extensive experience with SSRIs in geriatrics, the clinical view regarding side effects has evolved. Expected problems with nausea, diarrhea, anorexia, and overactivation have often proven transient or dose-related. On the other hand, sleep disturbances and daytime somnolence have been more persistent, and sexual dysfunction and weight gain have turned out to be much more common and problematic than predicted by premarketing studies (Sussman and Ginsberg 1998). SSRIs are not associated with significant orthostasis or ventricular conduction defects (Roose and Suthers 1998), but fluoxetine has been implicated in sinus node slowing and heart block alone and when co-administered with the β-blocker propranolol. Abnormal gastrointestinal bleeding, bruising, and nosebleed have been reported both with SSRI use and as a result of drug interactions with anticoagulants.

Earlier concerns that SSRIs might be uniquely associated with suicidal or homicidal ideation and acts have not been substantiated by controlled studies (Rasmussen et al. 1993). In fact, data from the NIMH Collaborative Depression Study show that fluoxetine treatment is associated with nonsignificant reductions in the likelihood of suicide attempts and completions and that elevated suicide risk correlates instead with severity of psychopathology (Leon et al. 1999).

Monoamine Oxidase Inhibitors

Use of MAOIs in the elderly is generally limited by significant dietary and drug interactions. Ingestion of tyramine-containing foods can precipitate a hypertensive crisis. Serious drug interactions can occur with commonly used over-the-counter medications, narcotics (especially meperidine), and SSRIs. Significant orthostasis, which can appear after a delay as long as 6 weeks, is another limiting problem in using MAOIs in elderly patients. Pyridoxine deficiency is a potential side effect that can be prevented by co-administration of pyridoxine (vitamin B_6).

St.-John's-Wort

St.-John's-wort, an over-the-counter herbal supplement, has been associated with bleeding (subarachnoid hemorrhage and subdural hematoma), photosensitivity, gastrointestinal symptoms, allergic reactions, fatigue, dizziness, and xerostomia (LaFrance et al. 2000). It is also a significant inducer of the CYP3A4 enzyme and can be associated with greatly reduced levels of cyclosporine, protease inhibitors, and other co-administered drugs.

Electroconvulsive Therapy

ECT is often cited as being safer to administer to geriatric patients than antidepressant medications. In fact, evidence to support this claim is lacking, as there has yet to be a comparative study of first-line pharmacotherapy with ECT in this population. ECT is associated with significant cardiovascular risks in elderly patients, and in some cases these risks are minimized by pretreatment with a β-blocker or calcium channel blocker. In general, however, ECT is well tolerated in the elderly, even in patients with dementia.

ECT may be associated with transient posttreatment confusion and memory impairment. Those at increased risk for these side effects include the very old, those taking psychotropic medications at the time of ECT, and those with major medical illness or prior cognitive impairment. Side effects are minimized by the administration of unilateral, nondominant pulse treatment given at longer intervals than are used for younger patients, as described earlier (see "Clinical Use").

System-Specific Side Effects

Anticholinergic Effects

Anticholinergic effects can be central (delirium, memory, and other cognitive impairments) or peripheral (constipation, urinary retention, visual problems, and dry mouth). These effects are amplified by use of excessive initial doses and too-rapid titration of medications. They can occur, however, with low starting doses and slow titration, and then they are persistent. Since tolerance does not develop over time, a switch to another agent should be considered early. Constipation prophylaxis can be provided by regular use of a bulk laxative (Metamucil) or docusate sodium (Colace). Cathartics such as Milk of Magnesia should be used only intermittently. Chronic or frequently recurrent constipation may be ameliorated by bethanechol at dosages ranging from 10 mg po qd to 30 mg po tid (Rosen et al. 1993).

Urinary anticholinergic symptoms include urinary hesitancy, dribbling, reduced flow, atonic bladder, urinary retention, and, in severe cases, even renal failure (Pollack and Rosenbaum 1987). Before treating urinary retention, it is important to establish that outflow is not obstructed (e.g., by an enlarged prostate). If not, bethanechol 10–30 mg po tid may be useful (Cole and Bodkin 1990). With urinary retention of even moderate severity, the anticholinergic medication should ordinarily be discontinued and urological consultation should be obtained.

Visual blurring can be treated with 1% pilocarpine eye drops or bethanechol 10–30 mg po tid (Pollack and Rosenbaum 1987). For patients with narrow-angle glaucoma, TCAs and other medications with anticholinergic effects are contraindicated. For patients with open-angle glaucoma, these medications can be used, but close follow-up is indicated.

In the patient without swallowing difficulty, dry mouth can be treated with sugarless gum or candy to stimulate salivary flow or with artificial saliva preparations available over the counter (Pollack and Rosenbaum 1987). Oral or sublingual bethanechol can be helpful, but the patient must be monitored for signs of cholinergic excess, including diarrhea, intestinal cramping, tearing, and rhinorrhea.

Cardiac Effects

Cardiac dysrhythmias.　Several types of cardiac rhythm disturbances, including ventricular tachycardia, conduction delay, increased ventricular irritability, and supraventricular dysrhythmias, are associated with different classes of antidepressant medication (Glassman and Preud'homme 1993). In general, these problems are managed prospectively; patients considered at risk are not treated with medications known to be associated with particular dysrhythmias.

Specifically, no TCA is safe in an elderly patient with a preexisting conduction delay. Furthermore, when cardiac rhythm disturbances develop in the course of treatment, discontinuation of the implicated medication is recommended.

Ventricular tachycardia, associated with TCA use, is by far the most serious of these disturbances, since it can progress to ventricular fibrillation and death. TCAs have been found to be proarrhythmic under conditions of ischemia such as angina or myocardial infarction; for this reason, TCAs are relatively contraindicated in elderly patients with ischemic heart disease (Glassman et al. 1993). This includes patients with coronary artery disease, evidence of ischemia on ECG or other testing, history of angina, or history of myocardial infarction.

TCAs and their hydroxy metabolites are also associated with slowing of intraventricular conduction. Patients with preexisting bundle branch block (QRS duration more than 100 ms) or intraventricular conduction delay are at significant risk of progressing to a higher-degree block (Glassman and Roose 1994). Patients with first-degree atrioventricular block (PR greater than 200 ms) have been understudied but probably have a risk somewhat less than those with bundle branch block (Glassman and Roose 1994). Earlier claims that doxepin was safer than other TCAs with regard to conduction delay were based on studies using subtherapeutic doses of that medication. In fact, no TCA is safe in elderly patients at risk because of preexisting cardiac conduction delays.

Compared with TCAs, SSRIs have a more benign cardiac effect profile. Although published reports exist linking these medications to various supraventricular dysrhythmias, including sinus bradycardia, atrial fibrillation, atrial flutter, heart block, and supraventricular tachycardia, the overall incidence of these dysrhythmias is low (Glassman and Preud'homme 1993; Sheline et al. 1997; Spier and Frontera 1991). Patients likely to be at higher risk for the development of these problems include those with preexisting sinus node dysfunction or significant left ventricular impairment. On the other hand, SSRIs do have significant CYP drug interactions with other medications used to treat dysrhythmias and related conditions (e.g., encainide and β-blockers). For this reason, caution is advised in using SSRIs in elderly patients with these cardiac problems who require cotreatment with other medications.

Trazodone may be associated with increased frequency of premature ventricular contractions in patients with preexisting ventricular "irritability." Although no clear guidelines exist as to when this medication is contraindicated, caution should be used in administering trazodone to patients with frequent premature ventricular contractions on baseline ECG. Venlafaxine and bupropion have minimal if any effect on cardiac conduction, and nefazodone has only benign effects on the ECG, such as asymptomatic slowing of heart rate (Stoudemire 1996). Preliminary evidence suggests that mirtazapine's effects on cardiac rhythm are infrequent and consist mainly of bradycardia and premature ventricular contractions.

Hypertension. Venlafaxine is associated with elevated supine diastolic blood pressure, even at recommended geriatric doses. Mirtazapine and bupropion may also be associated with hypertension.

Orthostatic hypotension. Risk factors for the development of orthostatic hypotension with antidepressant therapy include pretreatment orthostasis and evidence of conduction abnormality on the ECG (Halper and Mann 1988). It is not clear whether orthostatic hypotension improves over time with continued treatment. With MAOI therapy, moreover, orthostasis can appear after 5–6 weeks of treatment. "Ambulatory hygiene" practices such as rising slowly from lying or sitting, dangling feet over the side of the bed for a full minute upon arising from sleep, and sitting down and crossing legs when light-headedness occurs can help to prevent injury for all medication-treated elders. Strength training can also result in better hemodynamic response to orthostatic challenge in geriatric patients. When symptomatic orthostasis does develop, some patients benefit from the use of elastic stockings, abdominal binders, or footboards (Cole and Bodkin 1990). Pharmacological interventions can include lowering or dividing the dose of the offending medication, switching to another class of medication not associated with orthostasis (e.g., the SSRIs), or adding another agent to treat orthostasis. Trazodone-associated orthostasis peaks with the blood level 1 hour after oral administration and then lessens over several hours (Glassman and Preud' homme 1993). It is more likely to occur when the drug is taken on an empty stomach. Administration of trazodone at bedtime makes the problem of orthostasis moot for some patients, but it should be considered in patients who are up going to the bathroom soon after retiring for the night.

In a minority of patients, orthostasis may resolve over time. More commonly, orthostasis is managed by switching agents. The drugs available to treat orthostasis are not benign, particularly in patients with conditions such as congestive heart failure, edema, sodium retention, renal insufficiency, and cirrhosis. For these reasons, pharmacological therapy added to treat orthostasis should be considered carefully and used judiciously. The following agents may be useful but are generally not used in combination: sodium chloride tablets, fludrocortisone, midodrine, methylphenidate, ephedrine, caffeine, T_3, and T_4 (Pollack and Rosenbaum 1987; Tan and Bransgrove 1998).

Endocrine Effects

SIADH has been associated with SSRI use in elderly patients in a number of cases (Liu et al. 1996). This syndrome is marked by the co-occurrence of low serum sodium (usually less than 130 mEq/L) and high urine sodium (usually more than 20 mEq/L) levels—abnormalities that resolve with discontinuation of the offending agent. Most cases occur within the first month of treatment with an SSRI, although later development has been noted. Time to normalization of sodium after discontinuation of medication varies from days to weeks.

Gastrointestinal Effects

The most commonly noted side effects of the SSRIs are gastrointestinal: nausea, loose stools, diarrhea, and, in some cases, vomiting. Nausea is a particular problem with fluvoxamine. With time and with slow dose titration, these effects are minimized and tolerance does develop. More rarely, gastrointestinal bleeding (melena, rectal bleeding) has been reported with SSRI use (see discussion on hematological effects below). Venlafaxine is associated with a high incidence of nausea, particularly with rapid initial titration.

Genitourinary Effects

Urinary retention was discussed earlier in the context of anticholinergic effects. Males treated with trazodone may develop a persistent nonsexual penile tumescence known as priapism. Among elderly men treated with trazodone, this is rarely reported. In any trazodone-treated patient, when erection lasts longer than 1 hour, the patient should be brought to the acute care clinic or emergency room for treatment.

Hematological Effects

Serotonergic antidepressants can deplete serotonin from platelets, possibly resulting in bleeding in susceptible patients. Spontaneous bleeding has been reported with SSRIs (melena, rectal bleeding, nosebleed, and bruising) and with St.-John's-wort (subdural hematoma and subarachnoid hemorrhage). The risk of upper gastrointestinal tract bleeding with SSRIs is about the same as that with low-dose ibuprofen, and the risk of such bleeding with trazodone may be even greater (de Abajo et al. 1999). Mild problems with bruising can, in some cases, be treated with daily vitamin C supplementation; anything more severe or even minor bleeding that is recurrent should prompt discontinuation of the offending agent.

Neuropsychiatric Effects

Anxiety.　A potential side effect of SSRI therapy is anxiety, which is more problematic in the early stages of treatment and is more problematic with fluoxetine and sertraline than with citalopram and paroxetine. This problem is best managed by slow initial titration and patient education, but short-term use of a benzodiazepine such as lorazepam is sometimes needed.

Cognitive impairment.　Antidepressant effects on cognition are probably mediated by cholinergic and antihistaminic receptor blockade. Tertiary-amine TCAs are particularly problematic. Newer antidepressants have generally been understudied in relation to cognitive effects.

Delirium.　Delirium can develop with any antidepressant in elderly patients, but strongly anticholinergic drugs (e.g., TCAs such as amitriptyline) are particularly implicated, even at therapeutic dosages. Often heralding the onset of anticholinergic delirium is a prodrome characterized by restlessness and nightmares. When fully developed, a central anticholinergic syndrome may be seen, marked by the triad of delirium, myoclonus, and choreoathetoid movements. Dilated pupils and flushed, dry skin may also be noted. The syndrome is usually diagnosed presumptively, although a physostigmine challenge confirms the diagnosis when the patient shows transient resolution of symptoms. Physostigmine must be used with caution because of the risk of inducing cardiac dysrhythmias.

Insomnia. Antidepressants associated with insomnia include desipramine, fluoxetine, sertraline, venlafaxine, bupropion, and MAOIs. In some cases, the problem abates with continued treatment, whereas in others it is persistent. Antidepressant-related insomnia can be treated with trazodone 25–200 mg 1 hour before bedtime (although not with MAOIs), with one of the newer benzodiazepine-like hypnotics zolpidem or zaleplon, or with gabapentin 300 mg qhs. SSRIs may further disrupt sleep by increasing the frequency of periodic limb movements (Armitage et al. 1997). Nefazodone has been touted as particularly beneficial for depression-related insomnia, but this use has not been studied in elderly patients. In our experience, mirtazapine is especially useful for elders with depression-related insomnia, with positive effects on sleep noted usually within the first few doses of 7.5 mg po qhs.

Mania. All antidepressants, including bright light therapy and ECT, can induce mania in predisposed patients. Antidepressants can also be associated with the induction of rapid cycling in bipolar patients. These conditions are treated by taper and discontinuation of the offending agent and either initiation or optimization of the dose of a mood stabilizer. ECT, followed by continuation therapy with a mood stabilizer, can also be an effective treatment. Certain antidepressants, such as bupropion and the SSRI antidepressants, may be less likely to induce mania or rapid cycling than other antidepressants.

Motor dysfunction. Case reports have brought attention to the potential of SSRIs to cause extrapyramidal syndromes, particularly in elderly or medically ill patients (Pies 1997). In patients treated concurrently with SSRIs and antipsychotics, significant parkinsonism can occur, although the incidence of this effect is not known. SSRIs and TCAs may also be associated with a fine, distal resting tremor that can be exacerbated by caffeine and nicotine, as well as anxiety (Pollack and Rosenbaum 1987). This tremor can be treated with propranolol 10–20 mg po tid or qid, but if lithium is coprescribed, the treatment may be ineffective.

Akathisia developing in the course of antidepressant therapy can be treated with propranolol 10–20 mg tid; if the problem persists, a switch to another agent should be considered.

Seizures.   All antidepressants can be associated with lowering of the seizure threshold. In SSRI-treated and bupropion-treated patients who have been screened to rule out predisposition to seizure, the rate of seizure with therapy is on the order of 0.1% at recommended doses.

Sedation.   A number of antidepressants, including TCAs, nefazodone, mirtazapine, paroxetine, and, to a lesser extent, other SSRIs, have sedation as a side effect. TCA-associated sedation is attributed to histamine (H_1) receptor binding. This problem is dose related and can be minimized by starting the drug at a low dose and titrating slowly. Tolerance to sedation does develop over time, but this process may be too slow to make the medication acceptable to outpatients. Trazodone is also highly sedating and is widely used specifically as a sedative in elderly patients, whether or not depression is present. Nefazodone's usefulness as a treatment for depression in elders is actually limited by its sedating effects. Clinical experience suggests that mirtazapine is less sedating at higher than at lower doses because of the emergence of noradrenergic effects at higher doses. Paroxetine is more sedating than other SSRIs and is usually prescribed to be taken at bedtime.

Sexual Dysfunction

Sexual dysfunction is encountered most frequently in patients treated with TCAs, SSRIs, MAOIs, and, probably to a lesser extent, venlafaxine. Pretreatment screening for sexual problems such as erectile dysfunction, anorgasmia, or vaginal dryness can reveal conditions that represent an indication for urological or gynecological consultation. Baseline assessment makes it less likely that sexual dysfunction will be misattributed to antidepressant therapy. When antidepressant-related dysfunction occurs, any phase of the sexual cycle can be affected. In some cases, symptoms remit over time, but this can take time. Several therapeutic options exist: the offending medication can be replaced by bupropion, mirtazapine, or nefazodone, agents less associated with adverse sexual side effects; the dose of antidepressant can be reduced (especially effective with SSRIs used at higher doses); or a low dose of bupropion or mirtazapine can be added to an established antidepressant regimen (Delgado et al. 1999). The use of drug holidays planned for a time that sexual activity is anticipated (e.g., stopping sertraline or paroxetine from Thursday to Sunday) carries the risk of withdrawal symptoms and probably contributes to noncompliance. Antidotes such as yohimbine, cyproheptadine, and ginkgo biloba can be used but are best avoided in elders because of adverse effects and potential drug interactions.

Toxic Effects

Serotonin syndrome. The serotonin syndrome is a severe systemic reaction to serotonin excess, with symptoms of confusion, hypertension, restlessness, "agitation," muscle rigidity, myoclonus, increased deep tendon reflexes, diaphoresis, shivering, and tremor (Sternbach 1991). It can result from the combination of an MAOI with an SSRI, the combination of an MAOI with tryptophan, less commonly with other drug combinations such as paroxetine and dextromethorphan (Skop et al. 1994), or with lithium augmentation of SSRI or MAOI antidepressants. The offending agents are discontinued, and treatment consists mainly of supportive measures. Case reports suggest that cyproheptadine 8 mg po results in rapid symptom resolution (Graudins et al. 1998). Propranolol or methysergide may also be helpful.

Tyramine reaction. When certain foods or medications are ingested by patients being treated with nonselective MAOIs, a tyramine reaction can result. The reaction is characterized by a marked rise in blood pressure within minutes to hours, severe occipital headache, flushing, palpitations, retro-orbital pain, nausea, and diaphoresis. The blood pressure elevation may be so severe as to result in intracerebral bleeding. Patients prescribed these medications are warned not to lie down if they feel any of these symptoms, since this can further elevate blood pressure. It is no longer recommended that patients carry their own supply of chlorpromazine or nifedipine for sublingual use; instead, patients are advised to report to the nearest emergency room. Treatment consists of acidification of the urine, intravenous phentolamine for blood pressure control, and supportive measures.

Weight Changes

Patients of mixed age undergoing treatment with fluoxetine and other SSRIs may initially experience a small weight loss (2–4 pounds in the first 6 weeks). With fluoxetine, weight loss peaks at 20 weeks. At 6 months, weight begins to be regained, and at 1 year, weight is at least equal to baseline (Sussman and Ginsberg 1998). In fact, weight gains with SSRIs of 20–30 pounds are common when these medications are used chronically. Significant weight gain in patients treated with TCAs and MAOIs is also common.

There has been debate in the literature about the mechanism of weight gain with SSRIs and other antidepressants, since mechanism is closely linked to treatment. Weight gain has been attributed to fluid retention, histamine (H_1) receptor blockade, change in glucose metabolism, hypothalamic dysfunction, and increased appetite (Pollack and Rosenbaum 1987). SSRI-related weight gain may be a function of effects on the 5-HT_{2C} receptor, which appears to function as a component of a fat control system. Recently, Sussman has argued that SSRI antidepressants alter caloric expenditure by changing basal metabolic rate, without any influence of caloric intake; the implication of this would be that dieting would not help the problem (Sussman and Ginsberg 1998).

Management of antidepressant-related weight gain is as follows: when weight gain in the first 4 months of treatment exceeds 5 pounds, a dietary consultation is obtained. Consideration is given to a switch in antidepressant therapy to nefazodone or bupropion, both of which are associated with less weight gain compared with other antidepressants. The patient is instructed to minimize carbohydrate and fat intake and to exercise regularly as tolerated. New-onset fluid retention (edema) is an indication for medical consultation; in some cases, this may be the first evidence of a significant drug interaction.

Treatment of Selected Syndromes and Disorders With Antidepressants

Anxiety Disorders

Generalized Anxiety Disorder

Several antidepressant medications are useful in the treatment of elders with generalized anxiety disorder (GAD); optimally, these medications are used in tandem with psychotherapy. In our experience, SSRI antidepressants, venlafaxine, and mirtazapine may be particularly beneficial in treating GAD. Venlafaxine and paroxetine have received FDA approval for this indication, and several other SSRIs are likely candidates for approval. As with other anxiety disorders, initial doses for GAD may need to be lower than usual, and titration may need to be even slower than usual, to avoid acute anxiogenic effects. More flexible dosing allowed by liquid preparations of SSRIs (citalopram, fluoxetine, paroxetine) is especially useful. A typical treatment regimen for a geriatric patient is paroxetine 10 mg po qd for 2 weeks, then 20 mg po qd, with further dosage increases as needed and tolerated up to 40 mg po qd.

Obsessive-Compulsive Disorder

Compulsive behaviors such as hoarding are commonly seen among elderly patients with dementia, and obsessional ruminations are common among those with depression. Primary OCD is seen less often and usually represents the persistence of illness that developed earlier in life. Little is known from systematic study about the interplay of this disorder with other diseases of old age. Multimodal treatment—pharmacological, behavioral, and psychosocial—is used with elderly OCD patients, as it is with younger patients. The drugs of choice for elderly patients are the SSRIs. The SSRI is started at half the usual dose, and the dosage is titrated upward as tolerated to clinical effect. No controlled studies of optimal dosage for elderly OCD patients have been performed, but our clinical experience suggests that the equivalent of fluoxetine 60 mg daily may be needed for symptom control in some elderly OCD patients. In many cases, the symptoms of hoarding and rumination are also responsive to SSRI therapy.

Panic Disorder

Isolated panic attacks that occur in elderly patients in medical settings such as the intensive care unit may be effectively treated with short-term use of a benzodiazepine. For panic disorder involving recurrent panic attack and associated phobic symptoms, SSRIs are the drugs of choice. When an SSRI is started for treatment of panic, a small test dose is administered to determine whether the patient has an anxiogenic response. Therapy is then started with small doses (e.g., fluoxetine or citalopram 1–2 mg daily, obtainable with liquid preparations) and titrated extremely slowly to effect, with small dose increases made every 2–4 weeks. With these agents, the target dose averages about 20 mg qd. An adjunctive benzodiazepine such as lorazepam 0.5–1 mg bid or tid may be used in the early stages of treatment for those unable to tolerate SSRI initiation. Nefazodone may also be helpful for panic disorder.

Posttraumatic Stress Disorder

In elders with posttraumatic stress disorder (PTSD), SSRI antidepressants are the pharmacological treatment of first choice, followed by other atypical antidepressants such as venlafaxine and nefazodone. These drugs are initiated and titrated in the same way as for major depression (see the specific drug summaries at the end of this chapter). Trazodone or gabapentin may be useful in treating PTSD-associated insomnia, and mood stabilizers may be useful for prominent irritability and anger.

Depressive Disorders

Atypical Depression

Atypical depression, a variant of major depression, is characterized by severe anxiety and neurovegetative symptoms of reversed polarity, including hypersomnia, hyperphagia with weight gain, psychomotor retardation, mood reactivity, and, in some cases, sensitivity to interpersonal rejection. Phobic symptoms can be present, as can a subjective sense of fatigue or heaviness in the limbs ("leaden paralysis"). This disorder does occur in elderly patients, although probably not as commonly as in younger cohorts. In general, atypical depression is more responsive to MAOIs than to TCAs. Although anecdotal reports and clinical experience suggest that SSRIs are useful for inducing remission of symptoms in atypical depression, they might not be as effective as MAOIs in maintaining remission over time (McGrath et al. 2000).

Bereavement-Related Depression

Bereavement is a process commonly experienced in late life and is characterized in the acute phases by a high prevalence of depressive symptoms. One-third of widows and widowers meet criteria for major depression in the first month of bereavement, and half of this group remains significantly depressed 1 year later. The questions of when to intervene with pharmacotherapy and with which patients are important, since major depression is associated with high morbidity and mortality, and the length of a depressive episode in part determines treatment responsiveness. Antidepressant medication treatment does not interfere with the grieving process, but rather facilitates grieving. Bereaved individuals with major depression are saddled with the additional burdens of excessive guilt, feelings of worthlessness, and sometimes persistent thoughts about suicide. Pharmacological intervention is appropriate for those with such symptoms lasting 2 months or longer; almost all clinicians would treat these patients by 6 months. Although nortriptyline has been specifically studied and found efficacious in this population, any first-line antidepressant would likely be of benefit. In addition, psychotherapy is usually an integral part of treatment.

Bipolar Depression

The first-line treatment for bipolar I depression is a mood stabilizer (valproate, lithium, or lamotrigine). For nonresponse or breakthrough symptoms in patients with a history of rapid cycling, a second mood stabilizer is added. For patients without a history of rapid cycling, an antidepressant such as bupropion or an SSRI is added instead, usually for a limited period. Considering the risk of inducing rapid cycling or a switch into mania, however, any use of antidepressant medication in the bipolar patient should be undertaken with caution. (Some experts discourage the use of antidepressants in almost all bipolar patients, given these risks.) Patients with bipolar depression refractory to treatment are considered for ECT or other pharmacotherapy such as the MAOI tranylcypromine (Thase and Sachs 2000). The need for co-administration of a mood stabilizer with the antidepressant for a patient with bipolar II depression is determined in part by the frequency and severity of past hypomanic episodes, and the same caveat about induction of rapid cycling applies.

Dementia With Depression

The syndromes of dementia and depression overlap in several ways: depression can represent a prodrome to dementia, can occur in the context of an established dementia, or can be associated with reversible cognitive impairment in the "dementia of depression" (Alexopoulos et al. 1993). "Psychological" symptoms of excessive guilt, low self-esteem or self-loathing, and persistent suicidal ideation are important warning signs of depression and can help to distinguish depression from dementia in the geriatric population. In established dementia, patients may meet criteria for major depression or for more minor degrees of depression. When the latter are associated with behavioral disturbances, significant improvement can be seen with antidepressant therapy.

There is some evidence that elderly patients with dementia should be treated with lower antidepressant doses and lower target serum levels than those used with elderly patients without dementia (Streim et al. 2000). In general, antidepressants devoid of anticholinergic effects, such as the SSRIs, venlafaxine, bupropion, and nefazodone, are preferred.

Dysthymic Disorder

Dysthymic disorder is a milder but more chronic depressive illness that is a relatively common syndrome in the elderly. It is often misattributed to "growing old" but in fact is amenable to combined pharmacotherapy and psychotherapy in many cases. For risk-benefit reasons, SSRI antidepressants are often selected for this indication. Dosing and titration are the same as for major depression, but the latency to effect may be considerably longer.

Major Depression

Major depression is a neurochemical derangement occurring with or without precipitating stressors that is severe enough to cause significant disability in occupational and social functioning. Symptoms include depressed mood or anhedonia (particularly the latter, in elderly patients), sleep difficulties, appetite disturbances, low energy, psychomotor agitation or retardation, poor concentration, excessive guilt, and suicidal ideation or plan. Psychotic symptoms can occur, and significant cognitive impairment can develop that improves with treatment of the depression.

Melancholic depression is a subtype characterized by prominent neurovegetative signs, including persistent insomnia, lack of appetite with weight loss, complete loss of libido, and severely depressed mood. For melancholia, depression with psychotic features, or any severe depression in elderly patients, ECT should be considered for acute treatment, followed by continuation therapy with antidepressant medication. Alternatively, an antidepressant medication could be prescribed for acute as well as continuation treatment. As noted previously, some clinicians prefer to use non-SSRIs (e.g., nortriptyline or venlafaxine) for severe depression. Patients are often admitted for initiation of pharmacotherapy, not only to monitor for the emergence of adverse effects but also to observe for suicidality and to assist with daily care. Information about initiating therapy with recommended drugs is included in the specific drug summaries at the end of this chapter.

For the elderly patient with major depression associated with significant insomnia, the drugs of choice are mirtazapine or nefazodone, both of which improve sleep, although they have opposite effects on amount of REM sleep (Thase and Sachs 2000). For mirtazapine, tolerance develops after several days to sedative effects, but not to sleep-promoting effects (Winokur et al. 2000). Mirtazapine is also useful in depressed elders with significant anorexia; in our experience, its appetite-stimulating effects are similar to those of megestrol acetate (Megace).

Medical Illness With Depression

Terminal cancer. Major depression occurs in 5%–15% of cancer patients, and aggressive treatment of this condition is critical. The suicide rate among cancer patients is twice that of the general population (McDaniel et al. 1995). Treatment of depression in this population increases survival rates by processes that may be mediated by changes in immune function (McDaniel et al. 1995). In addition, treatment of depression ameliorates problems with sleep and pain.

All antidepressants have been tried and found to be effective in treating depression in cancer patients, at least as reported anecdotally. In choosing a particular agent, issues of concern in this population include anticholinergic effects, nausea, weight loss, and medication interactions (especially with narcotics). Mirtazapine may be a drug of choice because of associated sleep-promoting and appetite-stimulating effects. Alternatively, methylphenidate may be favored because it is associated with rapid resolution of symptoms such as apathy and depressed mood. SSRIs are effective but can provoke nausea and weight loss, and certain SSRIs are associated with significant CYP interactions with narcotic analgesics such as codeine. MAOIs impose dietary and medication restrictions likely to be problematic in cancer patients, such as the injunction against co-administration of meperidine.

Cardiac conditions and cardiovascular disease. Depression is common in patients with cardiovascular disease, and its presence heralds a poor prognosis for several groups of patients. After myocardial infarction, major depression is the best predictor of a future adverse event such as a second infarction, angioplasty, coronary artery bypass graft, or death (Roose et al. 1991). Among patients with significant dysrhythmias, depression and death are significantly associated (Roose et al. 1991). It is now clear that the risk of not treating patients with cardiac disease is far greater than the risk of treating them (Roose and Glassman 1994).

The only caveat here involves TCAs, which are dangerous for patients with ischemic heart disease, preexisting bundle branch block, or intraventricular conduction defect (with QRS widened to more than 110 ms) (Glassman and Preud'homme 1993; Roose and Dalack 1992). No individual TCA is safer than any other TCA (Glassman and Preud'homme 1993), including doxepin and nortriptyline, in this regard.

In general, SSRIs have a more benign cardiac effect profile than TCAs and are well tolerated in cardiac patients. In addition, SSRIs may confer additional positive effects on platelet-mediated coagulation indices. However, several case reports have implicated fluoxetine in the development of atrial arrhythmias (Sheline et al. 1997), and a case of complete heart block was reported in a patient given fluoxetine in combination with propranolol (Drake and Gordon 1994).

Antidepressants of choice in treating depressed cardiac patients include bupropion, venlafaxine, and SSRIs (Roose and Glassman 1994). Significant CYP interactions between SSRIs and antiarrhythmic agents as well as other cardiac medications are listed in Table 1–1 in Chapter 1.

Medication-induced depression. A number of commonly prescribed medications have been implicated as causes of depression in susceptible patients (Reynolds 1995). A list of these drugs is shown in Table 3–6. The onset of depression can often be linked temporally to initiation of the offending medication. In such cases, if the medical condition permits and suitable alternative treatments exist, the medication should be withdrawn. If depression persists, antidepressant therapy is indicated.

Pain syndromes.   Neuropathic pain and other chronic pain syndromes may be treated adjunctively with SSRIs and other serotonergic antidepressants, whether or not significant depression is present. Although first-generation TCAs are still often used for this indication, there is no compelling evidence that these medications are more effective than SSRIs. Newer atypical antidepressants with serotonergic effects are likely to be effective for pain syndromes in elderly patients but as yet are inadequately studied.

Parkinson's disease.   Among patients with Parkinson's disease (PD), approximately one-third suffer from major depression or dysthymic disorder (Cummings 1992). Neurotransmitter derangements in PD prominently affect the dopaminergic system but also involve the serotonergic and noradrenergic systems. Treatments include ECT and antidepressant medication. ECT results in rapid improvement in depressive as well as motor symptoms, but the latter may be short-lived (Cummings 1992).

In theory, the antidepressant of first choice for PD would be bupropion, a dopaminergic agent that is associated with motor as well as mood improvement (Cummings 1992). In fact, however, superior efficacy of bupropion or any other antidepressant in PD has yet to be demonstrated in controlled trials. On the basis of anecdotal evidence, other drugs recommended include nortriptyline and the SSRIs (Richard and Kurlan 1997), with the exception of fluoxetine. In a number of case reports, fluoxetine has been implicated in the exacerbation of extrapyramidal symptoms. Recent reports of the use of the dopamine agonist pramipexole (Mirapex) to treat bipolar depression (Goldberg et al. 1999) raise the possibility that this drug might be useful in PD-

Table 3–6.   Medications reported to cause depression

acyclovir	estrogen
anabolic steroids	fluoroquinolone antibiotics (ciprofloxacin)
anticonvulsants	H_2-receptor blockers
baclofen	interferon-α
barbiturates	isotretinoin
benzodiazepines	levodopa
β-blockers	mefloquine
bromocriptine	methyldopa
calcium channel blockers	metoclopramide
cholesterol-lowering drugs ("statins")	metronidazole
clonidine	narcotics
corticosteroids	NSAIDs
cycloserine	pergolide
dapsone	sulfonamides
digitalis	thiazide diuretics
disopyramide	vinblastine
disulfiram	

Note.   NSAIDs = nonsteroidal anti-inflammatory drugs.

associated depression. Bromocriptine has also been used in the past for depression in patients with PD, with some benefit.

The specific MAOI selegiline is often used in combination with L-dopa and may confer some antidepressant benefit despite the low doses usually employed. Nonselective MAOIs should be avoided in combination with L-dopa, and even low-dose selegiline should be avoided in combination with SSRIs because of the risk of serotonin syndrome.

Vascular disease and stroke.   Depression can occur as a consequence of stroke (large-vessel disease) or significant ischemia (small-vessel disease). The 2 years after stroke represent the period of greatest risk for depression, which can exacerbate neurological and cognitive deficits and significantly interfere with rehabilitation efforts. Particularly when depression has its onset more than 7 weeks after stroke, spontaneous remission is unlikely; the depressive symptoms are treated regardless of whether all criteria for major depression are met.

Antidepressants used for poststroke depression include nortriptyline, SSRIs, psychostimulants, and venlafaxine. In one study, nortriptyline was found to be more effective for this indication than fluoxetine, and the latter was associated with significant weight loss (Robinson et al. 2000). Bupropion is avoided because of seizure risk. Trazodone and amitriptyline have been found to slow recovery after stroke (Alexopoulos et al. 1996). When delusions or hallucinations are present, adjunctive antipsychotic medication should be used. For stroke patients unable to tolerate antidepressant medication, ECT should be considered.

Depression secondary to ischemic brain disease ("vascular depression") may have a more insidious onset and be more difficult to treat. It is often true that patients with this syndrome require antidepressant combination therapy or ECT for symptom remission.

Depression in the context of vascular disease can be a persistent and recurrent problem for patients in whom vascular events (both large and small) continue to occur. For this reason, prophylaxis with aspirin and other platelet aggregation inhibitors, treatment of hypertension and hypercholesterolemia, and management of other risk factors such as smoking are indicated.

Psychotic Depression (Delusional Depression)

Psychotic depression appears to be a distinct disorder, different from depression without psychotic features, which usually remains "true to form" from one episode to the next in a given individual. Psychotic symptoms can be either delusions or hallucinations. Delusions need not be mood congruent for the diagnosis to be made. Psychotic depression in the elderly is the foremost indication for ECT. If pharmacotherapy is used for acute treatment, an antipsychotic must be used in tandem with the antidepressant. When the psychotic symptoms have remitted (either with ECT or with antipsychotic medication), the antidepressant often can be used as sole continuation therapy. Subsequent relapse of psychotic symptoms suggests a schizoaffective process requiring maintenance therapy with an antidepressant-antipsychotic combination.

Seasonal Depression

Seasonal depression may be particularly common in elderly "shut-ins," who have virtually no outside light exposure, and among elders in northern climates, insofar as they are likely to spend more time indoors. To date, seasonal depression has been insufficiently studied in the geriatric population. Features of this disorder show a high degree of overlap with those of atypical depression as well as bipolar II disorder.

For mild to moderately severe seasonal depression in outpatients, bright light therapy can be used as the sole intervention. Exposure to a 10,000-lux lamp for 30 minutes every morning is sufficient to maintain normal mood for many patients (Rosenthal 1993). Intervention prior to the usual onset of depressive symptoms is preferred (e.g., in September for those with usual onset in October) (Meesters et al. 1993). Light sessions are continued on a daily basis for a minimum of 2 weeks and may need to be continued for the duration of the low-light season. For more severe seasonal depression, bright light therapy should be considered an adjunct to other standard antidepressant treatments. Among elderly patients, bright light therapy has also been used to treat insomnia and other disturbances of the sleep-wake cycle and to treat evening or nighttime agitation in those with dementia (Satlin et al. 1992).

Chapter Summary

- The elderly are at risk for undertreatment of depression because of low expectations regarding recovery and fears about aggressive pharmacotherapy as well as ECT.

- The presence of recent stressors, rather than arguing against pharmacotherapy in the seriously depressed patient, argues for cotreatment with medication and psychotherapy.

- For melancholia, depression with psychotic features, or any severe depression in elderly patients, ECT should be considered.

- Age-related changes in renal clearance of many drugs and metabolites result in higher drug concentrations for a given dose in older compared with younger patients.

- With some exceptions, CYP interactions are very significant for antidepressants.

- A CYP interaction between a substrate and an inhibitor does not prohibit the coprescription of those medications, but it does dictate that the clinician use caution in prescribing, particularly when substrates with narrow therapeutic indices are prescribed.

- A CYP interaction between a substrate and an inducer may significantly complicate therapy.

- Antidepressants generally preferred for elders include the SSRIs citalopram, fluoxetine, paroxetine, and sertraline; the atypical agents bupropion, venlafaxine, mirtazapine, and, possibly, reboxetine; and the TCA nortriptyline.

- In view of concerns about the safety of administering TCAs to elderly patients, most clinicians now consider SSRIs or selected atypical agents to be the first-line treatment for depression in this population.

- In general, a minimum of 6 weeks of antidepressant treatment should be undertaken in an elderly patient before any prediction about "nonresponse" is made for that trial.

- Continuation antidepressant therapy for elders should last for a minimum of 6 months, with 2 years being optimal for those with particularly severe episodes.

- For continuation as well as maintenance therapy, full acute doses of antidepressant medication are recommended, as is continuation of any adjunctive treatment such as lithium.

- A significant proportion of patients with conditions labeled "treatment resistant" respond to a simple increase in dose.

- In switching antidepressants in an elderly patient, the first drug is withdrawn gradually (over 1–2 weeks) as the second drug is titrated.

- Except when toxicity is suspected, antidepressant medications should be tapered rather than abruptly discontinued.

- Tolerance does not develop to orthostasis, cardiac rhythm disturbances, or delirium; these problems usually do not go away with time.

- All TCAs affect cardiac conduction and are relatively contraindicated in patients with ischemic heart disease, preexisting bundle branch block, or intraventricular conduction delay.

- TCAs have been found to induce arrhythmias under conditions of ischemia such as angina or myocardial infarction.

- Co-administration of SSRIs and antipsychotics may be associated with parkinsonism.

- With some exceptions, antidepressant medications are associated with significant weight gain when used long term.

References

Alexopoulos GS: The treatment of depressed demented patients. J Clin Psychiatry 57 (suppl 14):14–20, 1996

Alexopoulos GS, Meyers BS, Young RC, et al: The course of geriatric depression with "reversible dementia": a controlled study. Am J Psychiatry 150:1693–1699, 1993

Alexopoulos GS, Meyers BS, Young RC, et al: Recovery in geriatric depression. Arch Gen Psychiatry 53:305–312, 1996

Armitage R, Yonkers K, Cole D, et al: A multicenter, double-blind comparison of the effects of nefazodone and fluoxetine on sleep architecture and quality of sleep in depressed outpatients. J Clin Psychopharmacol 17:161–168, 1997

Blumenthal JA, Babyak MA, Moore KA, et al: Effects of exercise training on older patients with major depression. Arch Intern Med 159:2349–2356, 1999

Cole JO, Bodkin JA: Antidepressant drug side effects. J Clin Psychiatry 51 (1, suppl):21–26, 1990

Cummings JL: Depression and Parkinson's disease: a review. Am J Psychiatry 149:443–454, 1992

de Abajo FJ, Rodriguez LA, Montero D: Association between selective serotonin reuptake inhibitors and upper gastrointestinal bleeding: population based case-control study. BMJ 319:1106–1109, 1999

Delgado PL, McGahuey CA, Moreno FA, et al: Treatment strategies for depression and sexual dysfunction, in Antidepressants and Sexual Dysfunction: A Patient-Centered Approach—Proceedings of a Clinical Conference (J Clin Psychiatry Monograph, Vol 17, No 1). Memphis, TN, Physicians Postgraduate Press, 1999, pp 15–21

Dietch JT, Fine M: The effect of nortriptyline in elderly patients with cardiac conduction disease. J Clin Psychiatry 51:65–67, 1990

Drake WM, Gordon GD: Heart block in a patient on propranolol and fluoxetine. Lancet 343:425–426, 1994

Fava M, Borus JS, Alpert JE, et al: Folate, vitamin B_{12}, and homocysteine in major depressive disorder. Am J Psychiatry 154:426–428, 1997

Fawcett J, Barkin RL: A meta-analysis of eight randomized, double-blind, controlled clinical trials of mirtazapine for the treatment of patients with major depression and symptoms of anxiety. J Clin Psychiatry 59:123–127, 1998

Flint AJ: Recents developments in geriatric psychopharmacotherapy. Can J Psychiatry 39(8, suppl 1):S9–S18, 1994

Flint AJ: Pharmacologic treatment of depression in late life. Can Med Assoc J 157:1061–1067, 1997

Flint AJ, Rifat SL: The effect of sequential antidepressant treatment on geriatric depression. J Affect Disord 36:95–105, 1996

Flint AJ, Rifat SL: Maintenance treatment for recurrent depression in late life. Am J Geriatr Psychiatry 8:112–116, 2000

Folstein MF, Folstein SE, McHugh PR: "Mini-Mental State": a practical method for grading the cognitive state of patients for the clinician. J Psychiatr Res 12:189–198, 1975

Frommer DA, Kulig KW, Marx JA, et al: Tricyclic antidepressant overdose. JAMA 257:521–526, 1987

Glassman AH, Preud'homme XA: Review of the cardiovascular effects of heterocyclic antidepressants. J Clin Psychiatry 54 (2, suppl):16–22, 1993

Glassman AH, Roose SP: Risks of antidepressants in the elderly: tricyclic antidepressants and arrhythmia—revising risks. Gerontology 40 (suppl 1):15–20, 1994

Glassman AH, Roose SP, Bigger JT: The safety of tricyclic antidepressants in cardiac patients. JAMA 269:2673–2675, 1993

Goldberg JF, Frye MA, Dunn RT: Pramipexole in refractory bipolar depression (letter). Am J Psychiatry 156:798, 1999

Graudins A, Stearman A, Chan B: Treatment of the serotonin syndrome with cyproheptadine. J Emerg Med 16:615–619, 1998

Greenblatt DJ, von Moltke LL, Harmatz JS, et al: Drug interactions with newer antidepressants: role of human cytochromes P450. J Clin Psychiatry 59 (suppl 15):19–27, 1998

Halper JP, Mann JJ: Cardiovascular effects of antidepressant medications. Br J Psychiatry 153:87–98, 1988

Heeren TJ, Derksen P, van Heycop Ten Ham BF, et al: Treatment, outcome, and predictors of response in elderly depressed in-patients. Brit J Psychiatry 170:436–440, 1997

Hirschfeld RMA, Schatzberg AF: Long-term management of depression. Am J Med 97 (suppl 6A):33S–38S, 1994

Kitanaka I, Ross RJ, Cutler NR, et al: Altered hydroxydesipramine concentrations in elderly depressed patients. Clin Pharmacol Ther 31:51–55, 1982

LaFrance WC, Lauterbach EC, Coffey CE, et al: The use of herbal alternative medicines in neuropsychiatry. J Neuropsychiatry Clin Neurosci 12:177–192, 2000

Leon AC, Keller MB, Warshaw MG, et al: Prospective study of fluoxetine treatment and suicidal behavior in affectively ill subjects. Am J Psychiatry 156:195–201, 1999

Liu BA, Mittmann N, Knowles SR, et al: Hyponatremia and the syndrome of inappropriate secretion of antidiuretic hormone associated with the use of selective serotonin reuptake inhibitors: a review of spontaneous reports. Can Med Assoc J 155:519–527, 1996

Manly DT, Oakley SP, Bloch RM: Electroconvulsive therapy in old-old patients. Am J Geriatr Psychiatry 8:232–236, 2000

McDaniel JS, Musselman DL, Porter MR, et al: Depression in patients with cancer. Arch Gen Psychiatry 52:89–99, 1995

McEvoy GK, Litvak K, Welsh OH, et al: AHFS Drug Information. Bethesda, MD, American Society of Health-System Pharmacists, 2000

McGrath PJ, Stewart JW, Petkova E, et al: Predictors of relapse during fluoxetine continuation or maintenance treatment of major depression. J Clin Psychiatry 61:518–524, 2000

Meesters Y, Jansen JHC, Beersma DGM, et al: Early light treatment can prevent an emerging winter depression from developing into a full-blown depression. J Affect Disord 29:41–47, 1993

Menza MA, Kaufman KR, Castellanos A: Modafinil augmentation of antidepressant treatment in depression. J Clin Psychiatry 61:378–381, 2000

Nelson JC: Combined drug treatment strategies for major depression. Psychiatric Annals 28:197–203, 1998

Nelson JC, Mazure CM, Jatlow PI: Characteristics of desipramine-refractory depression. J Clin Psychiatry 55:12–19, 1994

Nelson JC, Mazure CM, Jatlow PI: Desipramine treatment of major depression in patients over 75 years of age. J Clin Psychopharmacol 15:99–105, 1995

Pies RW: Must we now consider SSRIs neuroleptics? J Clin Psychopharmacol 17:443–445, 1997

Pies RW: Handbook of Essential Psychopharmacology. Washington, DC, American Psychiatric Press, 1998

Piscitelli SC, Burstein AH, Chaitt D, et al: Indinavir concentrations and St. John's wort. Lancet 355:547–548, 2000

Pollack MH, Rosenbaum JF: Management of antidepressant-induced side effects: a practical guide for the clinician. J Clin Psychiatry 48:3–8, 1987

Pollock BG, Everett G, Perel JM: Comparative cardiotoxicity of nortriptyline and its isomeric 10-hydroxymetabolites. Neuropsychopharmacology 6:1–10, 1992

Pollock BG, Perel JM, Paradis CF, et al: Metabolic and physiologic consequences of nortriptyline treatment in the elderly. Psychopharmacol Bull 30:145–150, 1994

Rasmussen SA, Eisen JL, Pato MT: Current issues in the pharmacologic management of obsessive-compulsive disorder. J Clin Psychiatry 54 (6, suppl):4–9, 1993

Reynolds CF: Recognition and differentiation of elderly depression in the clinical setting. Geriatrics 50 (suppl 1):S6–S15, 1995

Reynolds CF, Perel JM, Frank E, et al: Three-year outcomes of maintenance nortriptyline treatment in late-life depression: a study of two fixed plasma levels. Am J Psychiatry 156:1177–1181, 1999

Richard IH, Kurlan R: A survey of antidepressant drug use in Parkinson's disease. Parkinson Study Group. Neurology 49:1168–1170, 1997

Robinson RG, Schultz SK, Castillo C, et al: Nortriptyline versus fluoxetine in the treatment of depression and in short-term recovery after stroke: a placebo-controlled, double-blind study. Am J Psychiatry 157:351–359, 2000

Roose SP, Dalack GW: Treating the depressed patient with cardiovascular problems. J Clin Psychiatry 53 (9, suppl):25–31, 1992

Roose SP, Glassman AH: Antidepressant choice in the patient with cardiac disease: lessons from the Cardiac Arrhythmia Suppression Trial (CAST) studies. J Clin Psychiatry 55 (9, suppl A):83–87, 1994

Roose SP, Suthers KM: Antidepressant response in late-life depression. J Clin Psychiatry 59 (suppl 10):4–8, 1998

Roose SP, Dalack GW, Woodring S: Death, depression and heart disease. J Clin Psychiatry 52 (6, suppl):34–39, 1991

Roose SP, Glassman AH, Attia E, et al: Comparative efficacy of selective serotonin reuptake inhibitors and tricyclics in the treatment of melancholia. Am J Psychiatry 151:1735–1739, 1994

Rosen J, Pollock BG, Altieri LP, et al: Treatment of nortriptyline's side effects in elderly patients: a double-blind study of bethanechol. Am J Psychiatry 150:1249–1251, 1993

Rosenbaum JF, Fava M, Hoog SL, et al: Selective serotonin reuptake inhibitor discontinuation syndrome: a randomized clinical trial. Biol Psychiatry 44:77–87, 1998

Rosenthal NE: Diagnosis and treatment of seasonal affective disorder. JAMA 270:2717–2720, 1993

Rouillon F, Gorwood P: The use of lithium to augment antidepressant medication. J Clin Psychiatry 59 (5, suppl):32–39, 1998

Ruschitzka F, Meier PJ, Turina M, et al: Acute heart transplant rejection due to St. John's wort. Lancet 355:548–549, 2000

Salzman C: Monoamine oxidase inhibitors and atypical antidepressants. Clin Geriatric Med 8:335–348, 1992

Satlin A, Volicer L, Ross V, et al: Bright light treatment of behavioral and sleep disturbances in patients with Alzheimer's disease. Am J Psychiatry 149:1028–1032, 1992

Schneider LS, Cooper TB, Staples FR, et al: Prediction of individual dosage of nortriptyline in depressed elderly outpatients. J Clin Psychopharmacol 7:311–314, 1987

Schneider LS, Cooper TB, Suckow RF, et al: Relationship of hydroxynortriptyline to nortriptyline concentration and creatinine clearance in depressed elderly outpatients. J Clin Psychopharmacol 10:333–337, 1990

Sheline YI, Freedland KE, Carney RM: How safe are serotonin reuptake inhibitors for depression in patients with coronary heart disease? Am J Med 102:54–59, 1997

Skop BP, Finkelstein JA, Mareth TR, et al: The serotonin syndrome associated with paroxetine, an over-the-counter cold remedy, and vascular disease. Am J Emerg Med 12:642–644, 1994

Spier SA, Frontera MA: Unexpected deaths in depressed medical inpatients treated with fluoxetine. J Clin Psychiatry 52:377–382, 1991

Stein G, Bernadt M: Lithium augmentation therapy in tricyclic-resistant depression. Br J Psychiatry 162:634–640, 1993

Sternbach H: The serotonin syndrome. Am J Psychiatry 148:705–713, 1991

Stoudemire A: New antidepressant drugs and the treatment of depression in the medically ill patient. Psychiatr Clin North Am 19:495–514, 1996

Streim JE, Oslin DW, Katz IR, et al: Drug treatment of depression in frail elderly nursing home residents. Am J Geriatr Psychiatry 8:150–159, 2000

Sussman N, Ginsberg D: Rethinking side effects of the selective serotonin reuptake inhibitors: sexual dysfunction and weight gain. Psychiatric Annals 28:89–97, 1998

Tan RS, Bransgrove L: Drugs and orthostatic hypotension in the elderly, Part II: reversing orthostatic hypotension with drug treatment. Clin Geriatrics 6:38–44, 1998

Thase ME, Sachs GS: Bipolar depression: pharmacotherapy and related therapeutic strategies. Biol Psychiatry 48:558–572, 2000

Tulloch IF, Johnson AM: The pharmacologic profile of paroxetine, a new selective serotonin reuptake inhibitor. J Clin Psychiatry 53 (2, suppl): 7–12, 1992

Wager SG, Klein DF: Treatment refractory patients: affective disorders. Psychopharmacol Bull 24:69–74, 1988

Winokur A, Sateia MJ, Hayes JB, et al: Acute effects of mirtazapine on sleep continuity and sleep architecture in depressed patients: a pilot study. Biol Psychiatry 48:75–78, 2000

Young RC, Alexopoulos GS, Dhar AK, et al: Plasma 10-hydroxynortriptyline and renal function in elderly depressives. Biol Psychiatry 22: 1283–1287, 1987

Generic name	bupropion
Trade name	Wellbutrin, Wellbutrin SR
Class	Atypical
Half-life	34 hours
Mechanism of action	Probably noradrenergic; inhibition of dopamine reuptake at doses > usual antidepressant doses
Available formulations	Tablets: 75, 100 mg SR tablets: 100, 150 mg
Starting dose	37.5 mg qd–37.5 mg bid SR: 100 mg daily
Titration	Increase by 37.5 mg (or 75 mg) every 3–4 days, as tolerated SR: Increase by 100 mg after 3–4 days
Typical daily dose	150 mg (divided bid or tid, with doses separated by 6 hours) SR: 100 mg bid
Dosage range	75–225 mg daily SR: 100–300 mg daily
Therapeutic serum level	Not established, although levels > 40 ng/mL may be poorly tolerated

Comments: A drug of choice for elderly patients because of relative lack of cardiovascular effects, cognitive effects, anticholinergic effects, and sedation. Well absorbed orally. Peak levels in 2 hours for immediate release and 3 hours for extended release (healthy adults). Metabolized by CYP2B6 enzyme. Two active metabolites: hydroxy-bupropion and threo-hydro-bupropion; metabolite levels may be much higher than levels of parent drug. Clearance decreased in the elderly and in those with renal or hepatic insufficiency, so lower dosesare used. Dosage adjustment not needed for dialysis patients. High metabolite levels are associated with poor response and psychotic symptoms. *Important drug interactions:* levodopa, potentially MAOIs; use therapeutic nicotine with caution. *Common adverse effects:* Agitation, dry mouth, insomnia, headache, nausea, constipation, weight loss or gain, and tremor. Hypertension may occur. *Serious but uncommon effect:* seizures.

Generic name	citalopram
Trade name	Celexa
Class	SSRI
Half-life	35 hours
Mechanism of action	Highly selective serotonin reuptake inhibition
Available formulations	Tablets: 20 mg (scored), 40 mg Oral solution: 10 mg/5 mL
Starting dose	10–20 mg qd
Titration	Increase by 10 mg after 7 days. Maintain at 20 mg (target dose) for 3–4 weeks; further titration as needed.
Typical daily dose	20 mg
Dosage range	10–40 mg daily
Therapeutic serum level	Not established

Comments: Probably a drug of choice for elderly patients because of its favorable side-effect profile and relative lack of significant medication interactions. Rapidly absorbed; not affected by food. Linear kinetics. Peak levels in 4 hours. 80% protein bound. Metabolized by CYP3A4, CYP2C19, and CYP2D6 enzymes. Parent drug shows no significant CYP inhibition, but desmethyl metabolite might be a weak CYP2D6 inhibitor. Clearance decreased in the elderly and in those with liver disease. *Adverse effects:* nausea, vomiting, dry mouth, headache, somnolence, insomnia, increased sweating, tremor, diarrhea, delayed ejaculation, and SIADH.

Generic name	desipramine
Trade name	Norpramin
Class	Tricyclic
Half-life	7 to >60 hours (varies directly with age)
Mechanism of action	Norepinephrine and (weak) serotonin reuptake inhibition
Available formulations	Tablets: 10, 25, 50, 75, 100, 150 mg Capsules: 25, 50 mg
Starting dose	25 mg qd
Titration	Increase by 25 mg every 7 days
Typical daily dose	100 mg (can be given in one dose after initial titration)
Dosage range	25–150 mg daily
Therapeutic serum level	>105 ng/mL

Comments: Not a drug of choice for elderly patients because of cardiac conduction effects and toxicity in overdose. Well absorbed orally, with peak concentration in 4–6 hrs. Hydroxylation yields active metabolite (2-hydroxy-desipramine), which is excreted intact by kidney. Substrate for CYP2D6 enzyme. Time to peak concentration delayed compared with imipramine, so less problematic acute side effects. *Serious adverse effect:* avoid using desipramine in patients with cardiovascular disease, particularly post–myocardial infarction patients, because of potential cardiotoxicity. *Other adverse effects:* orthostasis, urinary retention, precipitation of angle closure in glaucoma, tremor, agitation, insomnia, and occasional hypertension.

Generic name	dextroamphetamine
Trade name	Dexedrine, DextroStat
Class	Psychostimulant
Half-life	7–34 hrs
Mechanism of action	Blocks reuptake of dopamine and norepinephrine; causes release of catecholamines; inhibits monoamine oxidase
Available formulations	Tablets: 5, 10 mg Capsules (XR): 5, 10, 15 mg
Starting dose	2.5 mg qam (with breakfast)
Titration	Increase by 2.5–5 mg every 2–3 days
Typical daily dose	5 mg bid (with breakfast and lunch)
Dosage range	2.5 mg bid to 10 mg bid
Therapeutic serum level	Not established

Comments: Useful in treating medically ill, depressed elders needing urgent intervention for whom ECT is not an option. Often used as an "accelerator" to bridge the period of antidepressant latency, in which case it is discontinued after 2–3 weeks. As a sole antidepressant, efficacy is established for use of several months but not for longer periods. Well absorbed orally; not affected by food. Onset in 2–3 hrs; duration 4–24 hours. Extensively metabolized in liver. Dialyzable.
Contraindications: Contraindicated in patients with severe vascular or cardiovascular disease, hypertension, hyperthyroidism, diabetes, glaucoma, drug abuse, Tourette's disorder, or agitation. Potentially significant drug interaction with MAOIs, not often seen clinically.
Adverse effects: tachycardia, hypertension, restlessness, dizziness, insomnia, tremor, headache, psychotic symptoms, aggression, diarrhea, nausea/vomiting, constipation, anorexia, and blurred vision.

Generic name	fluoxetine
Trade name	Prozac
Class	SSRI
Half-life	Fluoxetine: 70 hours (3 days) Norfluoxetine: 330 hours (1–2 weeks)
Mechanism of action	Selective serotonin reuptake inhibition
Available formulations	Capsules: 10, 20 mg Liquid concentrate: 20 mg/5 mL
Starting dose	10 mg qd (depression and OCD) 2–5 mg qd (panic disorder)
Titration	In treating depression/OCD, increase dose to 20 mg after 1–2 weeks. Maintain at that dose 3–4 weeks before further dose increases, then only if response is partial.
Typical daily dose	20 mg
Dosage range	5–40 mg daily for depression 5–40 mg daily for panic 20–60 mg daily for OCD
Therapeutic serum level	Not established

Comments: Potentially a drug of choice for elderly patients, although side effects may limit use, and prolonged half-life is associated with accumulation of parent and metabolite on repeated dosing. Minimal age-related pharmacokinetic changes. Well absorbed orally, with peak levels in 4–8 hours. Food slows absorption. Hepatic demethylation yields norfluoxetine, an active metabolite. Half-lives of these compounds are approximately the same in elderly as in younger patients. 8–10 weeks to steady state of norfluoxetine. Long half-lives of parent and metabolite, so prolonged (5- to 6-week) risk of drug interactions after discontinuation. Nonlinear kinetics. *Dose:* Concentration is the same in elderly patients as in younger patients.

Inhibits CYP2D6 > CYP3A4 = CYP2C > CYP1A2; inhibits the metabolism of many drugs. *Adverse effects* (include): Nausea, vomiting, diarrhea, insomnia, nervousness, restlessness, "agitation," anxiety, light-headedness, drowsiness, fatigue, headache, tremor, initial weight loss (especially in those older than 75 years and underweight to begin with), possible long-term weight gain, hyponatremia, and sexual dysfunction. Rare SIADH, supraventricular arrhythmias, and synergistic effects in producing extrapyramidal symptoms when used with an antipsychotic.

Generic name	methylphenidate
Trade name	Ritalin, Ritalin-SR, Metadate ER
Class	Psychostimulant
Half-life	2–7 hours
Mechanism of action	Blocks dopamine reuptake; stimulates cerebral cortex and subcortical structures
Available formulations	Tablets: 5, 10, 20 mg Tablets (SR): 20 mg Tablets (ER): 10, 20 mg
Starting dose	2.5 mg qam (with breakfast)
Titration	Increase by 2.5–5 mg every 2–3 days
Typical daily dose	5 mg bid (with breakfast and lunch)
Dosage range	2.5 mg bid to 10 mg bid
Therapeutic serum level	Not established

Comments: Useful for medically ill, depressed elders needing urgent intervention for whom ECT is not an option. Often used as an "accelerator" to bridge the period of antidepressant latency, in which case it is discontinued after 2–3 weeks. As a sole antidepressant, efficacy is established for use of several months but not for longer periods. Absorption slow and incomplete. Peak effect in 2 hours; duration 3–6 hours. Eliminated in urine and bile. *Contraindications:* same contraindications as with dextroamphetamine, although effects on blood pressure and pulse in adults not well studied. *Drug interactions:* Significant drug interactions with warfarin and TCAs. Potentially significant drug interaction with MAOIs, not often seen clinically. *Adverse effects:* restlessness, behavior disturbances, hallucinations, slurred speech, ataxia, vertigo, Tourette's disorder, mania, hepatotoxicity, rash, rhabdomyolysis, physical dependence with withdrawal symptoms, and hypersensitivity.

Generic name	mirtazapine
Trade name	Remeron
Class	Tetracyclic
Half-life	20–40 hours
Mechanism of action	Noradrenergic and specific (postsynaptic) serotonergic antagonism
Available formulation	Tablets: 15, 30 mg (both scored), 45 mg (unscored)
Starting dose	7.5 mg qd (evening)
Titration	Increase by 7.5–15 mg every 1–2 weeks, as tolerated
Typical daily dose	30 mg (evening)
Dosage range	7.5–45 mg daily
Therapeutic serum level	Not established

Comments: Understudied in elderly patients. Rapidly and completely absorbed orally, with peak levels in 2 hours; not affected by food. 85% protein bound. Extensively metabolized in the liver via the CYP1A2, CYP2D6, and CYP3A4 enzymes. Clearance reduced in elderly (especially men) and in patients with hepatic or renal dysfunction. *Common side effects* (include): Sedation, dizziness, increased appetite with weight gain, increases in serum cholesterol and triglyceride levels, significant elevations in ALT levels without compromise of liver function, and hypertension. Associated with decreased heart rate variability, but less than with imipramine. Lower doses may be more sedating than higher doses, presumably because at higher doses noradrenergic effects balance histaminergic effects.

Generic name	nefazodone
Trade name	Serzone
Class	Phenylpiperazine
Half-life	2–4 hours (metabolites persist longer)
Mechanism of action	5-HT$_2$ antagonism Modest norepinephrine reuptake inhibition (minimal serotonin reuptake inhibition)
Available formulation	Tablets: 50, 100, 150, 200, 250 mg
Starting dose	25–50 mg bid
Titration	Increase by 50–100 mg every 1–2 weeks, as tolerated
Typical daily dose	100 mg bid
Dosage range	50–400 mg daily
Therapeutic serum level	Not established

Comments: Usefulness in the elderly limited by sedating effects. Food delays absorption and insignificantly lowers maximum concentration. Significant first-pass metabolism. Nonlinear kinetics. Peak concentrations in 30 minutes. Three active metabolites: m-CPP, triazolodione, and hydroxy-nefazodone. Potent CYP3A4 inhibitor; weak CYP2D6 inhibitor (see Table 1–1 in Chapter 1). Dose-to-concentration ratio different for elderly compared with younger patients, so dosing guidelines adjusted as noted above. Lower doses used in hepatic disease. *Adverse effects:* Orthostasis, sedation, nausea, constipation, headache, asthenia, dizziness, dry mouth, and visual symptoms (blurring and image trailing). At higher doses, cognition and motor function are affected. Effects on sleep include increased REM, increased total movement time, increased actual sleep time, and decreased wake after sleep onset. Early increases in oral temperature and serum prolactin levels that return to baseline with repeated administration. Nefazodone is associated with fewer reports of sexual dysfunction, weight gain, nervousness, insomnia, and tremor compared with other agents and may prove to be useful in treating depressed patients with prominent anxiety and sleep disturbances.

Generic name	nortriptyline
Trade name	Aventyl, Pamelor
Class	Tricyclic
Half-life	37–45 hours in elderly patients
Mechanism of action	Norepinephrine and serotonin reuptake inhibition
Available formulations	Capsules: 10, 25, 50, 75 mg Liquid concentrate: 10 mg/5 mL
Starting dose	10–25 mg qd (usually hs)
Titration	Increase by 10 mg (or 25 mg) every 7 days, as tolerated
Typical daily dose	50 mg (usually hs)
Dosage range	10–100 mg daily
Therapeutic serum level	50–150 ng/mL

Comments: A drug of choice for elderly patients with severe or melancholic depression. Substrate for CYP2D6 enzyme. Active metabolite 10-hydroxy-nortriptyline is excreted intact by the kidney. Metabolite may accumulate to toxic levels in patients with renal insufficiency. In general, a target dose of 1 mg/kg is adequate for patients 60–80 years. *Serious adverse effects:* warnings about use in patients with ischemic heart disease or preexisting cardiac conduction abnormalities (bundle branch block or intraventricular conduction delay) because of slowing of cardiac conduction. *Other adverse effects:* Delirium, weight gain, increased triglyceride levels, increased VLDL levels, increased heart rate (mean of 15 bpm), and decrease in creatinine clearance. Conflicting evidence regarding cognitive effects (impairments in free recall, verbal memory). Less likely than other TCAs to cause orthostasis or anticholinergic side effects; latter effects do occur and are persistent but are usually mild.

Generic name	paroxetine
Trade name	Paxil
Class	SSRI
Half-life	21 hours (may be longer in elderly patients)
Mechanism of action	Selective serotonin reuptake inhibition
Available formulations	Tablets: 10, 20, 30, 40 mg Liquid suspension: 10 mg/5 mL
Starting dose	10 mg qd
Titration	Increase to 20 mg after 1–2 weeks; maintain at that dose for 3–4 weeks before further dose increases, then increase only if partial response is seen
Typical daily dose	20 mg
Dosage range	5–40 mg daily for depression 20–60 mg daily for OCD
Therapeutic serum level	Not established

Comments: A drug of choice for elderly patients. The most potent SSRI in terms of serotonergic reuptake. No active metabolites. Prolonged half-life in the elderly. Higher plasma levels achieved in elders than in younger patients because of reduced clearance. Higher levels also in renal or hepatic disease. Nonlinear kinetics. Peak concentration in 7–8 hours; dinnertime administration avoids daytime drowsiness. Inhibitor of CYP2D6 enzyme. Withdrawal syndrome common with abrupt discontinuation. Minimal cardiovascular effects; relatively safe in overdose. Less likely than most other SSRIs to cause agitation. *Usual adverse effects:* Nausea, headache, insomnia or sedation, mild anticholinergic effects (one-fifth as anticholinergic as nortriptyline). Like other SSRIs, paroxetine has been associated with hyponatremia and SIADH.

Generic name	sertraline
Trade name	Zoloft
Class	SSRI
Half-life	36 hours in elderly patients
Mechanism of action	Selective serotonin reuptake inhibition
Available formulation	Tablets: 25, 50, 100 mg (all scored)
Starting dose	12.5–25 mg qd
Titration	Increase by 12.5–25 mg every 3–5 days, as tolerated
Typical daily dose	50–100 mg
Dosage range	12.5–200 mg daily (lower for panic, higher for OCD)
Therapeutic serum level	Not established

Comments: A drug of choice for elderly patients, particularly for outpatients with depression. Slowly but well absorbed orally, with peak concentrations in 4.5–8.4 hours. Food increases absorption, so sertraline must be given consistently with respect to meals. Linear kinetics. Extensively metabolized in the liver by multiple CYP enzymes. Capacity to inhibit CYP2D6 is dose dependent but weak. Prolonged half-life and increased concentrations in the elderly.
Adverse effects: Nausea, dyspepsia, headache, insomnia, sedation, and sexual dysfunction. Reported association with delirium.

Generic name	St.-John's-wort (*Hypericum perforatum*)
Trade name	Various
Class	Herbal
Half-life	16–36 hours
Mechanism of action	Serotonin reuptake inhibition, monoamine oxidase inhibition
Available formulation	Capsules: 150, 300 mg
Starting dose	
Titration	
Typical daily dose	300 mg tid
Dosage range	300 mg bid to 300 mg tid
Therapeutic serum level	Not established

Comments: Not a drug of choice for elderly patients because of significant drug interactions and a side effect of spontaneous bleeding. Available over-the-counter. As with other herbal formulations, concerns have been raised about product content and purity. Steady state in 4 days; onset of antidepressant effect after several weeks. *Drug interactions:* inducer of CYP3A4 enzyme and P-glycoprotein expression, so has significant interactions with antiviral agents (including indinavir), immunosuppressants (including cyclosporine), anticoagulants, and antiarrhythmic agents. *Adverse effects* (include): spontaneous bleeding (subarachnoid hemorrhage, subdural hematoma), photosensitivity, gastrointestinal symptoms, allergic reactions, fatigue, dizziness, xerostomia, and induction of mania.

Generic name	trazodone
Trade name	Desyrel
Class	Atypical
Half-life	Biphasic elimination: Initial: 4–8 hours Terminal: 12 hours
Mechanism of action	Antagonist at 5-HT$_2$ receptors > serotonin reuptake inhibition at usual doses; blocks norepinephrine reuptake presynaptically; down-regulates 5-HT$_2$ receptors with chronic use
Available formulation	Tablets: 50, 100, 150, 300 mg (all scored)
Starting dose	Depression: 12.5–25 mg bid or tid Insomnia: 12.5–25 mg hs
Titration	Increase by 25 mg every 3–7 days, as tolerated
Typical daily dose	Depression: 75–150 mg (divided tid) Insomnia: 25–50 mg hs
Dosage range	12.5–400 mg daily Depression: 50–400 mg daily (divided bid or tid) Insomnia: 12.5–300 mg hs
Therapeutic serum level	Not well established

Comments: Very effective hypnotic; modestly effective antidepressant. Absorption impeded by food, so must be given consistently with respect to meals. Onset of sedative effect in 20–30 minutes; earlier peak concentration when taken on an empty stomach (1 hour) than when taken with food (2 hours). Greatly increased volume of distribution in obese patients, resulting in prolonged half-life. 85%–95% protein bound. Extensively metabolized in the liver; m-CPP is an active metabolite and may be anxiogenic for some patients. Reduced clearance in elderly men necessitates dose reduction with chronic administration. Minimal muscarinic and histaminergic effects. *Drug interactions:* synergistic with other medications causing orthostasis or sedation. Wide therapeutic index. Usefulness as an antidepressant limited in many cases by sedation. *Adverse effects* (include): Hypotension (including orthostasis), ventricular irritability (increased premature depolarizations), sedation (associated with falls and cognitive dysfunction), myalgias, nausea, and dry mouth. The m-CPP metabolite may be anxiogenic in some patients. Priapism has rarely been reported in elderly men. Trazodone *not* recommended during the initial recovery phase from myocardial infarction.

Generic name	venlafaxine
Trade name	Effexor, Effexor XR
Class	Atypical
Half-life	5 hours (*o*-desmethyl metabolite: 11 hours)
Mechanism of action	Serotonin and norepinephrine reuptake inhibition (dopamine reuptake inhibition at doses > 350 mg daily)
Available formulations	Tablets: 25, 37.5, 50, 75, 100 mg (immediate release [IR]) Capsules 37.5, 75, 150 mg (extended release [XR])
Starting dose	IR: 25 mg qd XR: 37.5 mg qd
Titration	IR: Increase by 25 mg every 4–7 days, as tolerated, to 25 mg tid; if response is inadequate after 3 weeks at this dosage, increase slowly to 50 mg tid; if response is still inadequate after 3 more weeks, increase slowly to 75 mg tid XR: increase to 75 mg (target dose) after 4–7 days; may need to increase to 150 mg or 225 mg if response is inadequate
Typical daily dose	IR: 50 mg tid XR: 150 mg (given at the same time every day; swallowed whole)
Dosage range	IR: 150–225 mg daily (divided bid or tid) XR: 150–225 mg daily (one daily dose)
Therapeutic serum level	Not established

Comments: A drug of choice for elderly patients. May be particularly useful for those with treatment-refractory illness. Age does not affect pharmacokinetics, except for potential accumulation of metabolite with decreased renal function. Well absorbed orally, with peak levels in 2–3 hrs. 30% protein bound. Substrate for CYP2D6 enzyme. Major metabolite is *o*-desmethylvenlafaxine, which is active and has the same side-effect profile as the parent compound. Dose adjustments needed for mild to moderate renal dysfunction (decrease by 25%) and hepatic dysfunction (decrease by 50%). Stop TCAs, MAOIs, and SSRIs 2 weeks or more before initiating venlafaxine. *Adverse effects:* Nausea (very common, especially with fast titration), somnolence, dry mouth, dizziness (not orthostatic), nervousness, tremor, insomnia, constipation, sexual dysfunction, sweating, asthenia, and anorexia. Supine diastolic blood pressure elevation is a potential problem; blood pressure must be checked before and monitored during treatment. Low association with seizures, cardiac conduction changes, and orthostasis.

4

Mood Stabilizers

Mood stabilizers are used to lessen the frequency and severity of manic and depressive episodes in bipolar disorder and schizo-affective disorder and to treat mood lability in the context of dementia and personality disorders. In addition, particular anti-convulsant mood stabilizers are used to treat various pain syndromes, movement disorders, and alcohol and sedative withdrawal. Table 4–1 lists indications for mood stabilizers in the treatment of elderly patients.

Currently marketed drugs used as mood stabilizers include lithium, valproate, carbamazepine, gabapentin, lamotrigine, topiramate, and oxcarbazepine. The efficacy and safety of lithium and valproate are well established, and these are currently the drugs of choice among elderly patients, although many elders are unable to tolerate lithium. Despite demonstrated efficacy, carbamazepine is used as a second- or third-line agent because of side effects and drug interactions. It is not clear whether oxcarbazepine suffers from similar limitations, and insufficient data are

Table 4–1. Indications for mood stabilizers in elderly patients

Bipolar disorder

  Manic phase

  Depressed phase

  Maintenance therapy (prophylaxis)

Secondary mania

Schizoaffective disorder

Aggression in dementia

Adjunctive therapy in acute unipolar depression (lithium)

Prophylaxis of recurrent unipolar depression

Mood instability in other Axis I disorders (PTSD, personality disorders)

Alcohol or sedative-hypnotic withdrawal (carbamazepine, gabapentin)

Restless legs syndrome (carbamazepine, valproate, gabapentin)

Neuropathic pain (gabapentin)

Trigeminal neuralgia (carbamazepine)

Postherpetic neuralgia (gabapentin)

Note. PTSD = posttraumatic stress disorder.

available to support a recommendation for use of this drug in geriatric patients. Limited data from case reports and open studies suggest that gabapentin and lamotrigine may be useful in the treatment of geriatric patients. Topiramate as a mood stabilizer is unstudied in the geriatric population.

Atypical antipsychotics also have mood-stabilizing properties. Olanzapine and risperidone are preferred for this indication because of their efficacy and favorable side-effect profiles. Clozapine is clearly effective as a mood stabilizer, but it can cause significant side effects in elders, as noted in Chapter 2 ("Antipsychotics"). Insufficient data are available to support the use of quetiapine in this context. Benzodiazepines may be useful as adjunctive antimanic agents. Clonazepam is considered superior for the indication of mania and has a place in the geriatric pharmacopoeia despite concerns about its long half-life.

Pharmacokinetics

Mood stabilizer formulations and strengths are shown in Table 4–2. Information about absorption, distribution, metabolism, and clearance of selected mood stabilizers is included in the specific drug summaries at the end of the chapter.

Pharmacodynamics and Mechanism of Action

Lithium

Elderly patients are believed to be more sensitive to the effects of lithium, but in fact the pharmacodynamics of this drug are not well understood (Nelson 1998). In view of its multiple and complex neurotransmitter actions, lithium has been postulated to have fundamental effects on adenylate cyclase activity, cAMP (cyclic adenosine monophosphate) formation, receptor–G protein coupling, and phosphoinositol metabolism. In addition, it is known to alter the distribution and kinetics of sodium, potassium, calcium, and magnesium. At the neurotransmitter level, lithium affects GABA as well as cholinergic, serotonergic, adrenergic, and dopaminergic neurotransmission (Price and Heninger 1994).

Valproate

The mechanism of action of valproate has not been completely characterized, but effects probably relate in part to increased GABA levels, since valproic acid inhibits enzymes involved in GABA breakdown (McEvoy et al. 2000).

Carbamazepine

Pharmacological actions of carbamazepine are similar to those of phenytoin, primarily involving inhibition of synaptic transmission. This drug has many other actions, including sedative, anticholinergic, muscle relaxant, and antiarrhythmic actions (McEvoy et al. 2000).

Table 4–2.   Mood stabilizer formulations and strengths

Generic name	Trade name	Tablets (mg)	Capsules (mg)	Available formulations				
				Extended-release (XR) form	Oral suspension	Oral solution	Injectable form	
carbamazepine	Tegretol	200 100 (chewable)		100, 200, 300, 400	100 mg/5 mL			
clonazepam	Klonopin	0.5, 1, 2			0.1 mg/mL[a]			
gabapentin	Neurontin	600, 800	100, 300, 400		100 mg/mL[a]			
lamotrigine	Lamictal	25, 100, 150, 200 2,[b] 5, 25 (chewable)			1 mg/mL[a]			
lithium	various	300 (scored) (Eskalith, Lithotabs, Lithium Carbonate tablets)	150, 300, 600 (Eskalith, Lithonate, Lithium Carbonate tablets)	300, 450 (Lithobid, Eskalith-CR)		8 mEq/5 mL (300 mg/5 mL) (Lithium citrate syrup)		

Table 4–2. Mood stabilizer formulations and strengths *(continued)*

| Generic name | Trade name | Tablets (mg) | Capsules (mg) | Available formulations | | | | |
				Extended-release (XR) form	Oral suspension	Oral solution	Injectable form
olanzapine	Zyprexa	2.5, 5, 7.5, 10, 15					
	Zyprexa Zydis	5, 10					
oxcarbazepine	Trileptal	150, 300, 600 (all scored)					
topiramate	Topamax	25, 100, 200	15, 25, 50				
valproate	various	125, 250, 500 (Depakote)	250 (Depakene); 125 (Sprinkles)	500 (Depakote ER)		250 mg/5 mL	100 mg/mL (Depacon)

[a]Extemporaneous preparations, compounded according to instructions in Lacy CF, Armstrong LL, Goldman MP, et al.: *Drug Information Hand-book*, 8th Edition. Cleveland, OH, Lexi-Comp, Inc., 2000–2001.
[b]2-mg chewable tablet available directly from GlaxoWellcome.

Gabapentin

Although structurally related to GABA, gabapentin has no direct GABA-mimetic actions. It acts partly by inhibition of the GABA transporter, resulting in increased central nervous system (CNS) GABA levels (McEvoy et al. 2000).

Lamotrigine

Lamotrigine modulates release of the excitatory amino acids glutamate and aspartate by blocking presynaptic voltage-sensitive sodium channels (Kotler and Matar 1998).

Drug Interactions

Pharmacological interactions involving mood stabilizers are summarized in Table 4–3. The newer anticonvulsants gabapentin and lamotrigine have fewer reported interactions than other mood stabilizers, in part because they are renally excreted and undergo minimal hepatic metabolism.

Lithium has important interactions not only with medications but also with dietary modifications influencing salt concentrations, particularly sodium. The combination of lithium and haloperidol has been reported to be neurotoxic, although in practice this combination is often used safely. In fact, at least some case reports showing neurotoxicity involved excessive doses of these drugs.

Carbamazepine has been called "the great inducer" because of its capacity to induce various hepatic enzymes and thereby speed the processes of oxidation and conjugation for a large number of other drugs. In addition, carbamazepine itself is metabolized by a single enzyme—the cytochrome P450 (CYP) 3A enzyme—and thus is more susceptible to inhibition by agents such as antifungal agents, grapefruit juice, and nefazodone. Valproate has fewer problematic interactions than carbamazepine, since it is not an inducer, and is metabolized via several CYP pathways as well as noncytochrome mitochondrial pathways.

Table 4–3. Mood stabilizer drug interactions

Mood stabilizer	Interacting drug	Potential interaction
carbamazepine	clozapine	Increased risk of agranulocytosis
	isoniazid	Increased levels of both drugs
	lamotrigine	Carbamazepine metabolite toxicity
	lithium	Neurotoxicity, sinus node dysfunction
	TCA	Decreased antidepressant effect; accumulation of cardiotoxic metabolites of TCA
	theophylline	Two-way metabolic induction, with changes in half-lives and concentrations
	valproate	Increased level of carbamazepine epoxide metabolite, with neurotoxicity
	cimetidine, clarithromycin, danazol, diltiazem, erythromycin, fluconazole, fluoxetine, fluvoxamine, grapefruit juice, itraconazole, ketoconazole, propoxyphene, verapamil	Increased carbamazepine level; toxicity

Table 4–3. Mood stabilizer drug interactions (*continued*)

Mood stabilizer	Interacting drug	Potential interaction
carbamazepine (*continued*)	bupropion, clozapine, corticosteroids, cyclosporine, doxycycline, haloperidol, olanzapine, warfarin	Decreased level of interacting drug
gabapentin	Maalox	Reduced gabapentin absorption
lamotrigine	carbamazepine	Carbamazepine metabolite toxicity; decreased lamotrigine level
	valproate	Increased lamotrigine level; increased risk of serious skin rash
lithium	ACE inhibitors	Increased lithium level; toxicity; avoid co-administration, if possible
	phenothiazines	Unpredictable pharmacokinetics; neurotoxicity
	calcium channel blockers	Increased lithium clearance; pharmacodynamic interaction, with lithium toxicity at low serum concentrations
	carbamazepine	Additive neurotoxicity

Table 4–3. Mood stabilizer drug interactions (*continued*)

Mood stabilizer	Interacting drug	Potential interaction
	diuretics	Thiazide diuretics: reduced renal lithium clearance and increased serum levels, with toxicity
		Other diuretics: clearance reduced less consistently than with thiazide diuretics
	iodides	Hypothyroidism
	methyldopa	Lithium toxicity at low serum concentrations
	metronidazole	Lithium toxicity, with renal injury
	NSAID	Increased lithium concentrations; toxicity
	SSRI	Increased risk of toxicity/serotonin syndrome
	tetracycline antibiotics	Lithium toxicity
valproate	aspirin	Increased valproate level
	carbamazepine	Decreased valproate level; increased level of toxic valproate metabolite; carbamazepine toxicity
	cimetidine	Increased valproate level
	CNS depressants	Additive CNS depression

Table 4–3.   Mood stabilizer drug interactions (*continued*)

Mood stabilizer	Interacting drug	Potential interaction
valproate (*continued*)	erythromycin	Increased valproate concentration
	lamotrigine	Increased lamotrigine level; increased risk of serious skin rash
	phenobarbital	Increased phenobarbital level; decreased valproate level
	phenytoin	Unpredictable pharmacokinetic interactions
	zidovudine	Zidovudine toxicity

Note.   ACE = angiotensin converting enzyme; NSAID = nonsteroidal anti-inflammatory drug; SSRI = selective serotonin reuptake inhibitor; TCA = tricyclic antidepressant.

In anticipation of a course of electroconvulsive therapy (ECT), mood stabilizers may be discontinued, although this is by no means a universal practice. When stopped temporarily, they are often restarted at or near the end of the ECT course. With patients who require uninterrupted treatment with a mood stabilizer, however, some clinicians opt to reduce the level to the low end of the therapeutic range (Zarate et al. 1997). With lithium, for example, some lower the level to 0.2–0.4 mEq/L prior to ECT, while others discontinue it because of concerns about neurotoxicity.

ECT can also be useful for maintenance therapy in bipolar disorder. One prospective study of monthly ECT added to medications in 22 geriatric patients demonstrated good control of rapid cycling and delusional depression (Vanelle et al. 1994).

Efficacy

Most of what is known about the efficacy of mood stabilizers in geriatric populations was extrapolated from studies performed in younger patients. In general, the efficacy of these agents varies for different syndromes under treatment. Efficacy is highest for the manic phase of bipolar illness and is well established for lithium and valproate (Bowden et al. 1994). From extensive anecdotal experience, carbamazepine, olanzapine, and risperidone are known to be effective as well in the geriatric population. Neither these drugs nor any of the newer anticonvulsant mood stabilizers have been systematically studied for mania in this population. Furthermore, for reasons not yet understood, the efficacy of mood stabilizers is also, in part, individually determined; nonresponse to one agent does not predict nonresponse to another.

Certain subgroups of bipolar patients tend to be less responsive to lithium. These include patients with depression or "mixed" mania, rapid-cycling illness, or an episode sequence pattern of depressed–manic–well interval (as opposed to manic–depressed–well interval); those with more than three prior episodes before prophylaxis; those with no family history of bipolar disorder; and those with a history of substance abuse, head injury, or other complicating medical condition (Post et al. 1998). Valproate and other anticonvulsants may be more effective for some of these patients. For the depressed phase of bipolar illness, reduced efficacy is seen for all mood stabilizers except lithium and possibly lamotrigine (Calabrese et al. 1999).

For bipolar disorder prophylaxis, mood stabilizers are effective, but less so than for acute mania. In general, lithium is more effective for classical bipolar I disorder (without mood-incongruent delusions or comorbidity), whereas anticonvulsants such as valproate are superior for patients with nonclassical presentations common in geriatric populations, including secondary mania and mixed episodes.

Clinical Use

The acutely manic elder is often most safely treated in a hospital setting. As with younger patients, seclusion with close observation may be indicated for severe agitation. In general, it is best to avoid administering medications on a prn ("as needed") basis, and it is better to reexamine the patient at frequent intervals to make adjustments to standing medication regimens.

Choice of Drug

Lithium or valproate monotherapy is the standard first-line treatment for elderly patients with bipolar disorder. Lithium has been the mainstay of treatment for decades and remains the drug of choice for patients who have had a prior good response. There are, however, persistent concerns about the effects of prolonged lithium use on the kidney and other organ systems in old age. In addition, elderly patients are more sensitive to lithium's neurotoxic effects. Partly for these reasons, valproate is increasingly used as the mood stabilizer of first choice in treating elderly patients. The only patients for whom valproate is best avoided are those with significant hepatic dysfunction.

The atypical antipsychotics olanzapine and risperidone are increasingly used as first-line therapies for geriatric mania. Anecdotal experience suggests that these therapies are effective, although initial titration of risperidone may be too slow for practical purposes. In addition, both agents have been associated with mania induction among some treated individuals.

Little is known from controlled study about the use of carbamazepine in elderly patients. In general, this agent is considered a second- or third-line agent, for patients not responding to other treatments. This drug has a large number of highly significant drug interactions, as noted in Table 4–3. Newer mood-stabilizing agents such as lamotrigine, gabapentin, topiramate, and oxcarbazepine may prove useful in the treatment of elderly patients, but more systematic study and wider experience with these drugs are needed. Clinical experience suggests that gabapentin alone or in combination with other drugs is well tolerated by older patients in the treatment of insomnia, dementia with aggression, and bipolar disorder, although this use may be limited by excessive sedation. Controlled studies of gabapentin in bipolar disorder have not yet shown conclusive evidence of effiacacy.

ECT is safe and effective for the treatment of geriatric mania and results in rapid remission of symptoms, typically after four to six treatments. Bilateral electrode placement is usually preferred for bipolar patients but is associated with more confusion and memory impairment compared with unipolar placement. Follow-up treatment with a mood-stabilizing medication is often sufficient to maintain remission, although some patients do require maintenance ECT. In general, ECT is used for patients with very severe symptoms, those who prefer this initiation of treatment because of past positive experience, those intolerant of medication, or those who have a poor response to medication.

Alternative Formulations

Valproate is available as a capsule (Depakene), a capsule containing coated particles (Depakote Sprinkle), a delayed-release tablet (Depakote), an extended-release tablet (Depakote ER), an oral solution (Depakene Syrup), and in an injectable form (Depacon). Depakote and Depakote Sprinkles are less irritating to the gastrointestinal tract than the Depakene formulations. Compared with the delayed-release Depakote tablet, Depakote Sprinkles yield steadier serum levels, with reduced peak-level side effects (McEvoy et al. 2000). The new extended-release formulation shares this property but is available only as a 500-mg tablet, so it may have limited use in the geriatric population.

The preferred preparation of lithium for use in elderly patients is the regular-acting tablet, since it provides an adequately low trough level when the drug is administered once daily. The slow-release formulation may be useful for patients who do not develop tolerance to side effects related to peak drug level, such as nausea or tremor. The citrate formulation can be used to initiate lithium at very low doses (e.g., <75 mg) and for patients who are unable to swallow tablets.

Baseline Laboratory Studies and Clinical Evaluation

Elderly patients with elevated mood undergo a standard workup to assess for secondary causes and to establish baseline laboratory and clinical parameters. This workup minimally includes vital signs, physical and neurological examination, complete blood cell count (CBC) with platelets, electrolytes (including calcium and magnesium), liver function tests (aspartate transaminase [AST], alanine transaminase [ALT], alkaline phosphatase), creatinine clearance (usually calculated), thyroid function tests (thyroid-stimulating hormone [TSH]), and electrocardiogram (ECG). Correction of hypothyroidism and electrolyte derangements is essential for optimal lithium response. Electroencephalography can be useful in helping to distinguish mania from delirium, particularly in patients with dementia who are difficult to assess at the bedside (Jacobson and Jerrier 2000).

Dose and Dose Titration

Lithium is started in elderly patients at 75–150 mg qd in a single nightly dose. The dose is increased by 75–150 mg every 4–7 days. For "young-old" patients without concomitant medical disease or dementia, increments can be up to 300 mg every 4 days. Serum lithium levels are checked at steady state (7 days after a dose change), from 8–12 hours after the last dose administered. For reasons noted later in this section relating to renal protection (see "Side Effects"), lithium is best given in a single nightly dose (Plenge et al. 1982). When side effects necessitate splitting the dose during the early phase of treatment, it is important to consolidate the dose to a qd schedule as soon as possible. Every-other-day dosing is not recommended because of reduced prophylactic efficacy and compliance problems (Jensen et al. 1995).

Valproate is started at a dose of 125 mg qd to 250 mg bid. If the patient tolerates the initial dosing, the dose can be increased by 125 to 250 mg every 3–5 days, as tolerated. In the hospitalized manic patient, initial dosing can be higher, at least in "young-old" patients; a loading dose of 15 mg/kg can be used. Therapeutic levels are discussed below (see "Monitoring Treatment"). Although splitting the dose results in reduced peak-level side effects, valproate can be administered in a single daily dose at bedtime.

Dose and dose titration of other mood stabilizers are discussed in the specific drug summaries at the end of this chapter.

Course of Response

Time to response has not been studied in exclusively geriatric samples. In patients of mixed age, the response to lithium or valproate in acute mania occurs in as little as several days to as long as 2 weeks or more, depending on initial dose and rapidity of titration. It may be those patients who end up on small doses and who require little titration who respond early. The antidepressant response to lithium usually takes longer, on the order of 4 weeks or more.

Monitoring Treatment

Drug levels are routinely monitored for lithium, carbamazepine, and valproate. Serum levels are checked when the drug has reached steady state: after 5–7 days for lithium and after 3–4 days for val-proate. Serum level monitoring is more complicated for carbam-azepine because the half-life changes with autoinduction. In general, carbamazepine levels are checked 3–5 days after a dose change and are checked periodically until the level stabilizes at that dose (usually after several months). Levels for all mood sta-bilizers are drawn 12 hours after the last dose, even for once-daily regimens. Drug levels are obtained after initiating therapy, after any change in dose, after other medications that could affect levels are started or changed, or at any sign of toxicity. Lev-els are also checked at regular intervals during maintenance treatment, usually every 3–6 months in the stable patient.

For lithium, initial target serum levels for acute mania in the geriatric patient are in the range of 0.4 to 0.8 mEq/L (Schaffer and Garvey 1984). For patients who do not respond or who experi-ence significant side effects after 10 days in this range, the dose can be further titrated (Salzman 1998). Some elderly patients re-quire levels in the range of 0.8 to 1.0 mEq/L. For maintenance treatment, doses are reduced, and target levels are in the range of 0.2 to 0.6 mEq/L. When single nightly doses of short-acting lithium are used for elderly patients (as is recommended), the 12-hour level is approximately the same as for twice-a-day dosing, since the half-life in elders is greater than 36 hours.

Lithium dosing often requires adjustment downward as the patient ages. Dosage reductions are also indicated whenever there is a change in renal function, an electrolyte imbalance (particularly with sodium), or dehydration. As noted in Table 4–3, concurrent treatment with medications such as angiotensin converting en-zyme (ACE) inhibitors or nonsteroidal anti-inflammatory drugs may also necessitate lowering of the lithium dose. If a decline in renal function or significant polyuria occurs during lithium treat-ment, creatinine clearance should be measured or calculated (see Chapter 1) and compared with baseline, and urine osmola-lity and specific gravity should be obtained.

Other laboratory values monitored routinely with lithium therapy include serum creatinine, urinalysis, thyroid function tests (specifically, TSH), and ECG, performed roughly every 6 months (Eastham et al. 1998). For any complication of therapy (including co-administered interacting medication), more frequent monitoring may be required.

For valproate, target serum levels for acute mania in the geriatric patient are 50–100 µg/mL (McEvoy et al. 2000), usually achieved with doses in the range of 750 to 1,500 mg/day. Some patients with dementia manifesting agitation or secondary mania have been observed to respond to much lower levels, in the range of 13 to 52 µg/mL (Lott et al. 1995). Other laboratory values monitored routinely with valproate include liver function tests and CBC with platelets. As with younger patients, these laboratory tests are obtained every 1–4 weeks during the first 6 months of therapy, and then every 3–6 months, depending on the particular patient (McElroy et al. 1989).

For carbamazepine, target levels are less well established. Anecdotal support exists for a target level in the acutely manic geriatric patient of 4–8 µg/mL, although some patients require higher levels. One study of patients with dementia manifesting aggression found that levels in the range of 2.4 to 5.2 µg/mL (mean 4.13 µg/mL) were effective (Lemke 1995). Autoinduction complicates plasma level monitoring of carbamazepine, as noted earlier.

Other laboratory parameters routinely monitored with carbamazepine therapy include ECG, CBC with platelets, liver function tests, and serum levels of sodium and creatinine (Eastham et al. 1998). Blood is drawn weekly for the first 6 weeks of therapy, then monthly thereafter. An ECG is obtained when the therapeutic level of carbamazepine has been attained; if a disturbance of cardiac conduction is detected, the dose is reduced or the medication is withdrawn (Kasarskis et al. 1992).

Duration of Treatment

For the majority of elderly patients with primary bipolar disorder, long-term treatment with a mood stabilizer is indicated. This is particularly true for patients with frequent manic episodes (every

12 months or less) or any serious episode requiring hospitalization. Some patients with early-onset disease experience a cycle acceleration later in life, and morbidity is greatly minimized with appropriate prophylaxis.

In mania secondary to medical conditions or medication treatment, a slightly different treatment algorithm is used. In secondary mania, when the offending medication can be withdrawn or the medical condition can be treated, the mania often subsides. At that time, mood stabilizers are tapered and discontinued, since maintenance treatment is not needed. When definitive treatment is not possible (e.g., completed right hemisphere stroke), maintenance mood stabilization therapy may be advised.

Managing Treatment Resistance

Treatment is inadequate, either completely or partially, for a substantial subgroup of elderly bipolar patients. As with other types of medication, the options for management of nonresponse to mood stabilizers include switching and augmentation. Switching is used when the patient has had no response to an adequate trial, since it makes no sense to try to "augment" a nonresponse. In the interest of minimizing side effects, it is always best to taper and discontinue one agent before starting another in the geriatric patient. When this is not possible because of symptom severity, the drugs are cross-tapered such that the first drug is withdrawn when the second drug has reached the target level or dose. If the patient's symptoms recur as the first drug is withdrawn, dual therapy is considered. With elderly patients, compared with younger patients, changes in dose of both medications are smaller and are made at longer intervals. In addition, in general, the risk of polypharmacy is greater in elderly patients.

Pharmacological augmentation of mood stabilizers can involve other mood stabilizers, antidepressants, antipsychotics, benzodiazepines, thyroid hormone, clonidine, and folate. Combinations of mood stabilizers are often effective in treating patients who do not respond, and any combination could be used, with certain caveats. Valproate and carbamazepine have complicated pharmacokinetic interactions that result in increased levels of toxic metabolites. Although the combination is usually well tolerated in bipolar patients, it may be problematic for patients with secondary mania. Valproate and lamotrigine should also be co-administered with care, because this combination is associated with doubled serum levels of lamotrigine, as well as increased risk of lamotrigine-associated rash, which is potentially serious. For certain patients, the risks may be worth taking, since the lamotrigine-valproate combination has been reported to be effective for most patients with treatment-resistant conditions after 4 weeks (Kusumakar and Yatham 1997). Anecdotal reports indicate that when lithium is combined with an anticonvulsant, lower lithium doses can be used.

Antidepressants may be added to mood stabilizers when patients have significant breakthrough symptoms of depression. Antidepressant–mood stabilizer combinations generally are not used for prophylaxis because of the risk of inducing mania or rapid cycling (Altshuler et al. 1995) and because mood stabilizers alone are considered as effective as the combination for this purpose. Like younger patients, most elders who develop rapid cycling do so while taking antidepressants, and in some cases the rapid cycling does not remit when the antidepressant is discontinued. Antidepressants preferred for use with mood stabilizers in geriatric populations include bupropion and SSRIs, which apparently carry less risk of inducing mania. Antidepressants used for breakthrough depression while the patient is treated with a mood stabilizer are generally tapered and discontinued after 2–6 months.

Apart from the use of atypical antipsychotics as mood stabilizers, antipsychotic medications may be used to treat psychotic symptoms in acute mania. In this case, antipsychotics are withdrawn when the acute episode remits, usually after several weeks of treatment. Either an atypical antipsychotic or haloperidol could be selected for this purpose; haloperidol has the advantage of limited hypotensive and anticholinergic effects, whereas atypical agents are less likely to provoke extrapyramidal symptoms.

Benzodiazepines are also used with mood stabilizers in the manic elderly patient. In some elders, benzodiazepine–mood stabilizer combinations have undesired effects, including ataxia, oversedation, and disinhibition. In others, not only is the combination well tolerated, but cotreatment is required for long-term mood stabilization. Low-dose clonazepam is often very effective for this purpose.

Thyroid supplementation is crucial for patients with clinical or subclinical hypothyroidism, but thyroxine (T_4) augmentation may enhance response to mood stabilizers even for euthyroid bipolar patients, particularly those with rapid cycling. This therapy is not without risk, however; T_4 may be associated with induction of atrial arrhythmias, and long-term use of T_4 in postmenopausal women has been associated with an increased risk of osteoporosis.

Very limited data suggest that adjunctive clonidine can be useful for patients whose symptoms reflect high physiological arousal in the absence of prominent psychotic symptoms or motor hyperactivity. Clonidine dosages used in one study ranged from 450 to 900 µg/day in three divided doses (Hardy et al. 1986). With careful dosing, this treatment might be especially appropriate for a geriatric patient who also requires treatment for hypertension.

Daily supplementation of 300–400 µg of folic acid was found useful in one randomized controlled study in reducing affective morbidity during long-term lithium prophylaxis (Coppen et al. 1986). That study was limited by an excessive dropout rate, however, and has yet to be replicated.

Discontinuation of Mood Stabilizers

Abrupt discontinuation of lithium therapy is associated with an increased risk of early relapse (Suppes et al. 1991), so lithium is best tapered over at least a 2- to 4-week period (Faedda et al. 1993). Although not specifically studied in geriatric patients, discontinuation of other mood stabilizers is probably most safely done by slow taper as well, over several weeks.

Overdose/Overmedication

In the elderly patient treated with a mood stabilizer, toxic effects can occur with inadvertent overmedication, even when levels are in the "therapeutic" range, as well as with acute overdose. With lithium, toxicity at therapeutic levels may be associated with rapid dosage escalation, cotreatment with other psychotropic agents (antipsychotics, antidepressants, or anticonvulsants), preexisting electroencephalogram (EEG) abnormalities, or structural brain disease (Bell et al. 1993; Emilien and Maloteaux 1996). In addition, any derangement associated with reduction of the glomerular filtration rate will cause an increase in lithium levels and potential toxicity. Another mechanism of toxicity is dehydration and reduction of sodium levels through dietary restriction or other means.

Signs and symptoms of lithium intoxication can be gastrointestinal, neuropsychiatric, cardiac, renal, or systemic. Neuropsychiatric signs include lethargy, weakness, hyperreflexia, tremor and other abnormal movements, dysarthria, rigidity, ataxia, delirium, seizures, and coma (Bell et al. 1993). Characteristic EEG abnormalities are seen (Ghadirian and Lehmann 1980). A syndrome of disinhibition and giddiness that resembles mania can occur. Cardiac dysrhythmias, hypotension, renal failure, and fever can also be seen in the lithium-toxic patient (Jefferson 1991).

The goal of treatment of lithium toxicity is to minimize exposure to large lithium loads. This is accomplished by discontinuation of lithium and initiation of gastric lavage (repeated), continuous gastric suction, and restoration of normal fluid/electrolyte balance (Jefferson 1991). Administration of the ion exchange resin sodium polystyrene sulfonate (Kayexalate) may be helpful. Except in the mildest cases, patients are admitted to the hospital. Clinical examination and lithium levels are monitored serially and frequently. Hemodialysis is used for severe lithium intoxication (with coma, seizures, or respiratory failure), very high serum levels, rising serum levels, or progressive clinical deterioration (Jaeger et al. 1993). The rule of thumb for patients of mixed age is that hemodialysis should be considered when the lithium level drawn 12 hours after the last dose is 2.5 mEq/L or greater.

Clinical recovery after lithium intoxication may take several weeks, with neurological symptoms persisting long after lithium levels have normalized. Depending on the severity and duration of the toxic episode, a patient may demonstrate irreversible neurological injury, with dysarthria, nystagmus, ataxia, and intention tremor being most characteristic (Apte and Langston 1983; Donaldson and Cunningham 1983; Schou 1984).

Carbamazepine overdose produces gastrointestinal, neurological, and systemic signs, and anticholinergic excess that can be associated with urinary retention. Treatment consists of emesis induction or gastric lavage as well as general supportive therapy. The ECG is monitored for dysrhythmias (McEvoy et al. 2000).

Valproate overdose may result in somnolence, heart block, coma, and hepatic or pancreatic toxicity and has been associated with fatalities (McEvoy et al. 2000). Treatment is supportive, with an emphasis on maintaining urinary output. The effectiveness of gastric lavage or emesis is limited for immediate-release valproate because it is so rapidly absorbed, but these interventions may be of value for the delayed-release form if the time since ingestion is short enough (McEvoy et al. 2000). Hemodialysis removes significant amounts of valproate from the system. Naloxone can reverse CNS depressant effects of valproate toxicity but increases the risk of seizure (McEvoy et al. 2000).

Gabapentin absorption across the gut wall is limited at high doses by saturation of transport mechanisms (Elwes and Binnie 1996), rendering this drug safer in overdose than other mood stabilizers. The limited data available on lamotrigine suggest that this agent is also nonlethal in overdose but is associated with dizziness, headache, somnolence, and coma. Emesis and lavage are recommended, particularly for recent ingestions, since lamotrigine is rapidly absorbed. It is unclear whether hemodialysis is effective in removing lamotrigine from the system.

Side Effects

Side Effects of Specific Agents

Carbamazepine

The most common side effects of this drug are dizziness, drowsiness, nausea, skin reactions, and asthenia. The most serious side effects—hematological, cardiac, and gastrointestinal—make carbamazepine the last choice among mood stabilizers in the treatment of elderly patients. This medication is, in rare cases (1 in 200,000), associated with aplastic anemia, with an unquantified incidence in elders. Cardiac effects include bradycardia, exacerbation of existing sinus node dysfunction, and slowed atrioventricular node and His bundle conduction (Steckler 1994). Cardiac effects are especially common in elderly women and may be seen at therapeutic or only modestly elevated carbamazepine serum levels (Kasarskis et al. 1992). Gastrointestinal effects include significant elevations in liver function test values (AST, ALT, and γ-glutamyltranferase [GGT]) that may, in rare cases, be associated with hepatic insufficiency or failure.

Neuropsychiatric effects of carbamazepine (which may be due to its epoxide metabolite) include confusion, disorientation, sedation, dizziness, unsteadiness, ataxia, diplopia, lassitude, and weakness. Various dermatological reactions, including Stevens-Johnson syndrome, may be seen. Impaired water excretion with hyponatremia (syndrome of inappropriate antidiuretic hormone [SIADH]) is associated with carbamazepine and is more common in geriatric than in younger patients.

Gabapentin

The efficacy of gabapentin as monotherapy for major mood disorders has been disappointing, but this agent is still useful as an adjunct and possibly as sole therapy for secondary mood disorders in elderly patients. This drug is generally well tolerated, with side effects that are usually self-limiting. The most common adverse effects are neuropsychiatric: somnolence, dizziness, ataxia, fatigue, and nystagmus (McEvoy et al. 2000). Other adverse effects include nausea and vomiting, dry mouth, constipation, peripheral edema, rhinitis, pharyngitis, visual changes, and myalgia. Induction of rapid cycling has also been reported.

Lamotrigine

Lamotrigine is associated with numerous adverse effects, some of which are time limited and others of which are dose related (McEvoy et al. 2000). Common side effects include dizziness, ataxia, somnolence, headache, diplopia, blurred vision, nausea, vomiting, and rash. A relatively high discontinuation rate is seen for this drug and is associated with rash, dizziness, or headache. The rash, which has no distinguishing features, may herald the onset of Stevens-Johnson syndrome or toxic epidermal necrolysis and may ultimately be fatal. The risk of rash is increased by co-administration of valproate, by exceeding initial dosing recommendations, or especially by exceeding dose escalation recommendations. Other side effects include insomnia, incoordination, tremor, impairment in memory and concentration, constipation, and arthralgia.

Lithium

Although lithium is well known to cause frequent and sometimes serious side effects in elderly patients, it remains a drug of first choice because of efficacy and familiarity. In general, lithium's side-effect profile is the same for older as for younger patients (Eastham et al. 1998), but older patients are more likely to develop toxicity because of age-related renal and cerebral changes. Aging is associated with reduced ability to excrete lithium as well as hormonal changes affecting kidney function (Nelson 1998).

Adverse effects of lithium are largely dose- and level-dependent. The most frequent and bothersome side effects in elderly patients include excessive thirst, hand tremor, excessive urination, dry mouth, drowsiness, and fatigue (Chacko et al. 1987). Other common side effects include memory impairment, restlessness, constipation, and weight gain.

Whether lithium treatment causes structural (e.g., glomerular) changes in the kidney remains controversial, at least with regard to long-term treatment (Bendz et al. 1994; Conte et al. 1989; Hetmar et al. 1989). Episodes of lithium toxicity and multiple daily dosing appear to represent risks for renal injury, so both are avoided as far as possible (Hetmar et al. 1991). A separate problem is that lithium impairs the ability of the kidneys to concentrate urine in about one-third of elderly patients. The resultant polyuria, which may be manifest as incontinence, is also reduced with single daily dosing. When polyuria remains problematic, amiloride can be used; this medication paradoxically causes a reduction in urine volume (Price and Heninger 1994). More rarely, lithium treatment is associated with nephrogenic diabetes insipidus, with huge urine volumes and unquenchable thirst. This syndrome is usually reversible when lithium is discontinued, but we have seen at least one case in which symptoms were persistent.

Cardiac effects of lithium include ECG changes, conduction changes, and dysrhythmias (Steckler 1994). T wave depression on the ECG that is benign and reversible occurs in 20%–30% of lithium-treated patients (McEvoy et al. 2000). Sinus bradycardia, sinoatrial block, atrioventricular block, junctional rhythms, and ventricular premature depolarizations occur, although rarely. Sinus node dysfunction is most common in those with preexisting cardiac disease and in those taking blocking medications such as digoxin or propranolol (Steckler 1994). Ventricular tachycardia can occur during episodes of ischemia in lithium-treated patients with ventricular irritability or arteriosclerotic heart disease (Salzman 1998).

Neuropsychiatric effects of lithium are commonly reported by elderly patients with serum levels in the "therapeutic range" (Bell et al. 1993). These include fatigue, weakness, hand tremor, memory problems, dysarthria, balance problems, ataxia, neuromuscular irritability (fasciculations and twitching), lack of coordination, and nystagmus. In general, tolerance to these neuropsychiatric symptoms does not develop, but they may improve with reduction in dose. When lithium is discontinued because of the development of delirium or cerebellar dysfunction, symptoms can persist for weeks after serum levels are undetectable (Nambudiri et al. 1991). In some cases of more severe toxicity, irreversible cerebellar signs (ataxia and dysarthria) are seen (Kores and Lader 1997).

Among other effects, lithium is associated with reduced bone mineral content because of reduced uptake of magnesium, calcium, and phosphate (Ghose 1977). Associated abnormalities include elevated serum calcium and magnesium levels and elevated muscle magnesium and phosphate levels. The clinical significance of these findings in elderly patients is not known. Approximately half of lithium-treated patients gain weight, an average of about 10–20 pounds (Price and Heninger 1994).

Valproate

The most common side effects of valproate are gastrointestinal: dyspepsia, nausea, and vomiting (McEvoy et al. 2000). These effects are usually transient and can be minimized by giving the medication with food, using the enteric-coated formulation divalproex sodium (Depakote), and starting at a low dose and titrating slowly. Increased appetite and weight gain are also common. Many other gastrointestinal side effects, including fecal incontinence, have been reported. Hepatotoxicity is rare, idiosyncratic, and unrelated to dose. Pancreatitis has also been reported with therapeutic levels of valproate and may be more common in those with end-stage renal disease. Sedation is commonly seen upon initiation of therapy, with tolerance developing to this effect over 1–2 weeks. Tremor may also be seen. One underappreciated but potentially serious side effect of valproate is skeletal muscle weakness, which was associated with refusal to walk as well as ventilatory failure in a reported case (Trehan and Clark 1993). In our experience, this weakness can be significant in some cases and can interfere with the ability to transfer, stand, and walk without assistance. Other adverse effects of valproate include parkinsonism (especially tremor), elevated ammonia level, thrombocytopenia, rash, and SIADH.

System-Specific Side Effects

Cardiovascular Effects

Cardiovascular effects are found primarily with lithium and car-bamazepine and were discussed earlier in the sections on individual agents.

Dermatological Effects

Lamotrigine and carbamazepine have been associated with a syndrome first manifesting as a nonspecific rash that can progress to Stevens-Johnson syndrome or toxic epidermal necrolysis. Rarely, death has been a reported consequence. It is recommended that lamotrigine or carbamazepine be discontinued at the first sign of rash in a treated individual. Carbamazepine also has been associated with a generalized, pruritic, erythematous rash sometimes associated with a blood dyscrasia, including aplastic anemia (Cates and Powers 1998).

Lithium is known to exacerbate psoriasis, acne, and folliculitis. Although all may limit treatment, lithium exacerbation of psoriasis is potentially very serious, in some cases necessitating hospitalization for treatment with intravenous steroids. Lithium is also associated with the de novo development of rash, with hair loss and edema (Gitlin et al. 1989).

Valproate treatment may be associated with alopecia. It has been speculated that this might be a consequence of chelation of selenium and zinc in the gastrointestinal tract. Some clinicians supplement valproate treatment with a multivitamin containing selenium 150 mg and zinc 10 mg (Nelson 1998).

Endocrine Effects

Among other thyroid effects, lithium inhibits release of T_4 and T_3, resulting in decreased circulating levels of these hormones and a feedback increase in TSH (McEvoy et al. 2000). Approximately 8% of geriatric patients undergoing long-term treatment with lithium develop either symptomatic hypothyroidism or benign diffuse nontoxic goiter. Lithium-induced hypothyroidism more often develops in women. Symptoms include fatigue, weight gain, hair loss, coarse skin, hoarse voice, pretibial edema, sensitivity to cold, dementia, and depression. The syndrome usually comes on insidiously and, once developed, is associated with resistance to mood-stabilizing treatment. Treatment options include discontinuation of lithium or initiation of thyroid hormone replacement. Lithium-associated goiter more often develops in men, usually 1–2 years after treatment is initiated. It is often first detected when the patient reports difficulty swallowing (Salzman 1998). Less commonly, lithium may be associated with hyperthyroidism (Oakley et al. 2000).

Gastrointestinal Effects

Initiation of lithium is associated with mild, reversible gastrointestinal side effects (McEvoy et al. 2000). These include nausea, anorexia, epigastric bloating, diarrhea, vomiting, and abdominal pain—symptoms that usually resolve during continued therapy. Persistent effects may be associated with high peak serum concentrations and can be reduced by lowering the dose, giving the drug with food, or switching to a different preparation (capsule or tablet). When diarrhea is a problem, some patients benefit from a switch to the citrate preparation.

Lamotrigine is commonly associated with dose-related gastrointestinal effects, including nausea and vomiting (McEvoy et al. 2000). Other effects include diarrhea, dyspepsia, and abdominal pain. Rare fatalities with hepatic failure have been associated with lamotrigine. Gastrointestinal effects of carbamazepine, gabapentin, and valproate were discussed earlier in the context of the individual agents.

Hematological Effects

Carbamazepine is commonly associated with leukopenia and thrombocytopenia, dose-dependent phenomena associated at times with a rapid rate of dose escalation. For white cells, the reduction from baseline for patients of mixed age is on the order of 15%–20%. This cytopenia plateaus after several weeks and does not presage an aplastic episode (Gerner and Stanton 1992).

Much more rarely, carbamazepine is associated with agranulocytosis and aplastic anemia (1 in 200,000 cases). If the white blood cell count (WBC) falls to 3,000/mm^3, the dose of carbamazepine should be reduced and the WBC should be monitored weekly. If it falls to 2,500/mm^3 or less, the drug should be discontinued, and it should be restarted only after the cell count again exceeds 3,000/mm^3, after several weeks (Gerner and Stanton 1992).

The risk of leukopenia with valproate treatment is an order of magnitude less than with carbamazepine and at about the same level as with antidepressants (Tohen et al. 1995). The guidelines for monitoring and medication discontinuation outlined above for carbamazepine-associated leukopenia apply as well to valproate. Thrombocytopenia is relatively common with valproate treatment and most often is not clinically significant. The patient with low or declining platelet count should be monitored for bruising or bleeding, and serial platelet counts should be obtained.

Lithium is commonly associated with a mild to moderate leukocytosis involving mature neutrophils. It is important that this laboratory finding not be mistaken for infection or a more serious blood dyscrasia. This effect can be useful in preventing clozapine-induced leukopenia but does not prevent the development of agranulocytosis.

Hepatic Effects

Early in treatment, both carbamazepine and valproate can produce elevations in liver function tests (AST and ALT) (Gerner and Stanton 1992). These findings usually do not presage severe disease. If AST and ALT values are less than three times baseline values and alkaline phosphatase and bilirubin levels are normal, the patient is monitored with weekly liver function tests. When values plateau, longer testing intervals are permitted. If liver function test values rise to more than three times baseline (or more than twice the upper limit of normal), the drug should be discontinued or appropriate consultation should be obtained (Gerner and Stanton 1992). Another warning sign is elevation in either alkaline phosphatase or bilirubin levels; these laboratory abnormalities indicate that the anticonvulsant should be held, if not discontinued. Prothrombin time can also help determine functional hepatic effects. No laboratory test, however, should take precedence over clinical observations of malaise, nausea, anorexia, or jaundice, which can indicate significant hepatotoxicity. Since preexisting liver disease predisposes to hepatotoxicity, such patients are best treated with mood stabilizers other than carbamazepine or valproate.

Neuropsychiatric Effects

Sedation is common with all mood stabilizers, particularly on initiation of therapy or after a dose increase. For most patients, tolerance develops to this effect over 1–2 weeks, but in some cases the dose must be reduced. At the other extreme, lamotrigine has been associated with induction of mania, and gabapentin has been associated with induction of rapid cycling.

Cognitive impairment has long been recognized as a side effect of lithium therapy, but it is, in fact, unclear whether and to what extent bipolar illness itself is associated with progressive cognitive decline. Cognitive effects attributed to lithium include poor concentration, memory impairment, word-finding difficulty, cognitive "dulling," mental slowness, and loss of creativity (Gitlin et al. 1989; Lund et al. 1982). These effects can be seen during the early phases of treatment and at low doses, can continue during long-term treatment, and can persist when lithium is discontinued (Nelson 1998).

Anecdotal evidence suggests that valproate is less likely to cause cognitive impairment than is lithium, and that any impairment that occurs with valproate is evident by the time steady-state levels are achieved (Nelson 1998). A switch to valproate has been used to treat lithium-associated cognitive dulling and loss of creativity in a small series of younger patients.

Cognitive profiles of other anticonvulsants are beginning to be characterized. In a randomized study involving nongeriatric patients, neither gabapentin nor lamotrigine was found to have cognitive effects, but the newer anticonvulsant topiramate was associated with declines in attention and word fluency (Martin et al. 1999).

Extrapyramidal effects of mood stabilizers are not uncommon in geriatric patients. With lithium treatment, hand tremor occurs in up to 50% of patients of mixed age (McEvoy et al. 2000). The tremor is described as a distal resting or intention tremor that is less coarse than a parkinsonian tremor. In many patients, this tremor diminishes with time, but severe cases can be treated with dose reduction and/or administration of a β-blocker such as propranolol at a dosage up to 40 mg/day in divided doses. A similar tremor can also be seen with valproate, carbamazepine, lamotrigine, and topiramate, and this is treated in the same way. In addition, worsening of preexisting Parkinson's disease and de novo appearance of parkinsonism have been associated with lithium therapy (Mirchandani and Young 1993).

The development of seizures is a rare complication of mood stabilizer therapy, since most of these agents are anticonvulsants and are associated with seizure development only at toxic levels. The one exception to this is lithium, which can be associated with generalized seizures if the patient has clinical toxicity, regardless of serum level (McEvoy et al. 2000). Withholding lithium and resuming therapy at a lower dose usually eliminates this complication.

Other neurotoxic signs and symptoms attributed to lithium include cerebellar dysfunction (ataxia, incoordination, dysarthria, nystagmus), weakness, and myoclonus (Gitlin et al. 1989). Ataxia and incoordination are particularly problematic in elderly patients because of the risk of falls. Skeletal muscle weakness associated with valproate therapy was discussed previously. Carbamazepine has been associated with ataxia, and lamotrigine has been associated with dizziness and headache.

Sexual Effects

The combination of lithium and benzodiazepines has been associated with various symptoms of sexual dysfunction. It is not known whether these problems are more common in the elderly. Gabapentin has been associated with sexual side effects in nongeriatric patients.

Treatment of Selected Syndromes and Disorders With Mood Stabilizers

Clinical features of late-life mania include a combination of mood, motor, cognitive, and psychotic symptoms. Mood symptoms may resemble those of an agitated depression, with prominent dysphoria or irritability, labile or mixed affect, and morbid or depressive content of thought and speech. Increased motor and psychomotor activity is seen, with pressured speech and "agitation," especially repetitive vocalization. A reversible dementia syndrome of mania can occur, with prominent impairment in attention and memory. Delusional symptoms, usually persecutory, are common, but overt hallucinations may be less common than in younger patients with mania (Young and Klerman 1992).

Mania in the elderly can represent primary bipolar disorder or be secondary to medical or neurological disease. Secondary mania is more likely in an elderly patient who has a first episode in late life, has cerebrovascular disease, has no family history of mood disorder, responds poorly to lithium or develops toxicity at low lithium levels, or is treated with a mania-inducing medication such as an antidepressant (Young and Klerman 1992). Prominent symptoms of secondary mania include irritability, psychosis, pressured speech, and insomnia (Carroll et al. 1996). Causes of secondary mania are listed in Table 4–4.

In mania secondary to medical conditions or medication treatment, a slightly different treatment algorithm is used, as noted previously. In secondary mania, when the cause can be treated, the mania often subsides. A mood stabilizer may be used for a period of weeks to months and then be tapered and withdrawn. In other cases, when definitive treatment is not possible, maintenance mood stabilization therapy may be needed.

The prognosis for elderly patients with mania depends largely on perseverance until effective treatment is established. Irritable, uncooperative patients are often undertreated, and those with concomitant alcoholism or cognitive impairment are often non-compliant. In addition, elderly patients with mania can be extremely slow to regain insight, so continuation of treatment beyond the acute phase is not often achieved (Young and Klerman 1992). The need for long-term stabilization of symptoms is critical, since those who continue cycling may experience shorter cycles with more severe symptoms as they age (Young and Klerman 1992). Long-term treatment (at least with lithium) actually extends survival by reducing excess suicide risk as well as excess cardiovascular mortality (Ahrens et al. 1995).

Frontal lobe syndromes involving orbitofrontal dysfunction with consequent disinhibition are sometimes mistaken for mania in the elderly patient. The differential diagnosis of these entities can be difficult; in our experience, the most reliable indicator of mania, as opposed to frontal lobe dysfunction, is severe sleep disruption. A subset of patients with frontal lobe dysfunction will respond to mood stabilizer therapy. Other uses for mood stabilizers beyond bipolar disorder and related syndromes, including several pain syndromes, are discussed briefly below.

Aggression in Dementia

Mood stabilizers are among the agents of first choice for aggressive and certain agitated behaviors in elderly patients. Valproate at dosages of 250–1,500 mg/day (with levels of approximately 30 to 100 µg/mL) and carbamazepine 300 mg/day (with a level around 5 µg/mL) have been found to be effective for this indication (Hermann 1998; Porsteinsson et al. 1997; Tariot et al. 1998). Anecdotal reports suggest that gabapentin 300 mg bid may also be useful in treating agitation associated with Alzheimer's disease (Regan and Gordon 1997). The role of lamotrigine in dementia-associated aggression is not yet known, but this agent is being tried as a neuroprotective drug in Alzheimer's disease and thus may prove to have multiple beneficial effects in this population (Tekin et al. 1998). Dementia-associated aggression is discussed further in Chapter 8 ("Treatment of Dementias and Other Cognitive Syndromes").

Alcohol/Sedative Withdrawal

Although benzodiazepines remain the treatment of choice for acute withdrawal of alcohol and related sedatives, anticonvulsants are increasingly used as adjuncts. Carbamazepine, gabapentin, and valproate may reduce the amount of benzodiazepine needed acutely and facilitate abstinence as the benzodiazepine is tapered and discontinued in the subacute period.

Bipolar Depression

The first-line treatment for bipolar I depression is a mood stabilizer: valproate, lithium, carbamazepine, or lamotrigine. These medications are initiated and titrated as described in the specific drug summaries at the end of this chapter. Lamotrigine 200 mg daily as monotherapy was found to be effective and well tolerated in the treatment of bipolar depression in a randomized, controlled trial involving nongeriatric patients (Calabrese et al. 1999). The time to antidepressant effect with these agents is similar to that seen for antidepressants. For nonresponse or breakthrough depressive symptoms in patients with a history of rapid cycling, a second mood stabilizer is added. In our experience, the combination of lithium and valproate is particularly effective in elders and allows for a lower therapeutic serum level of lithium (0.4–0.6 mEq/L). For severely depressed patients without a history of rapid cycling, an antidepressant such as bupropion or an SSRI (citalopram or paroxetine) is added instead. Patients with conditions refractory to this treatment are considered for ECT or other pharmacotherapy such as an atypical antidepressant, venlafaxine, or the MAOI tranylcypromine in conjunction with the mood stabilizer (Thase and Sachs 2000). When an antidepressant is used for bipolar depression, it is tapered and discontinued after 2–6 months, depending on the duration and severity of the depressive episode. For the geriatric bipolar patient already taking lithium who presents with major depression, the possibility that the patient has a hypothyroid condition should be considered and a serum TSH level should be obtained.

The need for co-administration of a mood stabilizer with the antidepressant for a patient with bipolar II depression is determined in part by the frequency and severity of past hypomanic episodes.

When psychotic symptoms (delusions or hallucinations) accompany a bipolar depressive or a bipolar manic episode, adjunctive antipsychotic medication is used. Generally, the antipsychotic is tapered and withdrawn when the acute episode is fully treated, from 2–6 months after remission of the psychotic symptoms. Clinical experience is greatest with high-potency conventional antipsychotics such as haloperidol, and these agents are useful because of fast onset of action and a favorable side-effect profile in elderly patients. There is no good evidence to support early claims of a high incidence of neurotoxicity with co-administration of lithium and haloperidol, and this combination is frequently used safely. Olanzapine, risperidone, and other atypical agents are also likely to be useful for this indication.

Bipolar Mania

Elderly patients in a manic prodrome show the familiar features of distractibility, increased activity, and decreased need for sleep. Unlike their younger counterparts, however, elderly patients with mania may display prominent hostility and dysphoria, repetitious speech lacking in versatility or creative content, and persecutory rather than grandiose delusions (Young and Klerman 1992). Treatment follows an algorithm like that for younger patients (McElroy and Keck 2000; Sachs et al. 2000). In the geriatric patient, valproate is often the first step in therapy, followed by an atypical antipsychotic used as a mood stabilizer. In patients with psychotic symptoms, valproate is started in tandem with the atypical antipsychotic, or ECT is considered early as an option. As noted above, when antipsychotics are used for this purpose, they are tapered and discontinued after 2–6 months. Lithium is the best alternative first-line mood stabilizer. Although carbamazepine is effective, drug interactions and side effects render it less useful for elders, as discussed earlier (see "Side Effects"). Considering efficacy as well as side effects, neither lamotrigine nor gabapentin is recommended as a first-choice agent for bipolar disorder in the geriatric patient.

Response to a first-line mood stabilizer in acute geriatric mania is usually seen within the first 1–3 weeks, although there is considerable variability in response time among individuals. Co-treatment with an atypical antipsychotic is associated in many cases with faster response. The mood stabilizer is continued for a period of 1 year beyond the onset of clinical remission. In practice, most elders with primary mania require maintenance therapy with the mood stabilizer (see below) because of a history of frequent recurrence of episodes.

Bipolar Mixed State

Bipolar presentations involving simultaneous manic and depressed features are seen more frequently in elderly patients than in younger patients. For this indication, valproate is known to be more effective than lithium. It is often necessary to use adjunctive agents such as antidepressants and antipsychotics for mixed states. ECT is also effective but may require more treatments than are required for either bipolar manic or bipolar depressed episodes (Devanand et al. 2000). Gabapentin as an adjunct to lithium has also been noted to be helpful in treating mixed states.

Bipolar Disorder Prophylaxis

As noted earlier, many elderly patients with primary bipolar disorder require long-term treatment with a mood stabilizer or an atypical antipsychotic that is used as a mood stabilizer. Neuroleptics, antidepressants, and benzodiazepines used in acute stabilization are withdrawn as the index episode subsides. In our experience, it is not uncommon for geriatric patients to require combinations of mood stabilizers for adequate prophylaxis. For breakthrough episodes during prophylaxis, it is often preferable to add a second mood stabilizer or an atypical antipsychotic rather than move to a higher therapeutic dosage of the first mood stabilizer. For example, an elderly patient undergoing maintenance treatment with valproate with a serum level of 70 µg/mL who has breakthrough symptoms of irritability, agitation, and insomnia may do well with the addition of olanzapine 5 mg qhs.

Pain Syndromes

Several anticonvulsant mood stabilizers have been found to be effective in relieving neuropathic pain, presumably via suppression of neuronal firing. Severe pain affecting primarily the feet and ankles can be associated with nerve damage resulting from either type 1 or type 2 diabetes in diabetic neuropathy. This condition can be effectively treated with carbamazepine 400–800 mg/day or with gabapentin 900–3,600 mg/day (Backonja et al. 1998). With appropriate titration, these large doses of gabapentin are generally well tolerated by elderly patients, with side effects consisting mainly of somnolence and dizziness.

Postherpetic neuralgia, which is more prevalent among the elderly, is defined by pain in the area affected by herpes zoster persisting 3 months or more after crusting of the rash. After it is established, the syndrome can persist for years, and the pain can be so severe that the patient considers suicide. Gabapentin has been found to be highly effective for this condition in geriatric patients, at doses up to 3,600 mg/day (Rowbotham et al. 1998).

Personality Disorders

Patients with personality disorders associated with prominent mood instability, aggression, or impulsivity may respond to treatment with a mood stabilizer such as lithium, valproate, carbamazepine, or lamotrigine. Some experts who construe borderline personality as a bipolar variant report high success rates in treating symptoms with lamotrigine (Pinto and Akiskal 1998). Doses used for all these agents are detailed in the specific drug summaries at the end of the chapter.

Posttraumatic Stress Disorder

Mood stabilizers such as valproate or lithium may be helpful for symptoms of irritability and anger that do not respond well to first-line therapies such as antidepressants in patients with posttraumatic stress disorder.

Rapid Cycling

The first step in pharmacotherapy for rapid-cycling bipolar illness (defined by four or more major mood episodes per year) is discontinuation of antidepressant medication. Monotherapy with a mood stabilizer is indicated. In general, patients with rapid cycling respond better to valproate, and possibly to carbamazepine, than to lithium. In a patient already treated with a mood stabilizer who develops rapid cycling, either an atypical antipsychotic or a second mood stabilizer can be added. Levothyroxine may also be a useful adjunct, at a target dose of 100–200 µg/day.

Restless Legs Syndrome

As noted in the chapter on treatment of movement disorders (see Chapter 7), both restless legs syndrome and periodic limb movements of sleep may be treated with valproate, gabapentin, or carbamazepine.

Schizoaffective Disorder

Treatment of schizoaffective disorder in elderly patients increasingly focuses on the use of atypical antipsychotic agents, which appear to have particular efficacy for this indication. Mood stabilizers can be useful, however, and the general clinical impression is that anticonvulsants are superior to lithium. As with younger patients, the response tends to be more favorable and quicker in "schizomanic" elders than in "schizodepressed" elders. The treatment regimen for this population can become complicated, in that mood stabilizer combinations and other adjunctive therapies (e.g., antipsychotics, benzodiazepines, β-blockers) are needed to control symptoms.

Table 4–4. Selected causes of secondary mania

Medical conditions	Medications
Cerebrovascular disease and stroke	Anticholinergic agents
Brain neoplasms	Corticosteroids
HIV infection	Antidepressants (including St.-John's-wort)
Head trauma	Histamine$_2$ (H$_2$) receptor blockers
B$_{12}$ deficiency	Estrogen
Endocrine disorders	Levodopa
Neurosyphilis	Disulfiram
Normal-pressure hydrocephalus	Buspirone
Influenza	Folic acid
Epilepsy	Benzodiazepines (alprazolam, triazolam)
Basilar artery aneurysm	
Cryptococcosis	Amantadine
	Amphetamines, other sympathomimetic agents
	Baclofen
	Bromides

Secondary Mania

Table 4–4 lists selected causes of secondary mania. This syndrome may be more difficult to treat than primary mania when the cause is irreversible (e.g., stroke), or easier to treat when the cause is readily reversed (e.g., antidepressant medication-induced mania). It is generally believed that secondary mania is characterized by more irritable mood and less grandiosity than primary mania and that psychotic symptoms and cognitive dysfunction are more common in secondary mania (Carroll et al. 1996; Das and Khanna 1993). When mood stabilizers are required, anticonvulsants are generally superior to lithium, as noted at the opening of this section.

Unipolar Depression

Although not first-line agents for prophylaxis of true recurrent unipolar depression, lithium and other mood stabilizers (perhaps especially lamotrigine) may be effective for this purpose. Moreover, It has been noted that 10%–15% of patients of mixed age diagnosed with unipolar depression eventually have a manic episode, and mood stabilizers are also protective against mania in this subset (Price and Heninger 1994). The use of lithium to augment the antidepressant response in acute depression is discussed in Chapter 3 ("Antidepressants").

Chapter Summary

- ECT is safe and effective for the treatment of geriatric mania and results in rapid remission of symptoms, typically after four to six treatments.

- Among pharmacological treatments, valproate is currently the mood stabilizer of first choice in treating elderly patients.

- Target serum levels of mood stabilizers are generally lower for treating agitation in dementia than for treating primary mania in elderly patients.

- For the majority of elderly patients with primary bipolar disorder, long-term treatment with a mood stabilizer is indicated.

- In secondary mania, when the offending medication can be withdrawn or the medical condition can be treated, the mania often subsides.

- To minimize renal injury from lithium, avoid episodes of lithium toxicity as well as multiple daily dosing.

- Approximately 8% of geriatric patients undergoing long-term treatment with lithium will develop either symptomatic hypothyroidism or benign diffuse nontoxic goiter.

- Mood stabilizers occasionally may be associated with significant hepatotoxicity in elderly patients, as indicated by meaningful transaminase elevations or elevations in bilirubin or alkaline phosphatase levels or in prothrombin time; however, most liver function changes seen with mood stabilizer therapy are benign.

- Extrapyramidal effects of mood stabilizers are not uncommon in geriatric patients.

- The first-line treatment for bipolar I depression is a mood stabilizer.

- For nonresponse of bipolar depression or breakthrough depressive symptoms in patients with a history of rapid cycling, a second mood stabilizer is added.

- For severely depressed bipolar patients without a history of rapid cycling, an antidepressant such as bupropion or one of the SSRIs is added instead.

- When psychotic symptoms (delusions or hallucinations) accompany a bipolar depressed or bipolar manic episode, adjunctive antipsychotic medication is used.

References

Ahrens B, Berghofer A, Wolf T, et al: Suicide attempts, age and duration of illness in recurrent affective disorders. J Affect Disord 36:43–49, 1995

Altshuler LL, Post RM, Leverich GS, et al: Antidepressant-induced mania and cycle acceleration: a controversy revisited. Am J Psychiatry 152:1130–1138, 1995

Apte SN, Langston JW: Permanent neurological deficits due to lithium toxicity. Ann Neurol 13:453–455, 1983

Backonja M, Beydoun A, Edwards KR, et al: Gabapentin for the symptomatic treatment of painful neuropathy in patients with diabetes mellitus: a randomized controlled trial. JAMA 280:1831–1836, 1998

Bell AJ, Cole A, Eccleston D, et al: Lithium neurotoxicity at normal therapeutic levels. Br J Psychiatry 162:689–692, 1993

Bendz H, Aurell M, Balldin J, et al: Kidney damage in long-term lithium patients: a cross-sectional study of patients with 15 years or more on lithium. Nephrol Dial Transplant 9:1250–1254, 1994

Bowden CL, Brugger AM, Swann AC, et al: Efficacy of divalproex vs lithium and placebo in the treatment of mania. The Depakote Mania Study Group. JAMA 271:918–924, 1994

Calabrese JR, Bowden CL, Sachs GS, et al: A double-blind placebo-controlled study of lamotrigine monotherapy in outpatients with bipolar I depression. J Clin Psychiatry 60:79–88, 1999

Carroll BT, Goforth HW, Kennedy JC, et al: Mania due to general medical conditions: frequency, treatment, and cost. Int J Psychiatry Med 26:5–13, 1996

Cates M, Powers R: Concomitant rash and blood dyscrasias in geriatric psychiatry patients treated with carbamazepine. Ann Pharmacother 32:884–886, 1998

Chacko RC, Marsh BJ, Marmion J, et al: Lithium side effects in elderly bipolar outpatients. Hillside J Clin Psychiatry 9:79–88, 1987

Conte G, Vazzola A, Sacchetti E: Renal function in chronic lithium-treated patients. Acta Psychiatr Scand 79:503–504, 1989

Coppen A, Chaudhry S, Swade C: Folic acid enhances lithium prophylaxis. J Affect Disord 10:9–13, 1986

Das A, Khanna R: Organic manic syndrome: causative factors, phenomenology and immediate outcome. J Affect Disord 27:147–153, 1993

Devanand DP, Polanco P, Cruz R, et al: The efficacy of ECT in mixed affective states. J ECT 16:32–37, 2000

Donaldson IM, Cunningham J: Persisting neurologic sequelae of lithium carbonate therapy. Arch Neurol 40:747–751, 1983

Eastham JH, Jeste DV, Young RC: Assessment and treatment of bipolar disorder in the elderly. Drugs Aging 12:205–224, 1998

Elwes RDC, Binnie CD: Clinical pharmacokinetics of newer antiepileptic drugs. Clin Pharmacokinet 30:403–415, 1996

Emilien G, Maloteaux JM: Lithium neurotoxicity at low therapeutic doses: hypotheses for causes and mechanism of action following a retrospective analysis of published case reports. Acta Neurol Belg 96:281–293, 1996

Faedda GL, Tondo L, Baldessarini RJ, et al: Outcome after rapid vs gradual discontinuation of lithium treatment in bipolar disorders. Arch Gen Psychiatry 50:448–455, 1993

Gerner RH, Stanton A: Algorithm for patient management of acute manic states: lithium, valproate, or carbamazepine? J Clin Psychopharmacol 12 (1, suppl):57S–63S, 1992

Ghadirian AM, Lehmann HE: Neurological side effects of lithium: organic brain syndrome, seizures, extrapyramidal side effects, and EEG changes. Compr Psychiatry 21:327–335, 1980

Ghose K: Lithium salts: therapeutic and unwanted effects. Br J Hosp Med 18:578–583, 1977

Gitlin MJ, Cochran SD, Jamison KR: Maintenance lithium treatment: side effects and compliance. J Clin Psychiatry 50:127–131, 1989

Hardy MC, Lecrubier Y, Widlocher D: Efficacy of clonidine in 24 patients with acute mania. Am J Psychiatry 143:1450–1453, 1986

Hermann N: Valproic acid treatment of agitation in dementia. Can J Psychiatry 43:69–72, 1998

Hetmar O, Brun C, Ladefoged J, et al: Long-term effects of lithium on the kidney: functional-morphological correlations. J Psychiatr Res 23:285–297, 1989

Hetmar O, Povlsen UJ, Ladefoged J, et al: Lithium: long-term effects on the kidney. A prospective follow-up study ten years after kidney biopsy. Br J Psychiatry 158:53–58, 1991

Jacobson S, Jerrier H: EEG in delirium. Seminars in Clinical Neuropsychiatry 5:86–92, 2000

Jaeger A, Sauder P, Kopferschmitt J, et al: When should dialysis be performed in lithium poisoning? A kinetic study in 14 cases of lithium poisoning. Clin Toxicol 31:429–47, 1993

Jefferson JW: Lithium poisoning. Emerg Care Q 7:18–28, 1991

Jensen HV, Plenge P, Mellerup ET, et al: Lithium prophylaxis of manic-depressive disorder: daily lithium dosing schedule versus every second day. Acta Psychiatr Scand 92:69–74, 1995

Kasarskis EJ, Kuo C-S, Berger R, et al: Carbamazepine-induced cardiac dysfunction. Arch Intern Med 152:186–191, 1992

Kores B, Lader MH: Irreversible lithium neurotoxicity: an overview. Clin Neuropharmacol 20:283–299, 1997

Kotler M, Matar MA: Lamotrigine in the treatment of resistant bipolar disorder. Clin Neuropharmacol 21:65–67, 1998

Kusumakar V, Yatham LN: Lamotrigine treatment of rapid cycling bipolar disorder (letter). Am J Psychiatry 154:1171–1172, 1997

Lemke MR: Effect of carbamazepine on agitation in Alzheimer's inpatients refractory to neuroleptics. J Clin Psychiatry 56:354–357, 1995

Lott AD, McElroy SL, Keys MA: Valproate in the treatment of behavioral agitation in elderly patients with dementia. J Neuropsychiatry Clin Neurosci 7:314–319, 1995

Lund Y, Nissen M, Rafaelsen OJ: Long-term lithium treatment and psychological functions. Acta Psychiatr Scand 65:233–244, 1982

Martin R, Kuzniecky R, Ho S, et al: Cognitive effects of topiramate, gabapentin, and lamotrigine in healthy young adults. Neurology 52:321–327, 1999

McElroy SL, Keck PE: Pharmacologic agents for the treatment of acute bipolar mania. Biol Psychiatry 48:539–557, 2000

McElroy SL, Keck PE, Pope HG Jr, et al: Valproate in psychiatric disorders: literature review and clinical guidelines. J Clin Psychiatry 50 (3, suppl):23–29, 1989

McEvoy GK, Litvak K, Welsh OH, et al: AHFS Drug Information. Bethesda, MD, American Society of Health-System Pharmacists, 2000

Mirchandani IC, Young RC: Management of mania in the elderly: an update. Ann Clin Psychiatry 5:67–77, 1993

Nambudiri DE, Meyers BS, Young RC: Delayed recovery from lithium neurotoxicity. J Geriatr Psychiatr Neurol 4:40–43, 1991

Nelson JC: Geriatric Psychopharmacology. New York, Marcel Dekker, 1998

Oakley PW, Dawson AH, Whyte IM: Lithium: thyroid effects and altered renal handling. J Toxicol Clin Toxicol 38:333–337, 2000

Pinto OC, Akiskal HS: Lamotrigine as a promising approach to borderline personality: an open case series without concurrent DSM-IV major mood disorder. J Affect Disord 51:333–343, 1998

Plenge P, Mellerup ET, Bolwig TG, et al: Lithium treatment: does the kidney prefer one daily dose instead of two? Acta Psychiatr Scand 66:121–128, 1982

Porsteinsson AP, Tariot PN, Erb R, et al: An open trial of valproate for agitation in geriatric neuropsychiatric disorders. Am J Geriatr Psychiatry 5:344–351, 1997

Post RM, Frye MA, Denicoff KD, et al: Beyond lithium in the treatment of bipolar illness. Neuropsychopharmacology 19:206–219, 1998

Price LH, Heninger GR: Lithium in the treatment of mood disorders. N Engl J Med 331:591–598, 1994

Regan WM, Gordon SM: Gabapentin for behavioral agitation in Alzheimer's disease. J Clin Psychopharmacol 17:59–60, 1997

Rowbotham M, Harden N, Stacey B, et al: Gabapentin for the treatment of postherpetic neuralgia: a randomized controlled trial. JAMA 280:1837–1842, 1998

Sachs GS, Printz DJ, Kahn DA, et al: The Expert Consensus Guideline Series: Medication Treatment of Bipolar Disorder 2000. Postgrad Med April (Special No 1):1–104, 2000

Salzman C: Clinical Geriatric Psychopharmacology, 3rd Edition. Baltimore, MD, Williams & Wilkins, 1998

Schaffer CB, Garvey MJ: Use of lithium in acutely manic elderly patients. Clin Gerontol 3:58–60, 1984

Schou M: Long-lasting neurological sequelae after lithium intoxication. Acta Psychiatr Scand 70:594–602, 1984

Steckler TL: Lithium- and carbamazepine-associated sinus node dysfunction: nine-year experience in a psychiatric hospital. J Clin Psychopharmacol 14:336–339, 1994

Suppes T, Baldessarini RJ, Faedda GL, et al: Risk of recurrence following discontinuation of lithium treatment in bipolar disorder. Arch Gen Psychiatry 48:1082–1088, 1991

Tariot PN, Erb R, Podgorski CA, et al: Efficacy and tolerability of carbamazepine for agitation and aggression in dementia. Am J Psychiatry 155:54–61, 1998

Tekin S, Aykut-Bingol C, Tanridag T, et al: Antiglutamatergic therapy in Alzheimer's disease—effects of lamotrigine. J Neural Transm 105: 295–303, 1998

Thase ME, Sachs GS: Bipolar depression: pharmacotherapy and related therapeutic strategies. Biol Psychiatry 48:558–572, 2000

Tohen M, Castillo J, Baldessarini RJ, et al: Blood dyscrasias with carbamazepine and valproate: a pharmacoepidemiological study of 2,228 patients at risk. Am J Psychiatry 152:413–418, 1995

Trehan R, Clark CF: Valproic acid-induced truncal weakness and respiratory failure (letter). Am J Psychiatry 150:1271, 1993

Vanelle JM, Loo H, Galinowski A, et al: Maintenance ECT in intractable manic-depressive disorders. Convuls Ther 10:195–205, 1994

Young RC, Klerman GL: Mania in late-life: focus on age at onset. Am J Psychiatry 149:867–876, 1992

Zarate CA Jr, Tohen M, Baraibar G: Combined valproate or carbamazepine and electroconvulsive therapy. Ann Clin Psychiatry 9:19–25, 1997

Generic name	carbamazepine
Trade name	Tegretol, Tegretol-XR, and others
Class	Anticonvulsant (structurally related to TCAs)
Half-life	Initial: 18–55 hours; multiple dosing: 12–17 hours
Mechanism of action	Decreased synaptic transmission
Available formulations	Tablet: 200 mg Chewable tablet: 100 mg Suspension: 100 mg/5 mL XR tablets: 100, 200, 300, 400 mg
Starting dose	100–200 mg bid
Titration	Increase by 100–200 mg at 2- to 3-week intervals, as tolerated
Typical daily dose	Aggression in dementia: 300 mg (divided doses) Bipolar disorder: 800 mg (divided doses)
Dosage range	200–1,200 mg daily (divided doses)
Therapeutic serum level	Aggression in dementia: 2.4–5.2 µg/mL Bipolar disorder: 4–8 µg/mL

Comments: Not a drug of choice for mood stabilization in the elderly because of adverse effects and drug interactions. Nonlinear kinetics. Absorption slow; peaks unpredictably at 4–8 hours. Highly protein bound. Metabolized to active epoxide metabolite. Non–extended-release preparation must be given at least bid because of autoinduction. *Drug interactions:* Significant inducer of major CYP enzymes, associated with variably decreased concentrations of psychotropic, cardiac, and other drugs (see Table 4–3 and Table 1–1 in Chapter 1). Carbamazepine itself is metabolized mainly via CYP3A4 and induces its own metabolism via this enzyme, with decreased blood levels after 2–4 weeks. *Adverse effects* (include): hematological changes (e.g., leukopenia, thrombocytopenia), cardiovascular effects (including arrhythmias), abnormal liver function, increased urinary frequency, anticholinergic effects (including urinary retention, constipation, and blurred vision), renal failure, sedation, dizziness, vertigo, ataxia, diplopia, nystagmus, visual hallucinations, abnormal movements, nausea, vomiting, diarrhea, rash, and SIADH.

Generic name	clonazepam
Trade name	Klonopin
Class	Benzodiazepine
Half-life	19–50 hours
Mechanism of action	Potentiates effects of GABA by binding to GABA$_A$–benzodiazepine receptor complex
Available formulations	Tablets: 0.5, 1, 2 mg (scored 0.5-mg tablet available from Watson Laboratories, Inc.)
Starting dose	0.5–1 mg qd or bid
Titration	Increase by 0.5–1 mg, as tolerated
Typical daily dose	1 mg
Dosage range	0.5–8 mg daily
Therapeutic serum level	Not established

Comments: Useful as an adjunct in the initial treatment of mania. Long half-life must be taken into account in deciding dosing schedule. Rapidly and well absorbed orally. Onset of action in 20–60 minutes; duration 12 hours. 85% protein bound. Metabolized by nitro-reduction to an inactive metabolite. Clearance may be decreased in elders.
Common adverse effects: Sedation, ataxia, and hypotonia. In elders with mental retardation or brain injury, behavioral disturbances (aggressiveness, irritability, agitation, hyperkinesis) can occur.

Generic name	gabapentin
Trade name	Neurontin
Class	Anticonvulsant structurally related to GABA
Half-life	5–7 hours
Mechanism of action	No direct GABA-mimetic action; increases GABA levels by inhibiting the GABA transporter
Available formulations	Capsules: 100, 300, 400 mg Tablets (coated): 600, 800 mg Oral solution: 250 mg/5 mL
Starting dose	100 mg every 12 hours
Titration	Increase by 100 mg every 3 to 5 days, as tolerated
Typical daily dose	300 mg tid Dementia: 100 mg tid
Dosage range	300–1,800 mg daily in divided doses (higher for pain treatment)
Therapeutic serum level	Obtainable, but not used clinically

Comments: Anecdotal experience suggests efficacy of gabapentin for insomnia, anxiety, mood instability, certain pain syndromes, tremor, and some parkinsonian symptoms in elderly patients; controlled studies not performed to date. May have reduced bioavailability at higher dosages. Not protein bound; not appreciably metabolized (no CYP interactions); no pharmacokinetic interactions with other anticonvulsants. Renally excreted; clearance declines with age. Gabapentin dosage adjustment for renal failure (for treatment of seizures; not established for other indications) as follows: 30–60 mL/minute—dose is 300 mg bid; 15–30 mL/minute—dose is 300 mg qd; <15 mL/minute—dose is 300 mg qod; for hemodialysis patients, loading dose is 300–400 mg, and further doses are 200–300 mg following each 4 hours of dialysis. For all patients, short half-life necessitates tid dosing for indications such as anxiety and mood instability. May be administered at bedtime for insomnia. Generally well tolerated, with side effects that are mild to moderate in severity and self-limiting. *Most common adverse effects* are neuropsychiatric: somnolence, dizziness, ataxia, fatigue, and nystagmus. *Other adverse effects* (include): nausea/vomiting, dry mouth, constipation, peripheral edema, rhinitis, pharyngitis, visual changes, and myalgia. Induction of bipolar rapid cycling has been reported with this agent.

Generic name	lamotrigine
Trade name	Lamictal
Class	Anticonvulsant
Half-life	31 hours
Mechanism of action	Inhibits release of excitatory neurotransmitters by blocking presynaptic sodium channels
Available formulations	Tablets: 25, 100, 150, 200 mg Chewable tablets: 5, 25 mg Oral suspension can be compounded; see Table 4–2
Starting dose	12.5 mg qd
Titration	Increase by 12.5–25 mg every 2 weeks, as tolerated
Typical daily dose	50 mg bid
Dosage range	100–300 mg daily
Therapeutic serum level	Not used clinically

Comments: No randomized, controlled trials in elderly patients. Limited by need for slow titration of dose. Large therapeutic index. Rapidly and completely absorbed when taken orally; not affected by food. Peak concentration in plasma in 1.4–4.8 hours. 98% bioavailability. 55% protein bound. Major metabolite inactive. Linear kinetics. Kinetics affected by aging; drug exposure increased 55%, and clearance reduced 37% in elders. Some evidence of autoinduction, with half-life decreased by 25%. Predominantly renally excreted; half-life increased in renal insufficiency. Clearance 25% lower in non-Caucasians. Does not activate CYP enzymes, but lamotrigine levels are affected by carbamazepine and valproate. Adverse effects: rash develops in 3% of patients and may progress to Stevens-Johnson syndrome or toxic epidermal necrolysis; rash is nonspecific in appearance; current recommendation is to discontinue medication at the first appearance of any rash. *Other side effects* (include): headache, dizziness, ataxia, tremor, diplopia, drowsiness, and mild gastrointestinal upset (nausea, vomiting). When discontinuing this medication, taper over 2 weeks, except in the case of rash.

Generic name	lithium
Trade name	Cibalith-S, Eskalith, Lithane, Lithobid, Lithonate, Lithotabs
Class	Salt
Half-life	≥36 hrs in elderly or renally impaired
Mechanism of action	Unknown (affects GABAergic as well as cholinergic, serotonergic, adrenergic and dopaminergic neurotransmission; modulates phosphoinositol system)
Available formulations	Tablets: 300 mg (scored) Capsules: 150, 300, 600 mg Sustained release: 300, 450 mg Syrup: 300 mg/5 mL
Starting dose	75–150 mg qd
Titration	Increase by 75–150 mg every 4–7 days, as tolerated
Typical daily dose	300–900 mg
Dosage range	150–1,800 mg daily
Therapeutic serum level	Acute mania: 0.4–0.8 mEq/L Maintenance: 0.2–0.6 mEq/L

Comments: A drug of choice for mood stabilization in elderly patients despite its adverse side-effect profile. Initial dosing is divided (bid or tid) to minimize dose-related side effects (nausea, tremor); a switch is made to single nightly dosing as soon as tolerated to reduce long-term effects on the kidney. Absorption is complete, rapid, and not affected by aging. Peak plasma concentration in 1–2 hours after an oral dose. Peak brain concentration up to 24 hours later, so neurotoxic effects can be delayed. One of the only hydrophilic psychotropics. It is distributed to body water, which is proportionately decreased in elderly patients, particularly women, resulting in a decreased volume of distribution. Not metabolized, and no CYP interactions. Decreased glomerular filtration rate with aging has important effects on lithium clearance and half-life. Reduced clearance is exacerbated by renal disease, episodes of lithium toxicity, dehydration, changes in salt intake, extra-renal salt loss, and use of diuretic drugs. Blood level of lithium may not be equal to brain level. Lithium alters distribution and kinetics of sodium, potassium, calcium, and magnesium. *Drug interactions:* ACE inhibitors, phenothiazines, calcium channel blockers, carbamazepine, diuretics, iodides, MAOIs, metronidazole, neuromuscular blockers, narcotics, NSAIDs, and SSRIs. *Adverse effects:* renal dysfunction, diabetes insipidus, polydipsia, nausea, diarrhea, tremor, weakness, fatigue, weight gain, leukocytosis, hypothyroidism, muscle twitching, extrapyramidal symptoms, confusion, "dazed" feeling.

Generic name	oxcarbazepine
Trade name	Trileptal
Class	Anticonvulsant (carbamazepine derivative)
Half-life	2.5 hours (parent drug) 11 hours (10-hydroxy metabolite)
Mechanism of action	Decreased synaptic neurotransmission
Available formulation	Tablets: 150, 300, 600 mg
Starting dose	150 mg bid
Titration	Increase by 300 mg at 7-day intervals, at minimum, as tolerated
Typical daily dose	600 mg (divided doses)
Dosage range	300–1,200 mg daily (divided doses) (higher for pain treatment)
Therapeutic serum level	Not established

Comments: No data from controlled studies in bipolar disorder affecting elderly patients. Reportedly well tolerated by elders as an anticonvulsant. The parent drug (prodrug) is rapidly converted to the active 10-hydroxy metabolite. Rapidly absorbed; not affected by food. Extensively metabolized in liver; mono-hydroxy metabolite is active. Dose-dependent enzyme induction, with effects similar to those of carbamazepine. Maximum plasma concentrations 30%–60% higher in geriatric patients, mostly due to decreased creatinine clearance. *Drug interactions:* may inhibit CYP2C19 and/or induce CYP3A enzymes (see Chapter 1–1 in Chapter 1). *Adverse effects:* significant hyponatremia, headache, ataxia, dizziness, nausea, vomiting, constipation, diarrhea, anorexia, memory impairment, concentration difficulties, weight gain, and allergic skin reactions (including Stevens-Johnson syndrome and toxic epidermal neurolysis). With discontinuation, diplopia and abnormal vision may occur.

Generic name	topiramate
Trade name	Topamax
Class	Anticonvulsant
Half-life	21 hours
Mechanism of action	Blocks sodium channels, enhances GABAergic activity, and blocks glutamatergic activity
Available formulations	Tablets: 25, 100, 200 mg Capsules: 15, 25, 50 mg
Starting dose	25 mg qhs
Titration	Increase by 25 mg at 7-day intervals, as tolerated
Typical daily dose	50 mg bid
Dosage range	50–200 mg daily (divided bid)
Therapeutic serum level	Not established

Comments: Unstudied as a mood stabilizer for treating elderly patients. Unlike other mood stabilizers, associated with anorexia and weight loss. Well absorbed. Peak concentrations in 2–4 hours; food alters rate of absorption. Minimally metabolized in the liver. *Adverse effects:* leukopenia, thrombocytopenia, headache, alopecia, palpitations, cognitive dysfunction, psychotic symptoms, depression, paresthesias, sedation, dizziness, nystagmus, ataxia, tremor, speech disorders, psychomotor slowing, fatigue, weight loss, nausea, diarrhea, vomiting, flatulence, dyspnea, ocular effects, and urolithiasis. Dual action on GABAergic and glutamatergic systems confers both activating and sedating effects.

Generic name	valproate
Trade name	Depakote, Depakene
Class	Anticonvulsant (carboxylic acid derivative)
Half-life	8–17 hours in adults
Mechanism of action	Inhibits enzymes involved in GABA breakdown
Available formulations	Capsules: 250 mg Capsules with sprinkles: 125 mg Sustained release: 125, 250, 500 mg Extended release: 500 mg Syrup: 250 mg/5 mL Injectable: 100 mg/mL
Starting dose	125 mg qd–250 mg bid
Titration	Increase by 125–250 mg every 3–5 days, as tolerated
Typical daily dose	500–1,000 mg (divided doses)
Dosage range	250–1,500 mg daily (divided doses)
Therapeutic serum level	50–100 µg/mL 13–52 µg/mL (agitation in dementia)

Comments: A drug of first choice for mood stabilization in elderly patients. In plasma, all formulations (including enteric-coated, syrup, and sprinkles) exist as valproate. Rapidly absorbed after oral administration except for Depakote, which takes 2–4 hours. Absorption delayed by food. High bioavailability. Peak concentration in 1–4 hours; 3–5 hours with Depakote. Rapid distribution; reaches CNS within minutes. Many metabolites, some of which are active. Does have CYP interactions, but these are not as significant as those of carbamazepine. Clearance not affected by aging. *Drug interactions:* carbamazepine, CNS depressants, erythromycin, MAOIs, phenytoin, warfarin, zidovudine; substrate for CYP2D6 (see Table 1–1 in Chapter 1), although mainly metabolized outside cytochrome system. *Adverse effects:* Mostly gastrointestinal, including dyspepsia, diarrhea, nausea, vomiting, and anorexia. These effects are transient and can be minimized by giving the medication with food, using the enteric-coated formulation Depakote, and starting at a low dose and titrating slowly. Sedation is commonly seen on initiation of therapy, with tolerance developing to this effect over 1–2 weeks. One under-appreciated but potentially serious side effect of valproate is skeletal muscle (especially truncal) weakness. In our experience, this weakness can be significant in some cases and can interfere with the ability to transfer, stand, and walk without assistance. Valproate also associated with pancreatitis, fecal incontinence, weight gain, sedation, ataxia, tremor, elevated ammonia level, thrombocytopenia, rash, and SIADH. Hepatotoxicity rare, idiosyncratic, and unrelated to dose.

5

Anxiolytic and Sedative-Hypnotic Medications

Primary anxiety disorders are less prevalent in elderly cohorts than in younger cohorts. When encountered, they usually represent conditions that began earlier in life and persisted into old age. Secondary anxiety disorders, in contrast, are more prevalent among the elderly because conditions associated with these disorders (e.g., angina, emphysema) and the use of anxiogenic medications are more common in this population. In addition, other clinical indications for anxiolytic and sedative-hypnotic medications—including insomnia, periodic limb movements of sleep, agitation or aggression in the context of dementia, and sedation for brief diagnostic or surgical procedures—occur frequently among elders.

In this chapter, we focus on benzodiazepines but also include prescribing information for the nonbenzodiazepine hypnotics zolpidem and zaleplon, as well as for other agents useful as anxiolytics or sedative-hypnotics, such as buspirone, trazodone, gabapentin, mirtazapine, β-blockers, propofol, melatonin, and the herbal preparations kava and valerian. A number of drugs formerly used for treatment of anxiety or insomnia—including diphenhydramine, chloral hydrate, and barbiturates—are currently *not* recommended for geriatric patients, for reasons noted in this chapter.

Of all anxiolytic and sedative drugs, none is so controversial in geriatrics as the class of benzodiazepines. These medications are effective, are among the safest drugs marketed in terms of therapeutic index, and are associated with few significant drug interactions. There are, however, several ways that benzodiazepines can be misused in geriatric prescribing: the amount prescribed or taken can be too much or too little, the specific drug selected can be inappropriate, the duration of treatment can be too long, patient selection can be inappropriate, diagnosis can be wrong, or target symptoms can be so ill-defined that the endpoint of treatment is unclear (Burch 1990).

Excessive doses of benzodiazepines can be associated with serious adverse effects, including falls, motor vehicle accidents, and cognitive impairment. Inadequate doses can be associated with persistent anxiety symptoms or between-dose withdrawal. Benzodiazepines with long elimination half-lives such as diazepam accumulate in fatty tissues with repeated dosing and can lead to toxic effects, as noted later in this chapter. Treatment can continue beyond the time period indicated, as sometimes occurs after an acute hospitalization, or can be continued despite lack of efficacy.

Patient selection for benzodiazepine therapy must take into account any history of alcoholism or other substance abuse. Non–substance abusers typically adopt a pattern of benzodiazepine use that is *not* consistent with abuse. This pattern of medical use involves physician supervision of the treatment of a recognized clinical condition, with the goal of restoring normal function. For most of these patients, tolerance to anxiolytic effects does not develop over time, so escalation of dose does not occur. In contrast, substance abusers are likely to adopt a nonmedical or recreational use pattern that involves unsupervised use, a desire to "get high" rather than to achieve normal function, tolerance to mood-altering effects, and consequent escalation of dose (Farnsworth 1990).

Pharmacokinetics

The pharmacology of individual nonbenzodiazepine anxiolytic and sedative-hypnotic drugs is covered in the specific drug summaries at the end of this chapter. The pharmacology of benzodiazepines is covered here.

Although aging itself is associated with altered pharmacokinetics of benzodiazepines, these processes can be further altered by smoking, hospital diets, disease, and co-administration of other drugs (Greenblatt et al. 1991a, 1991b; Thompson et al. 1983). Benzodiazepines are well absorbed, with absorption enhanced by alcohol and delayed by antacids or food. When a faster effect is desired (as with initial insomnia), oral medication should be taken on an empty stomach, and a drug with a rapid onset of action (e.g., temazepam) should be chosen. With intramuscular use, lorazepam and midazolam are rapidly and completely absorbed, whereas chlordiazepoxide is not, and the rate of absorption of diazepam depends on the site of injection.

All benzodiazepines are lipophilic, and, with the exception of alprazolam, the volume of distribution for benzodiazepines increases with age. The most lipophilic drugs (e.g., diazepam) have a short duration of effect with single dosing because of rapid redistribution to adipose tissue (Greenblatt 1991). Less lipophilic drugs (e.g., lorazepam) have a longer duration of effect with single dosing (Greenblatt and Shader 1978; Greenblatt et al. 1977).

On the basis of metabolic pathway, benzodiazepines can be divided into two groups:

- *Oxidatively metabolized benzodiazepines.* This group includes alprazolam, chlordiazepoxide, clorazepate, diazepam, flurazepam, halazepam, quazepam, and prazepam. These drugs usually have active metabolites. In general, drugs in this group are *not* recommended for use in elderly patients.
- *Conjugated benzodiazepines* (those that undergo glucuronidation). This group includes lorazepam, oxazepam, and temazepam. These drugs have no active metabolites. These are drugs of choice in treating elderly patients for whom benzodiazepines are indicated.

Clearance of oxidatively metabolized benzodiazepines is reduced in old age, particularly in men (Greenblatt et al. 1991a, 1991b). Reduced clearance is associated with increased half-life, which, in turn, may be associated with significant daytime sedation and psychomotor impairment (Greenblatt 1991). Clearance of conjugated benzodiazepines is unaffected by age (Greenblatt et al. 1991a, 1991b). In general, conjugated benzodiazepines have shorter half-lives. Table 5–1 shows the half-lives of benzodiazepines and other anxiolytic and sedative-hypnotic drugs.

Pharmacodynamics and Mechanism of Action

Benzodiazepines act as classic agonists at the γ-aminobutyric acid$_A$ (GABA$_A$)–benzodiazepine receptor complex (Greenblatt 1992), located predominantly on postsynaptic neurons in the cerebral cortex, cerebellar cortex, and limbic regions (Bone et al. 1995). These drugs share sedative, anxiolytic, anticonvulsant, and muscle relaxant effects. The intensity of these effects depends on the degree of receptor occupancy, which is proportional to the concentration of the drug at the receptor site (Greenblatt 1992). For unknown reasons, elderly individuals appear to demonstrate a greater pharmacodynamic sensitivity to benzodiazepines at a given concentration at this site compared with younger patients (Greenblatt et al. 1991a, 1991b). In addition, any central nervous system (CNS) disorder, including Parkinson's disease,

Table 5–1. Pharmacokinetics of anxiolytic and sedative-hypnotic medications

Medication	Half-life (hours)	Active metabolites	Effects of age
Benzodiazepines			
alprazolam	12–20	—	+ (in men)
chlordiazepoxide	6.6–25	+ desmethyldiazepam	+
clonazepam	19–50	—	+
diazepam	90	+ desmethyldiazepam	+
estazolam	10–24	—	—
flurazepam	40–114	+ N-desalkylflurazepam	+
lorazepam	10–20	—	—
midazolam	1–10	+ 1-hydroxymethylmidazolam	+
oxazepam	5–20	—	—
quazepam	53	+ desalkylflurazepam	+
temazepam	10–20	—	—
triazolam	1.7–5	—	+

Table 5–1.   Pharmacokinetics of anxiolytic and sedative-hypnotic medications (*continued*)

Medication	Half-life (hours)	Active metabolites	Effects of age
Nonbenzodiazepines			
buspirone	2–11	+ 1-pyrimidinylpiperazine	—
chloral hydrate	8–11	+ trichloroethanol	+
gabapentin	5–7	—	+
kava	?	?	?
melatonin	0.5–1	—	+
mirtazapine	20–40	N-desmethylmirtazapine	+
propofol	Biphasic	—	+
propranolol	4–6	+ 4-hydroxypropranolol	+
trazodone	4–8; 12[a]	+ 1-m-chlorophenylpiperazine	+
valerian	?	?	?
zaleplon	1–2	—	+
zolpidem	3	—	+

Note.   + = present; — = none or negligible; ? = unknown. [a]Biphasic.

dementia, or stroke, can be associated with similarly increased sensitivity.

Neurotransmitter systems other than the GABAergic system are also involved in anxiolysis and sedation. Antidepressants useful as anxiolytic and sedative-hypnotic agents predominantly affect the serotonergic system.

Drug Interactions

Drug interactions involving benzodiazepines are mediated primarily by the cytochrome P450 (CYP) 3A4 enzyme system, for which certain benzodiazepines (alprazolam, clonazepam, diazepam, midazolam, and triazolam) are substrates. In the presence of CYP3A4 inhibitors such as antifungal agents, antibiotics, nefazodone, fluvoxamine, ritonavir, or grapefruit juice, levels of these drugs can be elevated. These elevations can be clinically important; for example, nefazodone is associated with a 34% increase in alprazolam level and a 500% increase in triazolam level (Rickels et al. 1998). In the presence of CYP3A4 inducers such as St.-John's-wort, carbamazepine, chronic alcohol consumption, and smoking, levels of these drugs can be reduced. Note that benzodiazepines recommended for elders (lorazepam, oxazepam, and temazepam) are not listed as CYP3A4 substrates. Diazepam undergoes metabolism via the CYP2C19 and CYP3A4 enzymes and is subject to drug interactions with inhibitors of these enzymes.

In addition to CYP450 interactions, benzodiazepines have additive sedative effects with other CNS depressants, including alcohol, opiates, and trazodone. See Table 5–2 for other anxiolytic and sedative drug interactions.

Indications

Benzodiazepines are used clinically for a variety of indications beyond the treatment of anxiety and insomnia, as shown in Table 5–3. Treatment approaches for selected problems are outlined later in this chapter.

Table 5–2. Anxiolytic and sedative-hypnotic drug interactions

Anxiolytic/sedative	Interacting drug	Potential interaction
All anxiolytics and sedatives	Other CNS depressants	Increased CNS depression
All benzodiazepines	Antacids	Delayed effect (slowed absorption)
	Anticholinergic medications	Increased cognitive impairment
	Clozapine	Sedation, hypotension, respiratory depression
	L-Dopa	Decreased effect of L-dopa
	Sympathomimetics (e.g., ephedrine, theophylline)	Antagonism of benzodiazepine effects
Buspirone	MAOIs	Hypertension
All benzodiazepines metabolized oxidatively by CYP3A4: alprazolam clonazepam diazepam midazolam triazolam Zolpidem	Ketoconazole and related antifungal agents Nefazodone Fluvoxamine Fluoxetine Erythromycin Clarithromycin Cimetidine Disulfiram Amiodarone Isoniazid Grapefruit juice Ritonavir	Increased benzodiazepine or zolpidem level (inhibition of CYP3A4 enzyme)

Table 5–2.   Anxiolytic and sedative-hypnotic drug interactions *(continued)*

Anxiolytic/sedative	Interacting drug	Potential interaction
All benzodiazepines metabolized oxidatively by CYP3A4: alprazolam clonazepam diazepam midazolam triazolam Zolpidem	Carbamazepine Rifampin Phenytoin Dexamethasone St.-John's-wort Chronic alcohol consumption (in absence of cirrhosis) Ritonavir	Decreased benzodiazepine or zolpidem level (induction of CYP3A4 enzyme)
Trazodone	Warfarin	Decreased anticoagulant effect

Note.   CNS = central nervous system; CYP = cytochrome P450; MAOI = monoamine oxidase inhibitor.

Efficacy

All benzodiazepines are effective for the short-term treatment of insomnia (Greenblatt 1991); continued long-term efficacy has not been systematically studied. All benzodiazepines are probably equally effective for the treatment of anxiety, although for anxiety occurring in the context of panic disorder, alprazolam and clonazepam are generally preferred. Buspirone is effective in the treatment of generalized anxiety disorder (GAD) and anxiety in dementia but not in panic disorder. Clinical failures with buspirone may relate to its long latency to effect, to inadequate dosage, or to lack of specificity in diagnosis. In addition, it has frequently been noted that patients already exposed to benzodiazepines may respond poorly to buspirone, although this is not true in all cases, particularly when the history of benzodiazepine use is remote (DeMartinis et al. 2000). Zolpidem and zaleplon are effective in the treatment of insomnia among elderly patients.

Table 5–3. Indications for anxiolytic and sedative-hypnotic medications

Anxiety (generalized, panic)

Insomnia

Alcohol and sedative withdrawal

Adjunctive use with mood-stabilizing medication for mania

Adjuntive use with antipsychotic medication for acute psychosis

Sedation for brief procedures (e.g., bronchoscopy, cardioversion, ECT, intubation, colonoscopy)

Ongoing sedation (e.g., patient on mechanical ventilation)

Anesthesia induction

Nausea/vomiting secondary to cytotoxic therapy (lorazepam)

Adjunctive use with antidepressant for phantom limb pain (clonazepam)

Seizures

Myoclonus

Akathisia

Periodic limb movements of sleep

Restless legs syndrome

REM sleep behavior disorder

Tinnitus (alprazolam)

Note. Some listed indications are off-label uses. ECT = electroconvulsive therapy; REM = rapid eye movement.

Clinical Use

Nonpharmacological Therapies

For anxiety, cognitive-behavioral therapy (CBT) is a well-established mode of treatment with proven efficacy. It may be used in conjunction with certain medications such as antidepressants, but there is some indication that cotreatment with benzodiazepines reduces its efficacy (van Balkom et al. 1996). Anxiety in the hospitalized patient can be reduced substantially through various environmental and psychological interventions, including increased physical activity, facilitated visits through more flexible visiting hours, familiarization of the setting with personal effects, skillful ventilator weaning, patient education about what to expect from procedures, frequent reassurance, maintenance of consistent staffing, distraction, and relaxation techniques (Bone et al. 1995).

For the treatment of initial insomnia (i.e., difficulty falling asleep), morning bright light therapy has been recommended (Lewy and Sack 1986) and, in our experience, is useful in some cases. For the treatment of middle insomnia or early morning awakening, evening bright light therapy can be useful. Side effects of bright light therapy are few and include headache, induction of mania, and skin rash. It is as yet an unsettled question as to whether bright light exposure increases the risk of retinopathy or maculopathy. Until more information is available, it is recommended that ophthalmological examination predate therapy. The duration of light therapy for the treatment of insomnia is not established.

For the long-term treatment of primary insomnia, effective interventions include restriction of time spent in bed, avoidance of daytime naps, maintenance of regular sleep and meal schedules, aerobic exercise early in the day, hot baths, relaxation exercises, bladder training, and a light snack at bedtime (Morin et al. 1994; Reynolds et al. 1998). Caffeine, nicotine, alcohol, and medications affecting sleep should be avoided, as should heavy meals, television, exercise, and other stimulating activities before bed (Reynolds et al. 1998).

Choice of Drug

When benzodiazepines are used in the treatment of elderly patients, small doses of short- or intermediate-acting drugs are preferred. For oral use, drugs of choice are lorazepam, oxazepam, and temazepam. If longer-half-life drugs such as clonazepam are prescribed ($t_{1/2}$ = 19–50 hours), frequency of use should be once

daily or every other day. For parenteral use, drugs of choice are lorazepam and midazolam. In general, oral or intravenous administration is preferred to intramuscular administration because the
latter is painful and, in some cases, associated with erratic absorption. Other routes of administration include rectal and sublingual. Other anxiolytic and sedative-hypnotic agents of choice
in the treatment of elderly patients with specific syndromes are
discussed later in this chapter.

For short-term pharmacological treatment of insomnia in the
geriatric patient, the nonbenzodiazepine hypnotics zolpidem
and zaleplon are often used in preference to benzodiazepines.
Both of these drugs effectively decrease sleep latency but have
little effect on sleep stages. Zaleplon is faster acting and less potent and has a shorter duration of effect than zolpidem. Accordingly, although zaleplon is not useful in treating early morning
awakening and, in general, does not increase total sleep time, it
does carry a lower risk of hangover effects, even when used in
the middle of the night ("Hypnotic Drugs" *The Medical Letter*
2000).

Since benzodiazepines are known to depress respiration, it
is generally believed that sleep apnea, chronic obstructive pulmonary disease (COPD), and congestive heart failure are contraindications to their use. However, with the possible exception
of sleep apnea, experimental data do not support this view
(Biberdorf et al. 1993; Camacho and Morin 1995; Guilleminault
et al. 1984). In general, benzodiazepines can be used safely in
patients with COPD, if used cautiously.

Antipsychotic medication is used for patients with anxiety or
insomnia coupled with positive psychotic symptoms (delusions
or hallucinations). Antipsychotics are *not* drugs of first choice in
the treatment of anxiety or insomnia in nonpsychotic elderly
patients.

Drugs formerly used but currently *not* recommended for
treatment of anxiety or insomnia in elders include antihistamines
such as diphenhydramine (Benadryl), chloral hydrate (Noctec),
barbiturates, meprobamate (Miltown), ethchlorvynol (Placidyl),

glutethimide (Doriden), and methyprylon (Noludar). Over-the-counter antihistamines such as diphenhydramine (e.g., Benadryl, Nytol) and doxylamine (e.g., Unisom) are FDA approved as hypnotics and are used by an estimated 11% of elders (Mellinger et al. 1985). Antihistamines may help with initiation of sleep but work poorly to maintain sleep. In addition, they are associated with the development of tolerance within days to weeks (Monane 1992). Side effects include anticholinergic effects (constipation, urinary retention, visual blurring, memory impairment, delirium), daytime sedation, and impairment of driving performance.

Chloral hydrate also has a low therapeutic index, with fatalities reported after 4-g doses ("Hypnotic Drugs" *The Medical Letter* 2000). This drug is associated with gastric irritation and interacts with the metabolism of warfarin. In addition, tolerance may develop to its hypnotic effects within 2 weeks, and physical dependence may occur with continued use. Withdrawal is associated with nightmares and significant insomnia. At present, chloral hydrate is used only for patients who do not respond to recommended drugs for insomnia, and for premedication prior to a sleep electroencephalogram (at doses of 125–500 mg).

Barbiturates and related sedatives are associated with serious side effects; significant drug interactions because of their role as CYP enzyme inducers; high physical dependence and abuse liability; low therapeutic index; high lethality in overdose; and seizures, nightmares, and insomnia on withdrawal (Thompson et al. 1983).

Patient Education

Before a benzodiazepine is prescribed for an elderly patient, informed consent should be provided detailing risks and benefits, the plan for frequency and duration of use, and the potential discontinuation symptoms. In particular, elderly patients who are motorists should understand that driving may be hazardous, with the hazard, in some cases, continuing as long as the day after taking a benzodiazepine for sleep.

Baseline Laboratory and Diagnostic Studies

For any patient presenting for the first time with GAD, panic disorder, or anxiety that is severe and disabling, a diagnostic workup for secondary causes of anxiety (e.g., hyperthyroidism, COPD, use of sympathomimetic agents) should be undertaken. In addition, the patient's existing medications should be reviewed. Table 5–4 lists medical conditions and medications that can cause anxiety or insomnia.

Table 5–4.   Causes of secondary anxiety or insomnia

Medical conditions	Medications and drugs
Depression	Sympathomimetics (including theophylline)
Dementia	
Substance abuse	Steroids (adrenal and gonadal)
Pain	Thyroid hormone
Hyperthyroidism	Anticholinergic agents
Hypothyroidism, hypoparathyroidism	L-Dopa
	Antidepressants
Chronic obstructive pulmonary disease (hypoxia)	Neuroleptics (akathisia)
	Antiarrhythmic agents (e.g., quinidine)
Asthma	Antibiotics (dyspepsia)
Angina	Phenytoin
Benign prostatic hypertrophy	Methyldopa
Parkinson's disease	Methysergide
Congestive heart failure	Caffeine
Left ventricular failure	Nicotine
Cardiac arrhythmia	Nicotine withdrawal
Hemolytic anemia	Alcohol withdrawal
Hypoglycemia	Diuretics (restless legs)
Hypovolemia	
Pneumothorax	
Pulmonary embolism	
Pneumonia	
Neoplasm	

For several reasons, it is important to determine whether the patient has a past or current history of alcohol or other substance abuse. As noted earlier, the problem of abuse of prescribed benzodiazepines with dose escalation over time is largely limited to populations with a substance abuse history. In addition, current use of alcohol can have sedative effects that are additive to those of prescribed benzodiazepines, and this may represent a danger for vulnerable elderly patients. A decision as to whether symptoms should be treated pharmacologically depends on a weighing of risk relative to benefit. Nonpharmacological options do exist, as outlined earlier in this section (see "Nonpharmacological Therapies").

Dose and Dose Titration

As with prescription of other psychotropic medications in treating elderly patients, the rule for benzodiazepines and other sedatives is to start at the lowest end of the therapeutic dose range and to increase the dose slowly, usually every few days (Shader and Greenblatt 1993). With oral benzodiazepines, anxiolytic, muscle relaxant, and anticonvulsant effects may be observed after the first dose; effects may then increase until steady state is attained. Most elderly patients respond to low doses of these medications. Since some require full doses for therapeutic effect, however, it is important to continue titrating until target symptoms are under control while monitoring for side effects.

When antidepressants are used to treat primary anxiety disorders in elderly patients, extremely low starting doses and very slow titration are often necessary to minimize anxiogenic side effects, as discussed earlier in the chapter on antidepressants (see Chapter 3). This is especially true with selective serotonin reuptake inhibitor (SSRI) antidepressants. Although antidepressants have not been systematically studied for anxiety disorders in elders, clinical experience suggests that their efficacy is comparable to that seen in younger patients.

Duration of Treatment

For most elderly patients, prescription of anxiolytic and sedative-hypnotic medications is time limited. In the treatment of anxiety disorders, benzodiazepines are used for 4 months or less, and then gradual taper and discontinuation are attempted (Shader and Greenblatt 1993). If the patient is unable to remain medication free after 4–6 weeks of not taking medication, benzodiazepine therapy may be resumed and the process repeated again after several months. In this way, a subset of elderly patients with chronic anxiety requiring chronic maintenance benzodiazepine treatment will be identified (Shader and Greenblatt 1993), and benzodiazepine therapy will be discontinued for all others.

In the treatment of insomnia, a benzodiazepine or one of the two related drugs zolpidem and zaleplon is used for 1–2 weeks, and then the need is reassessed. If insomnia persists for 2 weeks, a comorbid psychiatric or medical condition should be reconsidered, as noted below. Some patients do benefit from an extension to 4 weeks of treatment, but it is best if the medication is taken only intermittently, fewer than four times per week. When medication is to be discontinued, it should be tapered slowly to minimize withdrawal symptoms, and the patient should be informed about the nature of expected withdrawal symptoms. As with anxiety, some cases of insomnia are chronic, and the patients do respond to long-term therapy. Periodic review and attempts to taper medication will identify this subgroup of patients.

Monitoring Treatment

Response to anxiolytic and sedative-hypnotic drugs is monitored clinically, by changes in target signs and symptoms and development of adverse effects. The only drug for which meaningful serum levels might be drawn is alprazolam. In the treatment of panic disorder, alprazolam levels between 20 and 40 ng/mL are associated with therapeutic response in nongeriatric patients with spontaneous panic attacks (Greenblatt et al. 1993a). Therapeutic levels for geriatric patients have not been established.

Elderly patients who require chronic treatment with benzo-diazepines or related drugs should be evaluated at least every 6 months to assess cognitive and psychomotor function. Escalation of benzodiazepine dosage over time or concomitant excessive alcohol consumption should be understood as serious evidence of misuse. Anecdotal experience suggests that many patients treated with benzodiazepines chronically develop symptoms of toxicity as they reach old age. For this reason, it is important to reassess the need for treatment at regular intervals and to adjust the dose downward as indicated.

Management of Nonresponse

Nonresponse to anxiolytic and sedative-hypnotic drugs could be attributable to an incorrect diagnosis, the presence of a confounding medical or psychiatric disorder (e.g., substance abuse or depression), inadequate dose or duration, or inadequate concentration of active drug because of poor absorption or abnormal rate of metabolism. In using a benzodiazepine for brief sedation, initial nonresponse is best treated with larger doses of the original drug rather than by switching drugs; switching usually confers no advantage, since all benzodiazepines are equally effective for most patients. If the desired level of sedation is still not attained, a switch to another class of sedative is indicated (Bone et al. 1995).

Switching Drugs

When a switch from alprazolam to clonazepam is made, the following strategy has been found useful in nongeriatric patients: since clonazepam is approximately twice as potent as alprazolam, the patient takes half the usual daily alprazolam dose (mg) as clonazepam, divided bid, for 1 week. During the first week, alprazolam is taken as needed up to the usual dose. After the first week, if alprazolam is still required, the dose of clonazepam is increased instead (Pollack et al. 1987). To switch from a benzodiazepine to buspirone, the latter is added and titrated up to the target dose, the two medications are co-administered for 2–4 weeks, and then the benzodiazepine is tapered.

Overdose

In general, fatal overdose with oral benzodiazepines taken alone is rare unless the medication is ingested with alcohol or another CNS depressant (Martin and Chan 1986). Among benzodiazepines, oxazepam may be one of the safest in overdose, and temazepam is the least safe, as gauged by death rates per million prescriptions (Buckley et al. 1995). Symptoms of serious benzodiazepine toxicity include extreme sedation, falls, immobility, restlessness, incontinence, confusion, delirium, and coma (Buckley et al. 1995; Fancourt and Castleden 1986). A benzodiazepine antagonist such as flumazenil (Romazicon) can be used to reverse toxicity through competitive inhibition (Bone et al. 1995). Since sleep induction requires 60% benzodiazepine receptor occupancy, sedation and anticonvulsant effects require 30%–50% occupancy, and anxiolysis requires only 20% occupancy, flumazenil can usually reverse extreme sedation without affecting anxiolysis or anticonvulsant effects (Bone et al. 1995).

Tolerance and Abuse

Tolerance involves a change in receptor sensitivity with continued drug exposure (Miller et al. 1988), manifesting clinically as reduced effect from a constant drug dose. Tolerance may be seen with all benzodiazepines, as well as zaleplon and zolpidem. There is no good evidence that tolerance develops to anxiolytic or hypnotic effects of benzodiazepines, even with chronic use (Dubovsky 1990; Farnsworth 1990; Hollister et al. 1993; van Steveninck et al. 1997). Tolerance has been shown to develop to most adverse effects, including sedation, but not to amnestic effects (Hollister et al. 1993). How long it takes for tolerance to develop depends on the half-life of the particular benzodiazepine, as well as the specific effect in question (Byrnes et al. 1993).

Abuse denotes nontherapeutic use of a medication, involving

deliberate overuse despite contrary warnings. There is no evidence that medical use of benzodiazepines is a precursor of abuse in patients not already predisposed by a history of alcohol or substance abuse (or perhaps family history of alcohol abuse) (Ciraulo et al. 1997; Shader and Greenblatt 1993). This is true as well for chronic use of these medications (Geiselmann and Linden 1991). For patients with such a history, however, use of benzodiazepines is fraught with problems such as rekindling of craving, co-ingestion of alcohol with the prescribed medication, and increased risk of motor vehicle accidents (Graham et al. 1992). Similar problems could be anticipated with the benzodiazepine-like drugs zaleplon and zolpidem (Gericke and Ludolph 1994). Benzodiazepines with a fast onset of action—alprazolam, diazepam, and lorazepam—are believed, on the basis of anecdotal evidence, to have higher abuse potential (and greater street value) because of the rapid "kick" associated with ingestion (Griffiths and Wolf 1990).

Dependence, Discontinuation, and Withdrawal Syndromes

Physical dependence is defined by the appearance of an objective withdrawal syndrome after a drug is discontinued. The risk of dependence increases with dose and duration of therapy (Kruse 1990; Shader and Greenblatt 1993), but it is clear that dependence on benzodiazepines can occur at usual therapeutic doses (Shader and Greenblatt 1993) and after as few as 2 weeks of treatment (Ayd 1994). There is no evidence from controlled studies that some benzodiazepines are more likely than others to produce dependence.

Discontinuation of benzodiazepines can result in recurrence of symptoms, in rebound symptoms (in which symptoms are more intense than they were to begin with), or in withdrawal symptoms (in which physical effects of reduced GABA neurotransmission are seen). At times, these phenomena are difficult to distinguish. In general, however, interruption of therapeutic doses of benzodiazepines is associated with rebound, whereas interruption of high doses is associated with withdrawal (Pourmotabbed et al. 1996). Rebound symptoms include anxiety, restlessness, dysphoria, anorexia, nausea, vomiting, and insomnia (Jerkovich and Preskorn 1987); in elderly patients, disorientation and confusion can be prominent (Foy et al. 1986; Kruse 1990). Withdrawal symptoms include fever, tachycardia, postural hypotension, headache, sweating, photosensitivity, sensory distortion, delirium, tremor, myoclonus, and seizures (Fancourt and Castleden 1986); catatonia has also been reported in elderly patients (Rosebush and Mazurek 1996). In medically compromised elders, severe withdrawal could be life threatening.

How early withdrawal or other discontinuation symptoms develop depends on the half-life of the discontinued drug. In nongeriatric patients, withdrawal reactions peak at 2 days for short-half-life (<6 hrs) agents and 4–7 days for long-half-life agents (Rickels et al. 1990).

Symptoms of withdrawal are best avoided by slow taper of benzodiazepines, especially shorter-acting agents. Most patients tolerate a taper of 10%–25% of the total dose each week, although the last few dose decrements might require longer intervals (Schweizer et al. 1990; Shader and Greenblatt 1993). Patients unable to tolerate dose reductions may benefit from one of the following: carbamazepine 200–800 mg daily, with a plasma level of approximately 6 µg/mL (Schweizer et al. 1991); gabapentin 300–900 mg daily; controlled-release melatonin 2 mg qhs for withdrawal insomnia (Garfinkel et al. 1999); propranolol for autonomic symptoms; or a switch to a longer-acting agent, such as clonazepam, and subsequent taper of that agent.

Rebound insomnia usually lasting one to two nights occurs after discontinuation of benzodiazepines of short (<6 hours) or intermediate (6–24 hours) half-life (Roth and Roehrs 1992). This syndrome is dose related and can be prevented by the use of the lowest effective dose of benzodiazepine (Roth and Roehrs 1992). It probably also occurs with long-half-life benzodiazepines but, in that case, is less intense and more delayed in onset.

Side Effects

Adverse effects of anxiolytic and sedative-hypnotic drugs are extensions of therapeutic effects and in nongeriatric patients are usually mild and without serious sequelae (Mendelson et al. 1996). The most common side effects of benzodiazepines include drowsiness, fatigue, weakness, and incoordination. However, the severity of these effects is dependent on dose, and the clinical impact is greater for frail elderly individuals than for younger patients. As the dose increases, the risk of extreme sedation and weakness, confusion, depression, and ataxia increases. Among elderly patients treated with benzodiazepines, there is a significantly increased risk of falls, particularly with long-acting agents and in the first week after therapy is initiated (Ray et al. 2000), as well as motor vehicle accidents involving personal injury (Hemmelgarn et al. 1997).

Cognitive Effects

Amnesia may be regarded as a main (intended) effect of sedative-hypnotic therapy (as in sedation for patients in the intensive care unit [ICU] requiring ventilation or for patients undergoing brief medical procedures), or as an undesired side effect. Amnestic effects of benzodiazepines include impairment of information acquisition, impairment of consolidation and storage of memory, or both (Greenblatt 1992). The magnitude of these effects depends on drug dose, plasma concentration, and the time of information presentation relative to the time of dosing (Greenblatt 1992). Elders appear to be more sensitive to amnestic effects, even with single-dose administration (Pomara et al. 1989; Satzger et al. 1990). Amnestic effects may be more marked in heavy drinkers (Ashton 1995). Explicit (conscious) memory is thought to be affected by sedatives, whereas implicit memory is spared.

Chronic therapy with benzodiazepines may also be associated with deficits in sustained attention and visuospatial impairment that are insidious and not recognized by the patient (Ashton 1995; Ayd 1994). The benzodiazepine-treated elder with amnesia along with these other cognitive impairments will meet diagnostic criteria for dementia, which will turn out to be reversible on taper and discontinuation of the benzodiazepine.

In one controlled study, buspirone 20 mg was found to have no effect on memory (Lawlor et al. 1992). In another study, in younger subjects, neither propranolol nor atenolol was found to have cognitive effects on single-dose administration (Greenblatt et al. 1993b). Whether this latter finding holds true for elders on chronic therapy remains to be demonstrated.

Hemodynamic Effects

Benzodiazepines can be associated with hypotension and slowing of the heart rate, particularly when combined with other medications such as opiates (Bone et al. 1995). This effect is reportedly less pronounced than that seen with barbiturates. In combination with clozapine, benzodiazepines can be associated with cardiorespiratory collapse. Specific guidelines regarding co-administration of these medications appear in the chapter on antipsychotic medications (see Chapter 2).

Motor Effects

Motor side effects of benzodiazepines and other sedatives include weakness, postural sway, ataxia, dysarthria, and incoordination (Swift et al. 1984). Preexisting motor deficits can be unmasked or exacerbated by even minimal sedation (Thal et al. 1996). In addition, benzodiazepines, among many other drugs, impair motor recovery after stroke (Goldstein 1995) and are associated with an increased risk of falls. Among elderly benzodiazepine users, the risk of falls is highest in the first 7 days after initiation of the drug. Excessive dose, rapid rate of dose increase, and longer-half-life (>24 hours) agents are all associated with greater fall risk (Ray et al. 2000).

Psychiatric Effects

Benzodiazepines and other sedative-hypnotics have few psychiatric side effects. By way of their sedative effects, and possibly through other neurotransmitter effects, they are associated with exacerbation of depression in some patients.

In elderly patients with dementia, brain injury, or mental retardation who are administered benzodiazepines, behavioral disturbances (aggressiveness, irritability, agitation, hyperkinesis) can occur. These disturbances, sometimes referred to as "paradoxical reactions," may be more severe during the initiation of therapy and abate with continuation of therapy. Stimulants (methylphenidate or amphetamine) have been suggested as a possible treatment (McEvoy et al. 2000). The mechanism underlying this phenomenon remains unexplained, since there is no evidence from controlled study that benzodiazepines directly impair impulse control or lead to aggression in individuals without structural brain disease (Shader and Greenblatt 1993).

Similarly, there is no evidence that benzodiazepines specifically cause psychosis or depersonalization (Shader and Greenblatt 1993), symptoms once described in patients treated with certain hypnotics. In fact, these symptoms are as likely to be found among individuals with insomnia before treatment and in those who are untreated (Balter and Uhlenhuth 1992). Anecdotally, zolpidem at usual therapeutic doses has been associated with psychotic-like phenomena in several case reports.

Psychomotor Impairment

All benzodiazepines have the capacity to produce impairment in performance (Greenblatt 1992), including impairment of abilities critical to safe driving such as reaction time, tracking, hand-eye coordination, and judgment. With short-acting agents used at very low doses, impairment may be minimal in the "young-old" patient. With long-half-life agents used nightly, effects may persist throughout the following day, resulting ultimately in daytime impairment (Fancourt and Castleden 1986; Woo et al. 1991). Agents with a half-life of more than 24 hours confer a 45% increased risk of motor vehicle accident with injury in the first 7 days of use (Hemmelgarn et al. 1997). As with cognitive effects described earlier, neither propranolol nor atenolol was found to have psychomotor effects on single-dose administration in younger subjects (Greenblatt et al. 1993b), but, again, whether this holds true for elders undergoing chronic therapy remains to be demonstrated.

Respiratory Effects

As discussed earlier (see "Choice of Drug"), there is evidence that patients with COPD, as well as those with congestive heart failure, can safely be prescribed low doses of oral benzodiazepines. Even patients with mild sleep apnea have safely taken these agents, with close monitoring. Since anything more than mild apnea may represent a risk for exacerbation of breathing difficulties with any benzodiazepine treatment, these agents are better avoided altogether for patients with apnea. Respiratory depression is more likely to occur with high doses of benzodiazepine administered intravenously. Reportedly, midazolam causes more respiratory depression than diazepam, and lorazepam causes the least (Bone et al. 1995). When respiratory depression does occur, it is rapid in onset, usually of brief duration, and is exacerbated by co-administration of narcotics (Bone et al. 1995).

Sedation

All benzodiazepines have the capacity to produce dose- and concentration-dependent sedation that can manifest as tiredness, drowsiness, weakness, trouble concentrating, decreased visual accommodation, slowed thought, ataxia, balance problems (Shader and Greenblatt 1993), dysarthria, diplopia, vertigo, and confusion (Ashton 1995). Tolerance to these effects usually develops within the first 2 weeks of treatment (Ayd 1994; Shader and Greenblatt 1993).

Sleep Interference

Benzodiazepines are associated with decreased REM sleep (Bone et al. 1995) and decreased Stage 3 and Stage 4 (deep) sleep (Fan-

court and Castleden 1986). With prolonged use of benzodiazepines over several years, sleep architecture and quality can be
significantly affected. The clinical significance of these changes
is not established. Sleep effects of other anxiolytic and sedative-
hypnotic agents are described in the specific drug summaries at
the end of this chapter.

Treatment of Selected Syndromes and Disorders With Anxiolytics and Sedative-Hypnotics

Anxiety Disorders

Anxiety in Dementia

Symptoms of anxiety can further incapacitate patients with dementia. For some, treatment of the dementia itself with disease-
specific agents such as cholinergic drugs can be associated with
a reduction in anxiety. For treatment of acute anxiety, lorazepam or
oxazepam is recommended. For long-term treatment, buspirone
can be useful at dosages ranging from 5 mg bid to 20 mg tid. Alternatively, SSRI antidepressants can be useful, initiated at a low
dose (e.g., sertraline 12.5–25 mg or fluoxetine 2–10 mg suspension or capsule) and titrated to effects. For all these agents, a trial
of at least 12 weeks is needed to determine efficacy. When no
response is seen, a switch to another agent is indicated. An
emerging treatment for dementia-related anxiety is gabapentin
100–300 mg tid; this appears promising, but inadequate data are
available at this writing to recommend its use.

Anxiety in Depression

Anxiety may be a prominent feature of a major depressive episode. Treatment with antidepressant medication is often associated with resolution of anxiety along with other symptoms.
When an antidepressant is initiated for patients with depression
and comorbid panic attacks, very slow titration may be necessary. For a subset of depressed patients with intolerable anxiety,

a benzodiazepine is useful temporarily, at the start of therapy. Use of an anxiolytic alone for treatment of depression with anxiety is associated with a poor outcome. Novel antidepressant drugs—mirtazapine, venlafaxine, and nefazodone—appear to have particularly good anxiolytic efficacy. Caution should be exercised when nefazodone is coprescribed with benzodiazepines for the geriatric patient, however, since increased benzodiazepine levels can result, as noted earlier (see "Drug Interactions").

Anxiety in the Medically Ill Patient (Secondary Anxiety)

Significant anxiety in the ICU patient is an underappreciated and often mismanaged problem. It occurs in an estimated 70%–87% of ICU patients (Bone et al. 1995) and is a particular problem for patients on devices such as ventilators and intra-aortic balloon pumps. Nonpharmacological measures used to minimize anxiety in this patient population are discussed in an earlier section (see "Nonpharmacological Therapies"). Optimal pharmacological care for these patients includes standing doses of parenteral benzodiazepine sufficient to sedate, keep calm, and induce amnesia, along with analgesic and antipsychotic medications as indicated. For this purpose, intravenous lorazepam administered by bolus or continuous infusion, or intravenous midazolam administered by continuous infusion, can be used.

In the ventilator-dependent ICU patient, an alternative to benzodiazepines is propofol, which has been found in several controlled studies to be superior in facilitating patient-ventilator synchrony and faster weaning, as well as reducing time to wakefulness (Chamorro et al. 1996). Compared with midazolam, however, propofol is associated with greater hemodynamic impairment (Chamorro et al. 1996). In addition, propofol's association with prolonged periods of apnea may restrict its use to the ICU population. A combination of propofol and midazolam may be superior to monotherapy with either agent (Carrasco et al. 1998).

Many elderly patients with chronic medical illnesses associated with pain, insomnia, or anxiety benefit substantially from long-term treatment with benzodiazepines. These patients are not seen to escalate benzodiazepine use and experience few adverse effects. Others benefit preferentially from long-term treatment with antidepressants.

Generalized Anxiety Disorder

Several treatment options exist for GAD. For benzodiazepine-naive patients, buspirone 5 mg po bid to 20 mg po tid may be effective, although results may not be seen for 6 weeks or longer in elderly patients. Benzodiazepines are effective for generalized anxiety in the majority of patients. Among nonalcoholic patients with GAD who chronically use benzodiazepines, the use of such an agent is not seen to escalate with time, and anxiolytic efficacy persists (Dubovsky 1990; Farnsworth 1990). A typical benzodiazepine regimen for an elderly patient with GAD is lorazepam 0.5–1 mg po bid or tid or clonazepam 0.5–1 mg po qd. When tremor, tachycardia, or palpitations are prominent, β-blockers such as propranolol or atenolol can also be useful.

Increasingly, novel antidepressants such as venlafaxine and mirtazapine are used to control generalized anxiety in the absence of depression, and these agents appear to retain therapeutic efficacy over extended use.

Generalized anxiety can occur as a secondary syndrome (Table 5–4). When generalized anxiety is found in association with depression, it is best treated with an antidepressant. When it is secondary to a medical condition such as hyperthyroidism, treatment is directed first at the underlying cause.

Obsessive-Compulsive Disorder

Ideally, treatment of obsessive-compulsive disorder (OCD) consists of CBT in conjunction with pharmacotherapy and is usually lifelong. The medication of choice is an SSRI. Appropriate SSRI dosing for OCD in elderly patients has yet to be established, although clinical experience suggests that fluoxetine or paroxetine at total daily doses as high as 60 mg may be required for optimal effect. For nonelderly patients with OCD refractory to monotherapy, augmentation strategies include the addition of a second SSRI, buspirone, clonazepam, or carbamazepine. These combinations have not been systematically studied in elderly patients. Patients with OCD with concurrent tics or Tourette's disorder are treated with an adjunctive antipsychotic medication other than clozapine, which has been associated with worsening of OCD symptoms. Neither benzodiazepines nor buspirone has been found to be effective as monotherapy for OCD.

Panic Disorder

Ideally, treatment for panic disorder involves CBT in conjunction with antidepressant medication such as an SSRI. CBT may not be feasible for many geriatric patients, including those with cognitive impairment or low motivation.

High-potency benzodiazepines are effective for panic, but a large overlap of panic and alcohol dependence complicates this use. For selected patients, benzodiazepines used on either a standing or an as-needed basis may be the best choice of therapy. As of this writing, only alprazolam among the benzodiazepines is FDA labeled for treatment of panic, although lorazepam and clonazepam are also useful for this purpose. In one controlled study, clonazepam 1–2 mg daily was found to show the best balance of efficacy and tolerability in a partly geriatric sample of panic patients with and without agoraphobia (Rosenbaum et al. 1997). Standing alprazolam is effective in treatment of panic in nongeriatric patients at plasma levels of 20–40 ng/mL (Greenblatt et al. 1993). Alprazolam at doses of 0.25–1 mg may also be effectively used on an as-needed basis for patients with intermittent or provoked symptoms of panic. Most patients who discontinue benzodiazepines have recurrence of panic symptoms, and adjunctive CBT is known to help prolong remission in nongeriatric cohorts.

Posttraumatic Stress Disorder

The mainstay of pharmacological treatment for posttraumatic stress disorder (PTSD) is a serotonergic antidepressant. Appropriate SSRI dosing for PTSD in elderly patients has yet to be established, although clinical experience suggests that fluoxetine at total daily doses as high as 60 mg or sertraline at total daily doses as high as 150 mg may be required for optimal effect. Trazodone can be helpful for certain patients, but sedation often limits adequate dosing. The novel agents nefazodone, mirtazapine, and venlafaxine may be useful but have been understudied among geriatric patients for this indication. The required duration of treatment with any of these agents is not established. Benzodiazepines have little role in PTSD treatment and may be problematic for PTSD patients with comorbid substance abuse. For PTSD-associated nightmares, the adrenergic antagonist prazosin titrated to a daily dose of 5 mg was found to be helpful in one case series (Raskind et al. 2000); clonidine and cyproheptadine have also been reported to be useful. Psychotherapy remains an integral part of treatment for PTSD.

Social Phobia

For treatment of social phobia in elders, buspirone 15 mg tid or clonazepam 0.5 mg qd is effective for some patients. Other treatments include CBT and pharmacotherapy with SSRI antidepressants or monoamine oxidase inhibitors. Appropriate doses of these medications in elderly patients have not been established for this indication.

Sleep Disorders

Insomnia

In the geriatric patient, persistent insomnia associated with impairment in daytime performance warrants diagnostic testing and treatment. Before an extensive medical workup is undertaken, the patient is asked to keep a 1- to 2-week diary indicating time in bed (including naps), quality of sleep, time of exercise, and time of ingestion of meals, alcohol, caffeine, and nicotine. This diary can help identify appropriate environmental interventions. Other nonpharmacological therapies for insomnia, such as sleep restriction and bright light therapy, are discussed in an earlier section.

If these steps are not sufficient to remedy the problem, a medical workup is likely to identify some confounding factor. Overnight sleep laboratory (polysomnography [PSG]) study is indicated only if sleep apnea, abnormal limb movements, or other abnormal events in sleep are suspected, or if the patient fails to respond to the medical interventions listed below.

The first step in pharmacotherapy is to discontinue currently ineffective treatments. Over-the-counter hypnotics such as diphenhydramine are particularly likely to contribute to insomnia when used long term. As noted earlier, these agents have little value in maintaining sleep overnight and are associated with delirium and other anticholinergic side effects. Prescription hypnotics should also be tapered and discontinued. If insomnia persists for 4–6 weeks after the prescription hypnotic has been stopped and sleep hygiene measures have been implemented, another hypnotic should be considered.

For transient or short-term insomnia in elderly patients, pharmacological agents of choice include the following (with suggested doses indicated): zolpidem 5 mg qhs, gabapentin 300 mg qhs, mirtazapine 7.5 mg qhs, controlled-release melatonin 2 mg qhs, trazodone 25 mg qhs, zaleplon 10 mg qhs, nortriptyline 10 mg qhs, estazolam 1 mg qhs, or temazepam 15 mg qhs. In individual cases, doses may need to be adjusted upward or downward, depending on the main effect and side effects such as next-day sedation.

The same agents may be used for treatment of chronic insomnia, although the use of benzodiazepines for this purpose is more controversial. Some clinicians recommend their use only intermittently (three to four times per week) in patients who are closely followed and for whom a nonpharmacological plan is also in place (Monane 1992). Many patients report continued long-term effectiveness of benzodiazepines for insomnia, although this is not always verified by polysomnographic study.

Periodic Limb Movements of Sleep and Restless Legs Syndrome

Periodic limb movements of sleep (PLMS) involve complex involuntary limb movements occurring at regular intervals and associated with arousal from sleep. Restless legs syndrome (RLS) relates to a subjective sensation that legs "need to move" that occurs during wakefulness. Both syndromes are more prevalent in old age, and there is a large overlap of the two syndromes seen clinically. In addition, systemic conditions associated with neuropathy, such as anemia, vitamin B_{12} deficiency, and diabetes, may be linked to these abnormal movements. Use of medications such as SSRIs and TCAs or withdrawal from sedative-hypnotics or narcotics may also be associated with PLMS and RLS.

Many clinicians initiate treatment with vitamin and mineral supplements (folate, B_{12}, vitamin C, vitamin E, iron, and magnesium) when one of these conditions is diagnosed. Both conditions may be treated with clonazepam 0.5–1 mg po at bedtime. Duration of treatment has not been studied systematically, but tolerance to the arousal-suppressing effect over time has been noted (Nofzinger and Reynolds 1996). These disorders can be comorbid with sleep apnea, a condition for which sedatives may be contraindicated. Several case reports suggest that using a benzodiazepine in treating such patients is not associated with exacerbation of apnea (Morfis et al. 1997; Nofzinger and Reynolds 1996). For patients with PLMS or RLS treated with a TCA or an SSRI antidepressant, a switch to mirtazapine or nefazodone may be helpful. Movements can also be suppressed and sleep can be facilitated with ropinirole 0.5 mg qhs (Saletu et al. 2000) or levodopa/carbidopa (Sinemet), which is started at 25/100 mg and titrated to effect (Nofzinger and Reynolds 1996). When short-acting Sinemet is associated with worsening of leg movements during the day, the medication is given more than once daily and/or in sustained-release form (Brown 1997).

REM Sleep Behavior Disorder

Under normal circumstances, skeletal muscle atonia dampens movement during REM sleep. In individuals with REM sleep behavior disorder, atonia is incomplete, and dreams may be "acted out" physically. This disorder can be primary or can be associated with dementia, olivopontocerebellar degeneration, Guillain-Barré syndrome, or subarachnoid hemorrhage (Brown 1997). Elderly patients with loss of REM atonia are at risk for nighttime falls. In elders, the treatment for REM sleep behavior disorder is clonazepam 0.5–1 mg po qhs. In addition, the patient's sleep environment should be made safer by padding of the bed and removal of sharp objects (Brown 1997). Mirtazapine may prove to be an effective treatment for this condition as well, since it is known to reduce the amount of REM sleep.

Other Disorders

Agitation and Aggression in Dementia

As discussed in the chapter on the treatment of dementia (see Chapter 8), benzodiazepines have a relatively small role in the treatment of agitation and aggression in patients with dementia. Selected benzodiazepines are appropriately used for patients with prominent anxiety (e.g., lorazepam 0.5 mg po bid). For patients with insomnia, zolpidem is preferred.

Alcohol Withdrawal

Benzodiazepines have a specific and central role in the treatment of alcohol withdrawal, as discussed in the chapter on treatment of substance-related disorders (see Chapter 6).

Catatonia

Catatonia is optimally treated with lorazepam 1–2 mg im or iv, followed by a maintenance dose of lorazepam 1 mg po bid. Response is seen even in patients already treated with benzodiazepines. Patients who have been chronically catatonic may require a longer course or a higher dose of lorazepam. ECT is also highly effective and may be the treatment of choice for prolonged, debilitating catatonic states.

ECT-Induced Agitation

Usually appearing within minutes of an ECT-induced seizure, this syndrome is characterized by agitation, disorientation, and poor response to verbal command (Devanand and Sackeim 1992). It has traditionally been treated with intravenous diazepam. One study suggests that it can be prevented by administering an increased dose of methohexital prior to ECT (Devanand and Sackeim 1992).

Sedation for Brief Procedures

Cognitively impaired elderly patients may require conscious sedation for brief procedures such as gastrointestinal and radiological tests or interventions. For this purpose, propofol is increasingly used because of its rapid onset and rapid elimination (Carrasco et al. 1998), but this use has been challenged because of safety concerns (Marinella 1997; Van Der Auwera et al. 1990). Lorazepam and midazolam also are widely used. Midazolam has a faster onset than lorazepam, but the two have similar times to arousal. Lorazepam 1–2 mg given intravenously 15–20 minutes before a procedure has been found to be safe and effective, even for elders (Deppe et al. 1994). Midazolam 1 mg administered intravenously over 2 minutes can be given at the start of a procedure, with additional 1-mg increments given as needed up to 3.5 mg total; or a 2.5- to 10-mg dose can be given subcutaneously (Burke et al. 1991). Reversal of sedation can be accomplished with flumazenil.

Terminal Restlessness

Extreme restlessness may occur in the patient nearing death, usually in the context of delirium and often associated with multifocal myoclonus (Burke et al. 1991). Selected benzodiazepines used in conjunction with opiates for pain control may be useful in quieting the patient and in reducing myoclonus. For this purpose, diazepam may be given rectally as a suppository or by slow push into a rectal catheter (10 mg given over 5–10 minutes); this is repeated after 6–12 hours as needed (Burke et al. 1991).

An alternative in patients with fecal impaction, diarrhea, or other contraindication to rectal administration is midazolam. This can be given intravenously (1 mg over 2 minutes, waiting 2 or more minutes to observe effect, and giving additional 1-mg doses over 2 minutes as needed; >3.5 mg total dose rarely needed) or subcutaneously (2.5- to 10-mg bolus, repeated after 2 hours; or by continuous subcutaneous infusion with a syringe driver, with usual doses ranging from 20 to 60 mg daily) (Burke et al. 1991). Subcutaneous midazolam confers the advantage of more continuous effect than intravenous dosing and can be used in nonhospital settings.

Chapter Summary

- Patient selection for benzodiazepine therapy must take into account past or current history of alcoholism or other substance abuse.

- Less lipophilic drugs (e.g., lorazepam) have a longer duration of effect with single dosing because of limited tissue distribution.

- Compared with younger patients, elderly patients show a greater pharmacodynamic sensitivity to benzodiazepines at a given concentration at the postsynaptic receptor site.

- Benzodiazepines metabolized by conjugation—lorazepam, oxazepam, and temazepam—are preferred for use in elders.

- Benzodiazepines are effective for the short-term treatment of insomnia and anxiety.

- Drugs formerly used but currently *not* recommended for treatment of anxiety or insomnia in elders include antipsychotics, antihistamines, chloral hydrate, and barbiturates.

- In the treatment of anxiety disorders, benzodiazepines are optimally used for 4 months or less; then gradual taper and discontinuation are attempted.

- A subset of elderly patients with chronic anxiety require chronic maintenance benzodiazepine treatment.

- In the treatment of insomnia, benzodiazepines and related drugs are optimally used for 1–2 weeks, and then the need for such agents is reassessed.

- A subset of elderly patients with chronic insomnia require chronic pharmacological therapy.

- For many elderly patients treated with benzodiazepines chronically, the dose needs to be adjusted downward with advancing age.

- Symptoms of serious benzodiazepine toxicity include extreme sedation, falls, immobility, restlessness, incontinence, confusion, delirium, and coma.

- There is no good evidence that tolerance regularly develops to anxiolytic or hypnotic effects of benzodiazepines, even with chronic use.

- The risk of dependence increases with dose and duration of therapy.

- Interruption of therapeutic doses of benzodiazepines is associated with rebound, whereas interruption of high doses is associated with withdrawal; in severe cases, withdrawal can be medically serious in the frail elderly patient.

- Most patients tolerate a taper of 10%–25% of the total benzodiazepine dose each week, although the last few dose decrements might require longer intervals.

- Among elderly patients treated with benzodiazepines, there is a significantly increased risk of falls as well as motor vehicle accidents involving personal injury, particularly with long-acting agents and in the first week after therapy is initiated.

- Benzodiazepine use should be avoided as far as possible in patients with apnea syndromes.

References

Ashton H: Toxicity and adverse consequences of benzodiazepine use. Psychiatric Annals 25:158–165, 1995

Ayd FJ: Prescribing anxiolytics and hypnotics for the elderly. Psychiatric Annals 24:91–97, 1994

Balter MB, Uhlenhuth EH: New epidemiologic findings about insomnia and its treatment. J Clin Psychiatry 53 (12, suppl):34–39, 1992

Biberdorf DJ, Steens R, Millar TW, et al: Benzodiazepines in congestive heart failure: effects of temazepam on arousability and Cheyne-Stokes respiration. Sleep 16:529–538, 1993

Bone RC, Hayden WR, Levine RL, et al: Recognition, assessment, and treatment of anxiety in the critical care patient. Dis Mon 41:293–359, 1995

Brown LK: Sleep and sleep disorders in the elderly. Nurs Home Med 5: 346–353, 1997

Buckley NA, Dawson AH, Whyte IM, et al: Relative toxicity of benzodiazepines in overdose. BMJ 310:219–221, 1995

Burch EA Jr: Use and misuse of benzodiazepines in the elderly. Psychiatr Med 8:97–105, 1990

Burke AL, Diamond PL, Hulbert J, et al: Terminal restlessness—its management and the role of midazolam. Med J Aust 155:485–487, 1991

Byrnes JJ, Miller LG, Greenblatt DJ, et al: Chronic benzodiazepine administration, XII: anticonvulsant cross-tolerance but distinct neurochemical effects of alprazolam and lorazepam. Psychopharmacology (Berl) 111:91–95, 1993

Camacho ME, Morin CM: The effect of temazepam on respiration in elderly insomniacs with mild sleep apnea. Sleep 18:644–645, 1995

Carrasco G, Cabre L, Sobrepere G, et al: Synergistic sedation with propofol and midazolam in intensive care patients after coronary artery bypass grafting. Crit Care Med 26:844–851, 1998

Chamorro C, de Latorre FJ, Montero A, et al: Comparative study of propofol versus midazolam in the sedation of critically ill patients: results of a prospective, randomized, multicenter trial. Crit Care Med 24:932–939, 1996

Ciraulo DA, Barnhill JG, Ciraulo AM, et al: Alterations in pharmacodynamics of anxiolytics in abstinent alcoholic men: subjective responses, abuse liability, and electroencephalographic effects of alprazolam, diazepam, and buspirone. J Clin Pharmacol 37:64–73, 1997

DeMartinis N, Rynn M, Rickels K, et al: Prior benzodiazepine use and buspirone response in the treatment of generalized anxiety disorder. J Clin Psychiatry 61:91–94, 2000

Deppe SA, Sipperly ME, Sargent AI, et al: Intravenous lorazepam as an amnestic and anxiolytic agent in the intensive care unit: a prospective study. Crit Care Med 22:1248–1252, 1994

Devanand DP, Sackeim HA: Use of increased anesthetic dose prior to electroconvulsive therapy to prevent postictal excitement. Gen Hosp Psychiatry 14:345–349, 1992

Dubovsky SL: Generalized anxiety disorder: new concepts and psycho-pharmacologic therapies. J Clin Psychiatry 51 (1, suppl):3–10, 1990

Fancourt G, Castleden M: The use of benzodiazepines with particular reference to the elderly. Br J Hosp Med 35:321–326, 1986

Farnsworth MG: Benzodiazepine abuse and dependence: misconceptions and facts. J Fam Pract 31:393–400, 1990

Foy A, Drinkwater V, March S, et al: Confusion after admission to hospital in elderly patients using benzodiazepines. BMJ 293:1072, 1986

Garfinkel D, Zisapel N, Wainstein J, et al: Facilitation of benzodiazepine discontinuation by melatonin: a new clinical approach. Arch Intern Med 159:2456–2460, 1999

Geiselmann B, Linden M: Prescription and intake patterns in long-term and ultra-long-term benzodiazepine treatment in primary care practice. Pharmacopsychiatry 24:55–61, 1991

Gericke CA, Ludolph AC: Chronic abuse of zolpidem (letter). JAMA 272:1721–1722, 1994

Goldstein LB: Common drugs may influence motor recovery after stroke. The Sygen in Acute Stroke Study Investigators. Neurology 45:865–871, 1995

Graham AV, Parran TV, Jaen CR: Physician failure to record alcohol use history when prescribing benzodiazepines. J Subst Abuse 4:179–185, 1992

Greenblatt DJ: Benzodiazepine hypnotics: sorting the pharmacokinetic facts. J Clin Psychiatry 52 (9, suppl):4–10, 1991

Greenblatt DJ: Pharmacology of benzodiazepine hypnotics. J Clin Psychiatry 53 (6, suppl):7–13, 1992

Greenblatt DJ, Shader RI: Prazepam and lorazepam, two new benzodiazepines. N Engl J Med 299:1342–1344, 1978

Greenblatt DJ, Comer WH, Elliott HW, et al: Clinical pharmacokinetics of lorazepam, III. Intravenous injection: preliminary results. J Clin Pharmacol 17:490–494, 1977

Greenblatt DJ, Harmatz JS, Shader RI: Clinical pharmacokinetics of anxiolytics and hypnotics in the elderly: therapeutic considerations, Part I. Clin Pharmacokinet 21:165–177, 1991a

Greenblatt DJ, Harmatz JS, Shader RI: Clinical pharmacokinetics of anxiolytics and hypnotics in the elderly: therapeutic considerations, Part II. Clin Pharmacokinet 21:262–273, 1991b

Greenblatt DJ, Harmatz JS, Shader RI: Plasma alprazolam concentrations. Arch Gen Psychiatry 50:715–722, 1993a

Greenblatt DJ, Scavone JM, Harmatz JS, et al: Cognitive effects of beta-adrenergic antagonists after single doses: pharmacokinetics and pharmacodynamics of propranolol, atenolol, lorazepam, and placebo. Clin Pharmacol Ther 53:577–584, 1993b

Griffiths RR, Wolf B: Relative abuse liability of different benzodiazepines in drug abusers. J Clin Psychopharmacol 10:237–243, 1990

Guilleminault C, Silvestri R, Mondini S, et al: Aging and sleep apnea: action of benzodiazepine, acetazolamide, alcohol, and sleep deprivation in a healthy elderly group. J Gerontol 39:655–661, 1984

Hemmelgarn B, Suissa S, Huang A, et al: Benzodiazepine use and the risk of motor vehicle crash in the elderly. JAMA 278:27–31, 1997

Hollister LE, Muller-Oerlinghausen B, Rickels K, et al: Clinical uses of benzodiazepines. J Clin Psychopharmacol 13 (6, suppl 1):1S–169S, 1993

Hypnotic drugs. The Medical Letter, 42(August 7):71–72, 2000

Jerkovich GS, Preskorn SH: Failure of buspirone to protect against lorazepam withdrawal symptoms (letter). JAMA 258:204–205, 1987

Kruse WHH: Problems and pitfalls in the use of benzodiazepines in the elderly. Drug Safety 5:328–344, 1990

Lawlor BA, Hill JL, Radcliffe JL, et al: A single oral dose challenge of buspirone does not affect memory processes in older volunteers. Biol Psychiatry 32:101–103, 1992

Lewy AJ, Sack RL: Light therapy and psychiatry. Proc Soc Exp Biol Med 183:11–18, 1986

Marinella MA: Propofol for sedation in the intensive care unit: essentials for the clinician. Respir Med 91:505–510, 1997

Martin CD, Chan SC: Distribution of temazepam in body fluids and tissues in lethal overdose. J Anal Toxicol 10:77–78, 1986

McEvoy GK, Litvak K, Welsh OH, et al: AHFS Drug Information. Bethesda, MD, American Society of Health-System Pharmacists, 2000

Mellinger GD, Balter MB, Uhlenhuth EH: Insomnia and its treatment. Arch Gen Psychiatry 42:225–232, 1985

Mendelson WB, Thompson C, Franko T: Adverse reactions to sedative/hypnotics: three years' experience. Sleep 19:702–706, 1996

Miller LG, Greenblatt DJ, Barnhill JG, et al: Chronic benzodiazepine administration, I: tolerance is associated with benzodiazepine receptor downregulation and decreased gamma-aminobutyric acid–A receptor function. J Pharmacol Exp Ther 246:170–176, 1988

Monane M: Insomnia in the elderly. J Clin Psychiatry 53 (6, suppl):23–28, 1992

Morfis L, Schwartz RS, Cistulli PA: REM sleep behaviour disorder: a treatable cause of falls in elderly people. Age Ageing 26:43–44, 1997

Morin CM, Culbert JP, Schwartz SM: Nonpharmacological interventions for insomnia: a meta-analysis of treatment efficacy. Am J Psychiatry 151:1172–1180, 1994

Nofzinger EA, Reynolds CF: Sleep impairment and daytime sleepiness in later life. Am J Psychiatry 153:941–943, 1996

Pollack MH, Rosenbaum JF, Tesar GE, et al: Clonazepam in the treatment of panic disorder and agoraphobia. Psychopharmacol Bull 23:141–144, 1987

Pomara N, Deptula D, Medel M, et al: Effects of diazepam on recall memory: relationship to aging, dose, and duration of treatment. Psychopharmacol Bull 25:144–148, 1989

Pourmotabbed T, McLeod DR, Hoehn-Saric R, et al: Treatment, discontinuation, and psychomotor effects of diazepam in women with generalized anxiety disorder. J Clin Psychopharmacol 16:202–207, 1996

Raskind MA, Dobie DJ, Kanter ED, et al: The alpha$_1$-adrenergic antagonist prazosin ameliorates combat trauma nightmares in veterans with posttraumatic stress disorder: a report of 4 cases. J Clin Psychiatry 61:129–133, 2000

Ray WA, Thapa PB, Gideon P: Benzodiazepines and the risk of falls in nursing home residents. J Am Geriatr Soc 48:682–685, 2000

Reynolds CF, Regestein Q, Nowell PD, et al: Treatment of insomnia in the elderly, in Clinical Geriatric Psychopharmacology, Edited by Salzman C. Baltimore, MD, Williams & Wilkins, 1998, pp 395–416

Rickels K, Schweizer E, Case WG, et al: Long-term therapeutic use of benzodiazepines, I: effects of abrupt discontinuation. Arch Gen Psychiatry 47:899–907, 1990

Rickels K, Schweizer E, Case WG, et al: Nefazodone in major depression: adjunctive benzodiazepine therapy and tolerability. J Clin Psychopharmacol 18:145–153, 1998

Rosebush PI, Mazurek MF: Catatonia after benzodiazepine withdrawal. J Clin Psychopharmacol 16:315–319, 1996

Rosenbaum JF, Moroz G, Bowden CL: Clonazepam in the treatment of panic disorder with or without agoraphobia: a dose-response study of efficacy, safety, and discontinuance. J Clin Psychopharmacol 17:390–400, 1997

Roth T, Roehrs TA: Issues in the use of benzodiazepine therapy. J Clin Psychiatry 53 (6, suppl):14–18, 1992

Saletu B, Gruber G, Saletu M, et al: Sleep laboratory studies in restless legs syndrome patients as compared with normals and acute effects of ropinirole, 1: findings on objective and subjective sleep and awakening quality. Neuropsychobiology 41:181–189, 2000

Satzger W, Engel RR, Ferguson E, et al: Effects of single doses of alpidem, lorazepam, and placebo on memory and attention in healthy young and elderly volunteers. Pharmacopsychiatry 23:114–119, 1990

Schweizer E, Rickels K, Case WG, et al: Long-term therapeutic use of benzodiazepines. Arch Gen Psychiatry 47:908–915, 1990

Schweizer E, Rickels K, Case WG, et al: Carbamazepine treatment in patients discontinuing long-term benzodiazepine therapy. Arch Gen Psychiatry 48:448–452, 1991

Shader RI, Greenblatt DJ: Use of benzodiazepines in anxiety disorders. N Engl J Med 328:1398–1405, 1993

Swift CG, Swift MR, Hamley J, et al: Side-effect 'tolerance' in elderly long-term recipients of benzodiazepine hypnotics. Age Ageing 13:335–343, 1984

Thal GD, Szabo MD, Lopez-Bresnahan M, et al: Exacerbation or unmasking of focal neurologic deficits by sedatives. Anesthesiology 85:21–25, 1996

Thompson TL, Moran MG, Nies AS: Psychotropic drug use in the elderly, Part 1. N Engl J Med 308:134–138, 1983

van Balkom AJ, de Beurs E, Koele P, et al: Long-term benzodiazepine use is associated with smaller treatment gain in panic disorder with agoraphobia. J Nerv Ment Dis 184:133–135, 1996

Van Der Auwera D, Verborgh C, Loef B: Cardiovascular collapse after continuous infusion of propofol in elderly patients. Acta Anaesth Belg 41:13–16, 1990

van Steveninck AL, Wallnofer AE, Schoemaker RC, et al: A study of the effects of long-term use on individual sensitivity to temazepam and lorazepam in a clinical population. Br J Clin Pharmacol 44:267–275, 1997

Woo E, Proulx SM, Greenblatt DJ: Differential side effect profile of triazolam versus flurazepam in elderly patients undergoing rehabilitation therapy. J Clin Pharmacol 31:168–173, 1991

Generic name	alprazolam
Trade name	Xanax
Class	Benzodiazepine
Relative potency	High
Half-life	12–20 hours
Mechanism of action	Potentiates effects of GABA by binding to GABA$_A$–benzodiazepine receptor complex
Available formulations	Tablets: 0.25, 0.5, 1, 2 mg Oral concentrate: 1 mg/mL
Starting dose	0.125–0.25 mg bid
Titration	Increase by 0.125 mg every 4–5 days, as needed and as tolerated
Typical daily dose	0.25 mg bid
Dosage range	0.25–0.75 mg daily (divided bid or tid)
Therapeutic serum level	20–40 ng/mL (anxiety in panic disorder)

Comments: Not a drug of first choice in elderly patients, despite its short half-life and lack of active metabolites. Interdose anxiety may necessitate tid or qid dosing. Discontinuation is often problematic, requiring a switch to a longer-acting agent or to gabapentin or carbamazepine. Pharmacokinetics are independent of dose and are unchanged during multiple dosing. 80% protein bound. Volume of distribution decreased in elderly men but unchanged in elderly women. Metabolized extensively in liver via hydroxylation to less active metabolites. Peak plasma concentration in 1–2 hours. Delayed clearance (prolonged half-life) in elderly men. Withdrawal symptoms after abrupt discontinuation occur from 18 hours to 3 days later. *Adverse effects:* same as for other benzodiazepines (see text), except for a possibly increased risk of seizure and/or delirium on abrupt discontinuation.

Generic name	buspirone
Trade name	BuSpar
Class	Antianxiety
Half-life	2–11 hours
Mechanism of action	5-HT$_{1A}$ receptor antagonist/partial agonist
Available formulation	Tablets: 5, 10 mg
Starting dose	5 mg bid
Titration	Increase by 5 mg every 2–3 days
Typical daily dose	10 mg tid
Dosage range	5 mg bid to 20 mg tid
Therapeutic serum level	Not established

Comments: A drug of choice for generalized anxiety (but not panic) among elderly patients because of favorable adverse effect profile; not associated with psychomotor or cognitive impairment, dependence, withdrawal, abuse, or interaction with alcohol. Described as a "midbrain modulator" because of various effects on serotonergic, dopaminergic, cholinergic, and α-adrenergic neurotransmitter systems. Prior treatment with benzodiazepines, especially recent treatment, associated with reduced effectiveness of buspirone. Pharmacokinetics not related to age or sex, but considerable between-individual variation is seen. Extensive first-pass metabolism, leading to a major active metabolite. Food may decrease absorption, but also may decrease hepatic extraction, thus increasing bioavailability. 95% protein bound. Metabolized in the liver by CYP3A4 oxidation. Peak serum concentration in 40–60 minutes. Long latency to effect; may see some decrease in anxiety after 1 week, but full effect may take up to 6 weeks. Not effective when used prn (as needed). Not recommended for use in patients with hepatic or renal impairment; if used, reduced doses required. Not dialyzable. In changing from a benzodiazepine to buspirone, add buspirone; administer both for 2–4 weeks before starting benzodiazepine taper. Buspirone co-administration may allow lower doses of benzodiazepine, even if benzodiazepine cannot be discontinued. When buspirone is discontinued, extended taper not necessary. *Adverse effects:* Most common are dizziness, headache, drowsiness, and light-headedness. Nausea, insomnia, nervousness, and fatigue can also be seen. Less sedation and psychomotor impairment than with benzodiazepines. Doses greater than 60 mg daily may be associated with dysphoria. Laboratory test interactions: increased AST, ALT values.

Generic name	clonazepam
Trade name	Klonopin
Class	Benzodiazepine
Half-life	19–50 hours
Mechanism of action	Potentiates effects of GABA by binding to $GABA_A$–benzodiazepine receptor complex
Available formulation	Tablets: 0.5, 1, 2 mg (scored 0.5-mg tablet available from Watson Laboratories, Inc.)
Starting dose	Anxiety: 0.25 to 0.5 mg qd
Titration	Increase by 0.25–0.5 mg every 4–5 days, as needed and as tolerated
Typical daily dose	Anxiety: 1 mg
Dosage range	Anxiety: 0.5 mg qod to 2 mg qd
Therapeutic serum level	Not established for anxiety/sedation

Comments: A useful drug in the treatment of elderly patients, provided half-life is taken into account in deciding dosing schedule. Rapidly and well absorbed orally. Onset of action in 20–60 minutes; duration of action: 12 hours. 85% protein bound. Metabolized by nitro-reduction to an inactive metabolite. Clearance may be decreased in the elderly. *Common adverse effects* (include): sedation, ataxia, and hypotonia. As with other benzodiazepines, in elders with mental retardation or brain injury, behavioral disturbances (aggressiveness, irritability, agitation, hyperkinesis) can occur.

Generic name	estazolam
Trade name	ProSom
Class	Benzodiazepine
Half-life	10–24 hours
Mechanism of action	Potentiates effects of GABA by binding to GABA$_A$–benzodiazepine receptor complex
Available formulation	Tablets: 1, 2 mg
Starting dose	0.5–1 mg hs
Titration	Increase by 0.5 mg, as needed and as tolerated
Typical daily dose	1 mg hs
Dosage range	0.5–2 mg hs
Therapeutic serum level	Not established

Comments: Theoretically, a preferred drug for elderly patients because of its relatively short half-life and absence of active metabolites. Rapidly and well absorbed orally. Large inter-individual variation in concentration after a standard dose. Peak concentration in 0.5–1.6 hours, so should be administered just before bedtime. Rapidly and extensively metabolized to inactive metabolites. *Adverse effects:* same as for other benzodiazepines, as discussed in text.

Generic name	gabapentin
Trade name	Neurontin
Class	Anticonvulsant structurally related to GABA
Half-life	5–7 hours
Mechanism of action	No direct GABA-mimetic action; increases GABA levels by inhibiting the GABA transporter
Available formulations	Capsules: 100, 300, 400 mg Tablets (coated): 600, 800 mg Oral solution: 250 mg/5 mL
Starting dose	Sedation: 100 mg every 12 hours Insomnia: 100 mg qhs
Titration	Sedation: increase by 100 mg every 3–5 days, as tolerated Insomnia: increase to 200 mg on second night and 300 mg on third night
Typical daily dose	Sedation: 100 mg tid Insomnia: 300 mg qhs
Dosage range	100–1,800 mg daily in divided doses
Therapeutic serum level	Obtainable, but not used clinically

Comments: Anecdotal experience suggests efficacy for insomnia and anxiety, in addition to mood instability, certain pain syndromes, tremor, and some parkinsonian symptoms in elderly patients; controlled studies not performed to date. May have reduced bioavailability at higher doses. Not protein bound; not appreciably metabolized (no CYP interactions); no pharmacokinetic interactions with other anticonvulsants. Renally excreted; clearance declines with age. Dosage adjustment required for renal failure; administered after hemodialysis. For nondialysis patients, short half-life necessitates tid dosing for indications such as anxiety and mood instability. Administered at bedtime for insomnia. Generally well tolerated, with side effects that are mild to moderate in severity and self-limiting. *Most common adverse effects* are neuropsychiatric: somnolence, dizziness, ataxia, fatigue, and nystagmus. *Other adverse effects* (include): nausea/vomiting, dry mouth, constipation, peripheral edema, rhinitis, pharyngitis, visual changes, and myalgia. Induction of bipolar rapid cycling has been reported with this agent.

Generic name	kava extract (kava kava)
Trade name	Various
Class	Herbal (*Piper methysticum*)
Half-life	
Mechanism of action	Conflicting data regarding GABA receptor binding capacity
Available formulations	Various
Starting dose	
Titration	
Typical daily dose	100 mg po tid
Dosage range	300–600 mg daily (divided bid or tid)
Therapeutic serum level	Not established

Comments: May be useful as an anxiolytic in elders; understudied for this indication. Has skeletal muscle relaxant and analgesic and anesthetic properties. *Adverse effects:* dyspepsia, restlessness, drowsiness, tiredness, tremor, headache, extrapyramidal effects, and rash reminiscent of pellagra with heavy use. May potentiate effects of barbiturates and alprazolam.

Generic name	lorazepam
Trade name	Ativan
Class	Benzodiazepine
Half-life	10–20 hours
Mechanism of action	Potentiates effects of GABA by binding to GABA$_A$–benzodiazepine receptor complex
Available formulations	Tablets: 0.5, 1, 2 mg Oral concentrate: 2 mg/mL Injectable: 1 mg/0.5 mL, 2 mg/mL, or 4 mg/mL
Starting dose	0.5 mg daily
Titration	Increase by 0.5 mg every 4–5 days, as needed and as tolerated
Typical daily dose	Anxiety: 0.5–1 mg bid or tid
Dosage range	0.5 mg–4 mg daily (in divided doses)
Therapeutic serum level	20–80 ng/mL

Comments: A drug of first choice for anxiety in elderly patients because pharmacokinetics are little affected by aging. Not recommended for treatment of insomnia because of relatively short duration of effect. Promptly absorbed orally, and reliably absorbed with intramuscular use. Less lipophilic than fast-acting compounds such as midazolam; onset with intramuscular use in 20–30 minutes. 85% protein bound. Duration of effect: 6–8 hours. No active metabolites. Eliminated by glucuronidation; dose is reduced in renal insufficiency. *Adverse effects:* same as with other benzodiazepines, as discussed in text.

Generic name	melatonin
Trade name	Various
Class	Hormone (marketed as a dietary supplement)
Half-life	30–50 minutes
Mechanism of action	Mimics effects of endogenous melatonin; may normalize endogenous melatonin production
Available formulations	Various
Starting dose	2 mg qhs (CR preparation) 2 hours before bedtime
Titration	None
Typical daily dose	2 mg qhs (CR preparation) 2 hours before bedtime
Dosage range	Not established
Therapeutic serum level	Not established

Comments: Decreases sleep latency and increases sleep duration in melatonin-deficient individuals. Does not suppress REM sleep or delay its onset. Rapidly metabolized by the liver; 85% excreted in urine as 6-sulphatoxymelatonin. *Adverse effects:* nightmares, hypotension, sleep disorders, abdominal pain, and others. Purity and melatonin content of products sold in health food stores have been questioned; not FDA regulated.

Generic name	mirtazapine
Trade name	Remeron
Class	Tetracyclic
Half-life	20–40 hours
Mechanism of action	Noradrenergic and specific (postsynaptic) serotonergic antagonism
Available formulation	Tablets: 15, 30 (both scored), 45 mg (unscored)
Starting dose	Insomnia: 7.5 mg qhs
Titration	Increase by 7.5 mg after 1 week, if needed; may lose hypnotic efficacy at the higher dose
Typical daily dose	7.5 mg qhs
Dosage range	7.5–15 mg qhs
Therapeutic serum level	Not established

Comments: Understudied in elderly patients. Rapidly and completely absorbed orally, with peak levels in 2 hours; not affected by food. 85% protein bound. Extensively metabolized in the liver via CYP1A2, CYP2D6, and CYP3A4 enzymes. Clearance reduced in elderly patients (especially men) and in patients with hepatic or renal dysfunction. *Common side effects* (include): Sedation, dizziness, increased appetite with weight gain, increases in serum cholesterol and triglyceride levels, significant elevations in ALT levels without compromise of liver function, and hypertension. Can be associated with reduced heart rate variability. Lower doses are more sedating than higher doses because presumably at higher doses, noradrenergic effects balance histaminergic effects.

Generic name	oxazepam
Trade name	Serax
Class	Benzodiazepine
Half-life	5–20 hours
Mechanism of action	Potentiates effects of GABA by binding to GABA$_A$–benzodiazepine receptor complex
Available formulations	Capsules: 10, 15, 30 mg Tablets: 10, 15, 30 mg
Starting dose	Anxiety: 10 mg bid or tid Insomnia: 10 or 15 mg hs Alcohol withdrawal: 15 mg tid
Titration	Increase by 5–15 mg every 4–5 days, as needed and as tolerated
Typical daily dose	Anxiety: 10 mg tid Insomnia: 15 mg hs Alcohol withdrawal: 15–30 mg tid or qid
Dosage range	10 mg qd to 15 mg tid (anxiety) 10–30 mg hs (insomnia)
Therapeutic serum level	0.2–1.4 μg/mL

Comments: A drug of first choice in the elderly patients because of short half-life and absence of active metabolites. Pharmacokinetics are little affected by age. Completely but slowly absorbed orally, so not useful for prn dosing, and not useful for initial insomnia unless taken several hours before bedtime. 2–4 hours to peak serum concentration (faster for tablet than for capsule). 96%–99% protein bound. Metabolized in the liver to inactive compounds, mainly glucuronides. Wide variation in half-life; some individuals with anxiety require at least tid dosing for symptom control. Dosage reduced or interval increased in renal insufficiency. Not dialyzable. *Adverse effects:* same as with other benzodiazepines, as discussed in text.

Generic name	propofol
Trade name	Diprivan
Class	Phenolic compound
Half-life	Biphasic: 40 minutes/1–3 days (nongeriatric)
Mechanism of action	A general anesthetic and sedative unrelated to other sedatives
Available formulation	Injection: 10 mg/mL
Starting dose	0.5 mg/kg/hour (slow infusion)
Titration	Dose is decreased once sedation is established, adjusted to response; dose adjustments can occur at 3- to 5-minute intervals
Typical daily dose	Variable
Dosage range	Variable
Therapeutic serum level	Not established

Comments: Useful for sedation of ICU patients. Cardiac monitor, blood pressure monitor, and ventilator required. Serum triglyceride level should be checked before starting therapy and every 7 days thereafter. Rapid bolus injection associated with hypotension, desaturation, apnea, and airway obstruction. Onset of sedation/anesthesia in less than a minute. Metabolized in the liver to water-soluble sulfate and glucuronide conjugates. Hydroxylated by CYP2B6. Excreted mainly in urine. *Drug interactions:* increased toxicity of neuromuscular blockers; additive CNS and respiratory depression with benzodiazepines, opioids, phenothiazines, alcohol, and other anesthetics. *Adverse effects:* hypotension, apnea, and pain at injection site.

Generic name	propranolol
Trade name	Inderal, Inderal LA, Betachron
Class	β-Adrenergic blocker
Half-life	4–6 hours
Mechanism of action	Competitively blocks response to β_1- and β_2-adrenergic stimulation
Available formulations	Tablets: 10, 20, 40, 60, 80, 90 mg Solution: 20 mg/5 mL, 40 mg/5 mL Oral concentrate: 80 mg/mL Capsule, extended-release: 60, 80, 120, 160 mg Injectable: 1 mg/mL
Starting dose	5–10 mg bid or tid (anxiety)
Titration	Increase by 5–10 mg, as needed and as tolerated (monitor blood pressure and pulse)
Typical daily dose	10–20 mg every 8 hours (anxiety)
Dosage range	30–120 mg daily in divided doses (tid) (anxiety)
Therapeutic serum level	50–100 ng/mL

Comments: Useful in controlling anxiety in medically ill patients. Completely absorbed orally, with large between-individual variability in concentration attained with a standard dose. Readily crosses the blood-brain barrier. Onset of action: β blockade in 1–2 hours. Extensive first-pass metabolism, with bioavailability of 30%–40%. Metabolized in liver to active and inactive compounds. 4-Hydroxypropranolol (active) formed only during initial oral therapy and rapidly eliminated. A substrate primarily of CYP2D6. Dose decreased when hepatic disease is present. Eliminated primarily in urine. Not dialyzable. To discontinue, taper slowly (over 2 weeks). Contraindicated in patients with uncompensated heart failure, cardiogenic shock, bradycardia or heart block, asthma, hyperactive airway disease, COPD, Raynaud's syndrome, and diabetes. *Drug interactions:* Hypotension with phenothiazines, heart block with fluoxetine, hypotension with antihypertensive drugs and diuretics, potentiation of effects of neuromuscular blockers, increased hypoglycemic effects of antidiabetic agents. See Table 1–1 in Chapter 1 for CYP2D6 inhibitors and inducers. *Adverse effects:* Not dose-related and occur soon after initiation of therapy. Include bradycardia, hypotension, heart failure, fluid retention, lightheadedness, dizziness, ataxia, irritability, lethargy, hearing loss, visual disturbance, hallucinations, confusion, insomnia, vivid dreams, and depression.

Generic name	temazepam
Trade name	Restoril
Class	Benzodiazepine
Half-life	10–20 hours
Mechanism of action	Potentiates effects of GABA by binding to $GABA_A$–benzodiazepine receptor complex
Available formulation	Capsules: 7.5, 15, 30 mg
Starting dose	7.5 mg hs
Titration	Increase by 7.5 mg every 4–5 days, as needed and as tolerated
Typical daily dose	15 mg hs (given 1 hour before bedtime)
Dosage range	7.5–30 mg hs
Therapeutic serum level	26 ng/mL (24-hour level)

Comments: A drug of choice for the treatment of insomnia in elderly patients. Pharmacokinetics little affected by aging. Less lipid-soluble than other benzodiazepines, with onset in 30–60 minutes and peak in 1–3 hours. 96%–98% protein bound. Metabolized primarily by glucuronidation. Higher doses may be associated with impaired daytime performance in elders. *Adverse effects:* same as those for other benzodiazepines, as discussed in text.

Generic name	trazodone
Trade name	Desyrel
Class	Antidepressant
Half-life	4–8 hours; 12 hours (biphasic)
Mechanism of action	Potentiates serotonergic neurotransmission; antagonist at 5-HT_2 receptor
Available formulation	Tablets: 50, 100, 150, 300 mg (all scored)
Starting dose	Anxiety, agitation: 12.5–25 mg bid or tid Insomnia: 12.5–25 mg hs
Titration	Increase every 3–7 days, as needed and as tolerated
Typical daily dose	Anxiety, agitation: 25 mg tid Insomnia: 25–50 mg hs
Dosage range	Anxiety, agitation: 12.5 mg bid to 100 mg tid Insomnia: 12.5–300 mg hs
Therapeutic serum level	Not well established

Comments: Although marketed as an antidepressant, used primarily as a sedative-hypnotic. A drug of first choice for elderly patients with anxiety, agitation, aggression, or insomnia. Rapidly and completely absorbed orally; onset of sedative effect in 20–30 minutes. Peak concentration in 2 hours when taken with food and in 1 hour when taken on an empty stomach. 85%–95% protein bound. Extensively metabolized in the liver by various pathways, including oxidation by CYP3A4 (parent compound) and CYP2D6 enzymes (*m*-chlorophenyl-piperazine [m-CPP] metabolite). Not associated with dependence or withdrawal phenomena. *Drug interactions* (include): Risk of serotonin syndrome when given with other serotonergic drugs, additive hypotension with antihypertensive drugs, decreased antihypertensive effects of clonidine and methyldopa, decreased effect of warfarin and other anticoagulants, and increased levels of digoxin and phenytoin. See Table 1–1 in Chapter 1 for CYP drug interactions. *Adverse effects* (include): Hypotension (including orthostasis), ventricular irritability (increased premature depolarizations), sedation (associated with falls and cognitive dysfunction), myalgias, nausea, and dry mouth. The m-CPP metabolite may be anxiogenic in some patients. Priapism has rarely been reported in elderly men. Trazodone *not* recommended during the initial recovery phase from myocardial infarction.

Generic name	valerian
Trade name	Various
Class	Herbal supplement
Half-life	
Mechanism of action	Not established
Available formulations	Various
Starting dose	300–450 mg 30 minutes before hs
Titration	None
Typical daily dose	450 mg qhs
Dosage range	300–450 mg qhs
Therapeutic serum level	Not established

Comments: Mild hypnotic effects. Appears to increase slow-wave sleep and decrease Stage 1 sleep while not affecting sleep latency, REM sleep, or other sleep parameters. Does not appear to cause nightmares or hangover effect at recommended doses. *Adverse effects:* hepatotoxicity and sedation. Not regulated by the FDA, so product purity and content not guaranteed.

Generic name	zaleplon
Trade name	Sonata
Class	Pyrazolopyrimidine hypnotic (nonbenzodiazepine)
Half-life	1 hour
Mechanism of action	Potentiates effects of GABA by binding preferentially to the omega_1 (ω_1) subunit of the $GABA_A$–benzodiazepine receptor complex
Available formulation	Capsules: 5, 10 mg
Starting dose	5 mg hs (given immediately before bedtime)
Titration	Increase by 5 mg, as needed and as tolerated
Typical daily dose	5 mg hs (given immediately before bedtime)
Dosage range	5–10 mg qhs (given immediately before bedtime)
Therapeutic serum level	Not established

Comments: May be useful in reducing sleep latency in elders. Has sedative, anxiolytic, muscle-relaxant, and anticonvulsant properties. Food (especially with high fat content) may delay absorption. Bioavailability 30%. Peak serum levels in 1 hour. Extensively metabolized by CYP3A and aldehyde oxidase to inactive metabolites, mostly excreted in urine. Dose-dependent rebound insomnia may occur with discontinuation. Manufacturer recommends short-term (2–4 weeks) use. Abuse potential similar to that of benzodiazepines. *Adverse effects* (include): Depression, hypertonia, nervousness, amnesia, difficulty concentrating, myalgia, migraine, constipation, dry mouth, and rash. Cognitive side effects probably less than for benzodiazepines.

Generic name	zolpidem
Trade name	Ambien
Class	Imidazopyridine hypnotic (nonbenzodiazepine)
Half-life	2.9 hours
Mechanism of action	Potentiates effects of GABA by binding preferentially to the ω_1 receptor of the $GABA_A$–benzodiazepine receptor complex
Available formulation	Tablets: 5, 10 mg
Starting dose	5 mg hs (given immediately before bedtime)
Titration	Increase by 5 mg, as needed and as tolerated
Typical daily dose	5 mg hs (given immediately before bedtime)
Dosage range	5–10 mg hs (given immediately before bedtime)
Therapeutic serum level	80–150 ng/mL (not well established)

Comments: May be useful in the elderly for short-term treatment of insomnia. Enhances sleep without affecting sleep architecture. Reportedly lacks anxiolytic, anticonvulsant, and muscle-relaxant effects. Pharmacokinetics affected by age (increased AUC and half-life in the elderly) and sex (higher plasma concentrations in women). Rapidly absorbed. First-pass metabolism results in 70% bioavailability. Rapid onset (within 30 minutes), with peak levels in 2.2 hours and duration of 6–8 hours; useful to initiate and to maintain sleep. 92% protein bound. Metabolized to inactive metabolites in liver. Substrate for CYP3A4, CYP2C9, and CYP1A2 enzymes. Rapidly eliminated. Dose must be reduced when renal or hepatic disease is present. Half-life in cirrhosis increased to 10 hours. Although manufacturer recommends short-term (<1 month) use, drug may maintain hypnotic efficacy for long periods. Case reports of tolerance, with dose escalation. A withdrawal syndrome can occur, with symptoms of tachycardia, tachypnea, anxiety, tremor, sweating, nausea, and abdominal pain. *Most common adverse effects:* dizziness, lightheadedness, somnolence, headache, and gastrointestinal upset. *Other adverse effects:* Case reports of hallucinations occurring shortly after ingestion, apparently more severe and prolonged in patients concomitantly taking serotonergic antidepressants. Anecdotal reports of hypotension and falls among elderly patients taking this drug, especially at higher doses (>20 mg). Like benzodiazepines, zolpidem may worsen sleep apnea. Flumazenil may partially reverse sedation in cases of toxicity. Not dialyzable.

PART 2

Treatment of Other Geriatric Syndromes and Disorders

6

Treatment of Substance-Related Disorders

Substance abuse in the current elderly cohort involves mainly alcohol and tobacco. Abuse of drugs such as cocaine occurs less commonly. Of prescribed medications, benzodiazepines are most often implicated in dependence syndromes in elderly patients—an order of magnitude more frequently than prescribed narcotics (Holroyd and Duryee 1997).

In community samples, heavy alcohol use is found in up to 14% and problematic use in up to 17% of elderly individuals (Atkinson et al. 1990). Many are covert drinkers who do not come to legal or clinical attention because they do not work, do not drive, and live alone. Although different drinking patterns are seen, most elders who drink do so in small amounts on a daily basis. Because of aging-associated pharmacokinetic and pharmacodynamic changes, as well as coprescribed medication and comorbid illness, these small amounts can have significant effects.

In clinical populations, alcohol abusers are more heavily

represented, particularly among patients with hypertension, liver disease, dementia, depression, falls, motor vehicle accidents, and other sequelae of alcoholism. Alcohol abuse is associated with an increased risk of suicide. Psychiatric consequences of alcohol and drug dependence are shown in Table 6–1, and medical consequences of alcohol dependence are shown in Table 6–2. It is expected that future cohorts of elderly individuals will have higher rates of alcoholism, particularly among women. The economic burden of caring for this subpopulation of the medically ill elderly is enormous; in 1989, hospital charges to Medicare alone for alcohol-related admissions totaled $234 million (Adams et al. 1993). A move toward better preventive care is clearly needed, as is more widespread recognition that alcoholism is as treatable in elders as it is in younger patients.

Table 6–1. Psychiatric consequences of alcohol and drug dependence in the elderly

Anxiety/anxiety disorders	**Mood symptoms/disorders**
Generalized anxiety	Depression
Panic	Insomnia
Phobias	Mania
Cognitive disorders	Suicidal ideation/homicidal ideation
Amnesia	Violent behavior
Delirium	**Personality change**
Functional decline	Apathy
Frequent falls	Interpersonal difficulties
Legal problems	Irritability
Loss of capacity to perform ADLs	Social withdrawal
Noncompliance	**Psychotic symptoms**
Poor hygiene	Delusions (especially paranoid)
	Hallucinations

Note. ADL = activity of daily living.

Table 6–2. Medical consequences of alcohol dependence in the elderly

General/Systemic	Gastrointestinal
Anemia	Bleeding
Cardiomyopathy	Cirrhosis
Electrolyte disturbance	Esophageal varices
Hypercortisolemia	Gastritis
Hypovitaminosis	Hepatitis
Malignancy	Pancreatitis
Osteopenia	Ulcers
Susceptibility to infection	
Neuropsychiatric	
Amnestic disorder (Korsakoff's syndrome)	
Cerebellar degeneration	
Delirium tremens	
Dementia	
Peripheral neuropathy	
Wernicke's encephalopathy	

Tobacco dependence is the most common substance-related disorder among elderly individuals in the United States, although tobacco use is less prevalent in elders than in middle-aged adults because of smoking-related mortality and smoking cessation. Elderly patients are in fact able to overcome tobacco dependence; each year, 10% of elderly smokers are successful in quitting smoking (Salive et al. 1992). Medically based smoking cessation programs are an important intervention in this population.

Benzodiazepines prescribed for anxiolytic or hypnotic purposes are more likely to be continued long-term in elderly patients compared with younger cohorts, particularly in elders with lower education levels (Mant et al. 1988). Abuse of benzodiazepines is rarely a problem among elders, but long-term use may be associated with physical dependence.

In general, substance-related disorders are classified as either *substance use disorders* (dependence and abuse) or *substance-induced disorders* (intoxication, withdrawal, cognitive disorders, mood disorders, etc.).

Substance Use Disorders

Diagnosis of Abuse and Dependence

Substance abuse is a maladaptive pattern involving harmful consequences of repeated use of alcohol, a drug, or a medication. An elderly person who abuses alcohol, for example, may meet this criterion by failing to maintain adequate hygiene, by having repeated falls en route to the liquor store, or by alienating children through constant argument about the consequences of intoxication. *Substance dependence* is a maladaptive pattern involving the development of tolerance, withdrawal symptoms on discontinuation, compulsive use, restriction of activities, and/or continued use despite adverse physical or psychological effects. Applied to alcohol, substance dependence is more commonly known as "alcoholism."

The alcohol-abusing elder is most likely to present as an unmarried male with no close friends, a lifelong drinking history, and a positive tobacco use history (Bristow and Clare 1992; Nakamura et al. 1990). Alcoholism should be considered, however, in any elderly patient presenting because of a fall, trauma, seizure, hypertension, stroke, exacerbation of chronic obstructive pulmonary disease (COPD), cardiomyopathy, gastrointestinal bleeding, hepatic dysfunction, incontinence, malnutrition, repeated infection, self-neglect, unexplained functional decline, insomnia, depression, cognitive impairment, sexual dysfunction, or treatment resistance (e.g., refractory hypertension or depression). Among covert alcohol abusers, these problems are usually misattributed to other causes.

The weight of alcoholism diagnosis is carried by the history, and this is problematic for elderly patients because they are more likely to deny alcohol use. Several alcoholism screening instruments are used in elderly clinical populations, including the

AUDIT (Bradley et al. 1998), CAGE (Buchsbaum et al. 1992), and Michigan Alcoholism Screening Test—Geriatrics (MAST-G; Blow 1991). In our experience, even these instruments are not necessarily well suited for screening elderly alcohol abusers who intend to minimize a drinking problem. In screening this population, a simple (medical-appearing, nonjudgmental) approach consisting of the following two questions may be helpful:

- When was your last drink?
- Have you ever had a drinking problem?

Positive responses of "<24 hours ago" and "yes" have been found to have a 92% sensitivity compared with the MAST in detecting an alcohol problem (Cyr and Wartman 1988).

Laboratory tests useful in confirming alcohol consumption include breath analysis, urine alcohol, blood alcohol level (BAL), serum γ-glutamyltransferase (GGT), and percent serum carbohydrate-deficient transferrin (%CDT) (Spies et al. 1996). %CDT is a marker for high alcohol consumption and is more sensitive and specific than GGT (Lesch et al. 1996). GGT, mean corpuscular volume (MCV), AST (aspartate transaminase), and ALT (alanine transaminase) may be more affected by other substance use or comorbid medical conditions (Chang et al. 1990; Mowe and Bohmer 1996). Cortical atrophy (most prominent frontally) and cerebellar atrophy are commonly seen on head computed tomography (CT) or magnetic resonance imaging (MRI) in alcohol-abusing elders (Carlen et al. 1978, 1986; Pfefferbaum et al. 1988). Frontal atrophy may be associated with lack of motivation and social withdrawal, which could be expected to influence the success of alcoholism treatment (Rosse et al. 1997).

Treatment

Alcohol Dependence

In treating the elderly alcohol abuser, the clinician should adopt the attitude that every day of sobriety makes a difference in the physical and psychological health of the patient; complete abstinence may be an unachievable goal when imposed on a long-standing drinker. For all patients, nonpharmacological interventions are useful in initiating and maintaining abstinence. Physician counseling about alcohol overuse is associated with a significant decrease in alcohol consumption among hospitalized and clinic patients (Fleming et al. 1999; Moore et al. 1989).

In our experience, continued abstinence among elders depends on a fairly intensive program of regular attendance at Alcoholics Anonymous (AA) or other recovery group meetings, an ongoing one-to-one relationship with a supportive family/friend surrogate (usually a sponsor or counselor), regularly scheduled medical and psychiatric follow-up, and repeated reinforcement of abstinence. Some elders respond well to group therapy experiences, as long as they are with age-peers who also have a history of alcohol dependence. For many elders, the biggest obstacle to participation in such a program is transportation to and from appointments. For homebound elderly patients, identification and education of the "supplier" of alcohol may be a critical step.

There is limited evidence that biofeedback may reduce alcohol consumption in detoxified alcohol abusers (Denney et al. 1991), and this may be a useful adjunct when available, but it is not reimbursable under many insurance plans. One study of acupuncture appeared promising but suffered from an excessive rate of attrition from both the active and control groups (Bullock et al. 1989).

Pharmacological therapies for alcohol dependence include naltrexone, disulfiram, SSRI antidepressants, and possibly ondansetron and buspirone. Naltrexone (ReVia) is thought to act by antagonizing the reinforcing effects of alcohol and suppressing craving (Swift 1998). Its use is generally limited by low patient acceptance and compliance. Naltrexone is considered most appropriate for patients with severe alcohol dependence, high craving, and cognitive impairment, but must be avoided in patients who are opioid-dependent because of the risk of precipitating withdrawal. The efficacy and safety of naltrexone have been demonstrated in several studies, but only up to 12 weeks (Croop et al. 1997; Oslin et al. 1997). Side effects are minimal (nausea and headache), and no effect on liver function tests is seen at recommended doses. Naltrexone is initiated in elderly patients at a total dose of 25 mg daily, and the dosage is maintained there or increased to 50 mg daily. It is always administered in conjunction with appropriate nonpharmacological interventions noted earlier. Anecdotally, even at a daily dose of 50 mg, naltrexone is reputed to be effective for only a limited period of time, on the order of several months.

Use of disulfiram (Antabuse) in elderly patients is limited by cardiovascular and other serious effects when it is combined with alcohol (Swift 1998). This medication interferes with the second step of alcohol metabolism, resulting in a buildup of the toxic intermediate acetaldehyde, which has aversive properties. A randomized, controlled trial of disulfiram in a Veterans Administration population found this medication to be no more effective than placebo (Fuller et al. 1986), although anecdotal experience suggests that supervised administration of disulfiram (which ensures that it is taken) increases its effectiveness. When disulfiram is used in treating elders, the dose is maintained at 125–250 mg daily. There is some question as to whether this dose generates a blood level sufficient to produce an alcohol-disulfiram reaction if the patient drinks (Gorelick 1993), such that the deterrent might actually be the threat of reaction rather than an actual reaction. Despite all this, the drug has found a small niche in particular populations, where patients take it to keep a "slip" from turning into a binge, or in situations they know will pose a high risk for drinking (Duckert and Johnsen 1987). With regular users, disulfiram compliance can be determined by testing urine for diethylamine, a metabolite (Fuller and Neiderhiser 1980).

The SSRIs citalopram, fluoxetine, and sertraline have been found to reduce craving and drinking behavior during the first week or weeks of treatment in nongeriatric samples (Gorelick and Paredes 1992; Naranjo et al. 1995; Sellers et al. 1992), but limited follow-up suggests that these effects may not be sustained in all patients (Naranjo et al. 1995). In our experience, the SSRIs can be effective in alcohol-abusing elderly outpatients without major depression who are closely followed in structured abstinence programs, as described earlier (see "Alcohol Dependence").

Ondansetron, a selective serotonin$_3$ (5-HT$_3$) receptor antagonist marketed for treatment of nausea, has been shown to be effective in reducing alcohol consumption and increasing abstinence in a large, mixed-age cohort of patients with early-onset alcohol dependence (Johnson et al. 2000). The effective dosage of ondansetron in that study was 4 μg/kg twice daily.

Early data suggested that buspirone might be useful in reducing alcohol craving. In one controlled 8-week trial of 50 outpatients with mild to moderate alcohol abuse histories, buspirone was associated with reduced craving, reduced anxiety levels, and lower attrition from treatment (Bruno 1989). In an open trial, buspirone was associated with reduced craving and reduced anxiety in patients with high levels of anxiety, but had no effect on craving in those with low levels of anxiety (Kranzler and Meyer 1989). In general, clinical experience has been that buspirone's effect in reducing alcohol craving and consumption over the long term has been disappointing.

Acamprosate is an agent that decreases glutamatergic activity and increases GABAergic function in the central nervous system (CNS). This drug is reported to reduce alcohol craving associated with conditioned withdrawal and thereby to increase abstinence (Poldrugo 1997). Several randomized, controlled trials lasting 12 months in nongeriatric patients have demonstrated the longer-term effectiveness and safety of acamprosate (Paille et al. 1995; Whitworth et al. 1996). This drug is not yet marketed in the United States, but a multicenter controlled trial is under way.

Tobacco Dependence

Cigarette smoking involves more than nicotine dependence. There is some evidence that smoking increases brain dopamine levels and induces brain monoamine oxidase activity, thereby conferring antidepressant effects. In addition, hydrocarbons in cigarette smoke have complex pharmacokinetic effects as inducers of the activity of cytochrome P450 (CYP) enzymes 1A2 and 3A4, as noted in Chapter 1.

The antidepressant bupropion (Zyban), used in conjunction with behavioral interventions, has been reported to reduce withdrawal-related dysphoria, weight gain, and relapse in those who are attempting to quit smoking. In acute withdrawal, bupropion has similar efficacy to nicotine replacement therapies (discussed below), and the combination of bupropion and nicotine replacement is superior to monotherapy (Jorenby et al. 1999), although the safety of this combination has not been specifically studied in elders. When bupropion is started, a "quit date" is selected, usually 1–2 weeks later. Sustained-release (SR) bupropion is initiated in elderly patients at a dose of 100 mg daily; the dosage is increased to 100 mg bid after 4–7 days, as tolerated. SR doses must be separated by 8 hours. The antidepressant is continued for 7–12 weeks; at 7 weeks, if the patient has made no progress toward quitting, the medication is discontinued. The goal of therapy is complete cessation of smoking. Ideally, when this is achieved by 12 weeks, the medication is stopped; tapering is not necessary, although the patient should be monitored for the possible emergence of depressive symptoms.

Nicotine replacement therapies in the form of gum, patches, sprays, and inhalers are effective in 13% of smokers (Law and Tang 1995). In a partly geriatric cohort of patients with treatment-refractory tobacco dependence and significant medical comorbidity (e.g., COPD, cardiac disease) who underwent an intensive 2-week inpatient program that included use of the transdermal nicotine patch, 29% were still abstinent at 1 year (Hurt et al. 1992).

Nicotine equivalencies of various products are shown in Table 6–3. Although alternative delivery systems provide lower peak nicotine levels and slower onset compared with cigarette smoking, caution is advised in using these products in patients

Table 6–3. Nicotine equivalents

Form of nicotine	Nicotine content	Amount of nicotine delivered
Cigarette	6–11 mg	1–3 mg
Chewing gum	2 mg	1 mg
	4 mg	2 mg
Transdermal patch	15 mg/day (range 7–22 mg, depending on system)	1 mg/hour (variable)
Nasal spray	10 mg/mL	1 mg (0.5 mg/pulse × 2 nostrils)
Oral inhaler	10 mg/cartridge	4 mg total/cartridge

with coronary artery disease, recent myocardial infarction, uncontrolled hypertension, or cardiac dysrhythmias. Nicotine replacement therapies are analogous to benzodiazepine management of alcohol withdrawal; in themselves, they do not constitute a treatment. Moreover, it could be expected that these therapies would eventually have greatest utility in long-term maintenance of patients who cannot be weaned from nicotine.

Many elderly patients are unable to use nicotine in a gum form because of dentures or dental problems. For those who prefer this vehicle, nicotine gum (2 mg) is placed in the mouth and chewed slowly for 20–30 minutes and then discarded. Transdermal patches impregnated with smaller doses of nicotine (e.g., 7, 14, or 15 mg) are generally used for elderly patients. One patch is applied every 24 hours, and the area of the used patch is wiped clean. Insomnia can be alleviated by removing the patch before sleep. It is important that tobacco use not continue while the patch is in use, or nicotine levels can become toxic.

Benzodiazepine Dependence

Long-term use of benzodiazepines by elderly patients may, in some cases, be associated with depression, residual anxiety, cognitive impairment, daytime sedation, ataxia, and poor physical health (Mellinger et al. 1984; Rodrigo et al. 1988). With discontinuation, recurrence and rebound symptoms are sometimes seen; these include anxiety, irritability, insomnia, fatigue, headache, muscle twitching, tremor, sweating, dizziness, and difficulty concentrating. Somewhat less common are true withdrawal symptoms of nausea, anorexia, tinnitus, perceptual distortions, delusions, hallucinations, and seizures. Patients withdrawing from a combination of alcohol and benzodiazepines can show a later-onset, longer-lasting withdrawal syndrome characterized by greater autonomic and psychomotor signs than alcohol withdrawal alone (Benzer and Cushman 1980).

Data regarding the success of treatment for benzodiazepine dependence in elders are sparse. In general, very gradual withdrawal over a period of 1–4 months is preferred, with the final steps of the taper proceeding most slowly. Guidelines for discontinuation of short-acting benzodiazepines (e.g., alprazolam) by way of switching first to a longer-acting agent can be found in Chapter 5 ("Anxiolytic and Sedative-Hypnotic Medications"). β-Blockers may lessen the severity of benzodiazepine withdrawal; the use of atenolol in elders is described later in this chapter in the context of alcohol withdrawal (see "Alcohol-Related Syndromes"). The role of tertiary-amine tricyclic agents such as imipramine in treating elderly patients for benzodiazepine dependence is not yet clear. After benzodiazepine withdrawal is completed, most elderly patients will have significant residual anxiety, depression, and insomnia (Ashton 1987; Golombok et al. 1987; Higgitt et al. 1985). For these symptoms, an SSRI antidepressant with or without co-administered trazodone for insomnia is often helpful.

Barbiturate Dependence

Although prescription of barbiturates and related sedative-hypnotics has declined with the advent of safer drugs such as the benzodiazepines, there remain elderly patients in the community who have been treated long term with these medications. As noted in the chapter on sedative-hypnotics (Chapter 5), the therapeutic index of barbiturates is narrow, and these drugs have numerous side effects, including respiratory depression and induction of various CYP enzymes. When an elderly patient taking a barbiturate on a stable regimen is encountered clinically, a decision has to be made whether it is feasible to undertake a slow taper and discontinuation of that medication. This taper may need to done over a period of 3–6 months or longer.

Narcotic Dependence

In the elderly patient with a prior history of substance abuse, prescription use of narcotics can result in addiction, with escalation of use over time and drug-seeking behaviors. Patient and family education and regular outpatient follow-up are important components of treatment. The narcotic dose is tapered slowly, at a rate of 10% every 3–7 days, to avoid the emergence of the flulike discontinuation syndrome. Comorbid psychiatric conditions such as depression should be treated aggressively.

Substance-Induced Disorders

Alcohol-Related Syndromes

Intoxication

As noted earlier, as a consequence of kinetic and dynamic changes, elders may become intoxicated with smaller amounts of alcohol compared with younger people. Symptoms of intoxication are similar, although falls may be more common in elders. Blackouts—the forgetting of events occurring over several hours while intoxicated, even though consciousness appears normal to observers—can be seen in elders (Rubino 1992). Serious complications of intoxication include coma and death from respiratory depression. When an elderly patient presents in an intoxicated state, BAL can help guide treatment and placement decisions. For example, an alert and nondysarthric patient with a very high BAL (e.g., 250 mg%) is at risk for severe withdrawal because of demonstrated high tolerance (Rubino 1992); this patient should be monitored closely in a supervised setting.

Withdrawal

Symptoms of alcohol withdrawal are attributed to a sudden decrease in GABA neurotransmission and increase in sympathetic activity (Gorelick 1993), increase in activity of the hypothalamic-pituitary-adrenal axis (Merry and Marks 1972), and increased glutamatergic neurotransmission. Symptoms range in severity from tremulousness to hallucinosis, seizures, and delirium tremens. In patients of mixed age, tremor onset is usually within 6–8 hours, hallucinosis within 8–12 hours, seizures within 24 hours, and delirium tremens after 72 hours (Rubino 1992).

Severity of withdrawal is determined with the use of a scale such as the Clinical Institute Withdrawal Assessment for Alcohol—Revised (CIWA-Ar) (Sullivan et al. 1989). This instrument allows the clincian to score withdrawal severity in 10 areas: nausea and vomiting, tremor, paroxysmal sweating, tactile disturbance, auditory disturbance, visual disturbance, anxiety, agitation, headache/fullness in head, and orientation/clouding of sensorium. (The instrument is in the public domain and is readily available on the Internet.) A score of 10 or more on the CIWA-Ar indicates the need for benzodiazepine treatment as a supplement to supportive measures provided to all patients in withdrawal (discussed later in this section). It is worth noting that some specialists use a cut-off score of 8 on the CIWA-Ar to determine whether benzodiazepines are needed.

Patients with a prior history of withdrawal seizures or numerous prior detoxifications are at increased risk for the development of alcohol withdrawal seizures (Brown et al. 1988). The most sensitive predictor of delirium tremens is a history of heavy daily alcohol use; other predictors include a history of delirium tremens or seizures (but not a history of tremulousness or hallucinosis) (Cushman 1987). Older age is the most significant factor in the lethality of delirium tremens (Feuerlein and Reiser 1986), which usually results from cardiovascular events, metabolic disturbances, or infections. Elders going through moderate to severe withdrawal appear to be at higher risk of developing delirium, falls, and dependence in activities of daily living and for these reasons are best treated in a supervised environment (Kraemer et al. 1997). In such a setting, vital signs are monitored, and a scale such as the CIWA-Ar is administered serially to determine ongoing treatment needs.

Supportive measures for all patients in alcohol withdrawal include parenteral thiamine (100 mg/day); adequate nutrition and hydration (usually oral, unless the patient is significantly volume depleted from vomiting or bleeding); and the opportunity to rest in a quiet, supervised environment.

As noted earlier, benzodiazepines are used to prevent the development of severe withdrawal symptoms. For elderly patients, lorazepam is the drug of first choice because it can be given intramuscularly if needed, but equivalent doses of oxazepam may also be used (Hoey et al. 1994). For withdrawal prophylaxis, lorazepam 0.5–1 mg tid is given orally or intramuscularly or intravenously. When mild to moderate withdrawal symptoms are already present, lorazepam 0.5–2 mg im or iv every 3 hours is administered, and haloperidol 0.5–2 mg im or iv every 6–12 hours may be added for persistent hallucinations. The risk in using antipsychotics in this context is that these drugs lower the seizure threshold.

Adjunctive gabapentin is an emerging treatment for alcohol withdrawal that has been noted in a small case series to reduce the total amount of benzodiazepine used (Bonnet et al. 1999). The dose for elderly patients in withdrawal is not established, but in our experience, a dose of gabapentin 300 mg po every 8 hours may be sufficient for this indication.

The addition of a β-blocker (e.g., atenolol) to the benzodiazepine for withdrawal treatment is associated with more rapid resolution of withdrawal symptoms and shorter length of hospital stay (Kraus et al. 1985) and with reduced craving and lower rate of relapse among outpatients (Horwitz et al. 1989). Use of atenolol may obviate the need for an antipsychotic (Horwitz et al. 1989). The dose of atenolol for an elderly patient in withdrawal is 25–50 mg once daily (titrated to heart rate); some patients may require and tolerate a dose of up to 100 mg daily. β-Blockers can precipitate hypoglycemia in malnourished alcohol abusers with large alcohol loads and should be used with caution in patients with COPD or cardiomyopathy (Rubino 1992), as well as diabetes or preexisting bradyarrhythmias.

Clonidine has also been associated with faster resolution of withdrawal symptoms and reduced need for sedation (Baumgartner and Rowen 1987; Bjorkqvist 1975) at doses averaging 0.6 mg daily in nongeriatric samples (Rosenbloom 1988). Since clonidine is initiated in elders at 0.05 mg bid, the required titration period makes this medication less useful for acute withdrawal. In addition, clonidine use can be associated with hypotension in elderly patients.

Alcohol withdrawal seizures are of the generalized tonic-clonic type, with a short postictal period. Adequate treatment of alcohol withdrawal with a benzodiazepine prevents the development of seizures. When a seizure does occur, lorazepam 2 mg iv can prevent recurrence (D'Onofrio et al. 1999). Adjunctive anticonvulsant medications can be used but are usually not required unless the patient has a history of non–alcohol-related seizures.

The occurrence and severity of delirium tremens depends in large part on whether the patient suffers from an intercurrent medical disease (e.g., pneumonia) or injury (Wojnar et al. 1999). Delirium tremens is characterized by extreme autonomic activity (fever, tachycardia, tachypnea, hypertension, tremor, diaphoresis, anxiety, insomnia) and delirium. Delirium tremens represents a medical emergency best treated in a monitored setting with a continuous intravenous infusion of lorazepam or 1- to 3-mg boluses of lorazepam given intravenously every 1–3 hours. Patients with delirium tremens also require rehydration; correction of glucose, magnesium, and phosphate imbalances; supplementation with thiamine and multiple vitamins; and other supportive measures (Newman et al. 1995). Severely psychotic or agitated patients with delirium tremens may also be treated with haloperidol 3-mg boluses given intravenously every 1–2 hours (Newman et al. 1995). Carbamazepine has been used as an alternative to benzodiazepines for moderate to severe alcohol withdrawal (Butler and Messiha 1986; Malcolm et al. 1989; Stuppaeck et al. 1992), but this use has not been adequately studied in geriatric patients.

Alcohol-Induced Persisting Amnestic Disorder

The cardinal sign of alcohol-induced persisting amnestic disorder (alcoholic amnestic disorder, Korsakoff's syndrome) is severe anterograde amnesia that may be associated with retrograde amnesia of variable length. The patient may also be apathetic and demonstrate confabulation but lacks the global cognitive impairment of dementia and the impairment in consciousness of delirium. Amnesia persists beyond the period of alcohol intoxication and withdrawal.

Thiamine deficiency in combination with alcohol neurotoxicity is thought to underlie Wernicke's encephalopathy, the acute phase of the Wernicke-Korsakoff continuum. Untreated or recurrent episodes of encephalopathy provide the pathogenetic link to the persisting amnestic disorder (Korsakoff's syndrome). As in alcohol abusers without Korsakoff's syndrome, generalized brain atrophy with increased cerebrospinal fluid (CSF) volume is seen; in addition, however, patients with alcohol-induced persisting amnestic disorder show atrophy in anterior diencephalic structures such as the septal nuclei and hypothalamic gray (Jernigan et al. 1991). Patients with alcohol amnestic disorder have more severe memory impairment than chronic alcohol abusers that involves verbal as well as visual stimuli (Salmon and Butters 1985).

The core deficit of alcohol-induced persisting amnestic disorder is not currently treatable, although cholinergic enhancing drugs may prove useful for this indication. In addition, limited data suggest that SSRI antidepressants may improve memory function in this condition (Linnoila et al. 1987; Weingartner et al. 1983). For all patients showing signs of Wernicke's encephalopathy, aggressive measures are undertaken to achieve and maintain abstinence in order to prevent the development of the persisting amnestic disorder.

Slowly Resolving Cognitive Deficits (Intermediate Brain Syndrome)

Slowly resolving cognitive deficits (intermediate brain syndrome), a poorly defined and characterized category, refer to residual cognitive deficits still present after 4 weeks of abstinence that show variable improvement over a period of years (Atkinson 2000). This syndrome is seen clinically, possibly more commonly among elders. Deficits can be patchy, focal, or global in distribution. Scant literature suggests that impairments in areas such as psychomotor skill and short-term memory may resolve after 5 or more years of abstinence (Brandt et al. 1983). The relation of this syndrome to (or its overlap with) alcoholic dementia is unclear.

Alcohol-Induced Persisting Dementia

A subset of alcohol-abusing patients develop global cognitive impairment that persists beyond the period of intoxication and withdrawal. Such impairment has been termed *alcohol-induced persisting dementia* (dementia associated with alcoholism, alcoholic dementia). Little is known from systematic study about this diagnostic entity, particularly among elderly patients (Nakada and Knight 1984), and even its existence is controversial. Reported symptoms include amnesia, disturbance in other cortical functions (e.g., apraxia), and impairment in judgment and abstract thinking. Increased CSF volume disproportionate to age is found on head CT or MRI (Pfefferbaum et al. 1993). Among the institutionalized elderly, patients with presumed alcoholic dementia demonstrate milder cognitive deficits and are younger than patients with Alzheimer's disease (Carlen et al. 1994). One feature helpful in distinguishing alcoholic dementia from Alzheimer's disease is the presence of a language deficit (anomia, or inability to name) in the latter that is not a prominent feature of alcoholic dementia. In addition, cerebellar atrophy is much more likely to be found in alcoholic dementia (Ron 1983).

Cognitive function is variably recovered over time with abstinence, and anecdotal experience suggests that recovery takes longer in elderly alcohol abusers. Although the standard on neuropsychiatric units is generally to wait through 2 weeks of abstinence before undertaking neuropsychological testing (Page and Linden 1974), this period might not actually be long enough. Even nongeriatric alcohol abusers who have been abstinent for 4 weeks may have a subacute syndrome of impairment that resolves with further abstinence (Grant et al. 1984). It has been suggested that early improvement might reflect recovery of cortical function, whereas persistent deficits (e.g., in long-term memory) might reflect permanent injury to the diencephalon (Brandt et al. 1983).

Alcohol-Induced Mood Disorder

Elderly patients dependent on alcohol or benzodiazepines may present with a constellation of symptoms highly suggestive of major depression, including depressed mood, insomnia, poor appetite, apathy, disorientation, memory problems, paranoia, and hallucinations (Solomon et al. 1993). In one mixed-age sample, 42% of alcohol-abusing patients were significantly depressed on admission to a treatment unit, but only 6% were still depressed at 4 weeks (Brown and Schuckit 1988). The biggest change in depressive symptoms was seen in the first 2 weeks. For reasons such as these, the standard of care is to wait at least 2 weeks before treating depression in an abstinent alcohol abuser. When depression persists, pharmacological treatment is effective, even if the patient continues to drink (Oslin et al. 2000), although this combination is not advisable from the standpoint of liver function. Moreover, treatment with an SSRI may additionally help to reduce craving. For depression-related insomnia, trazodone can be used in combination with the SSRI.

Cerebellar Degeneration

Persons who chronically abuse alcohol may present with a wide-based stance and ataxia that is more prominent in the lower extremities. On head CT or MRI, cerebellar atrophy is seen, particularly in the anterior and superior vermis and adjacent folia. It is believed that this syndrome is a further consequence of thiamine deficiency (Rubino 1992). Although there is no specific treatment for this condition, symptoms may improve with abstention from alcohol (Nakada and Knight 1984).

Wernicke's Encephalopathy

Wernicke's encephalopathy represents a neurological emergency manifested by the clinical triad of confusion, ataxia, and ocular movement abnormalities (usually horizontal nystagmus) (Rubino 1992). Punctate hemorrhages develop in the gray matter surrounding the third and fourth ventricles, thalamus, hypothalamus, and mammillary bodies. This midline damage may extend to the midline cerebellum and basal forebrain (Willenbring 1988). Treatment consists of parenteral thiamine, glucose, and correction of magnesium deficiency (Nakada and Knight 1984), with avoidance of carbohydrate loading prior to thiamine administration. Most patients who do not recover completely with treatment within the first 48–72 hours will develop Korsakoff's syndrome (Nakada and Knight 1984). Untreated, the syndrome may result in coma and death.

Chapter Summary

- Alcohol abuse should be suspected in any elder presenting with treatment-refractory hypertension or depression, unexplained functional decline, frequent falls, or malnutrition.

- Percent serum carbohydrate-deficient transferrin is a marker for high alcohol consumption and is more sensitive and specific than GGT.

- In treating the elderly alcohol abuser, the clinician should adopt the attitude that every day of sobriety makes a difference in the physical and psychological health of the patient; complete abstinence may be an unachievable goal.

- Pharmacological therapies for alcohol dependence include naltrexone, disulfiram, SSRI antidepressants, and possibly ondansetron and buspirone.

- Caution is advised in using alternative nicotine delivery systems in patients with coronary artery disease, recent myocardial infarction, uncontrolled hypertension, or cardiac dysrhythmias.

- It is important that tobacco use *not* continue while a nicotine patch is in use, or nicotine levels could become toxic.

- In the benzodiazepine-dependent elder, very gradual withdrawal of the drug over a period of 1–4 months is preferred, with the final steps of the taper proceeding most slowly.

- As a consequence of kinetic and dynamic changes, elders may become intoxicated with smaller amounts of alcohol than would younger people.

- Severity of alcohol withdrawal is determined with the use of a scale such as the Clinical Institute Withdrawal Assessment for Alcohol—Revised (CIWA-Ar).

- A score of 10 or more on the CIWA-Ar indicates the need for benzodiazepine treatment in alcohol withdrawal.

- For withdrawal prophylaxis, lorazepam 0.5–1 mg tid is given orally, intramuscularly, or intravenously. When mild to moderate withdrawal symptoms are already present, lorazepam 0.5–2 mg is given intramuscularly or intravenously every 3 hours, and haloperidol 0.5–2 mg im or iv every 6–12 hours may be added for hallucinations.

- For the patient withdrawing from alcohol, the addition of atenolol 25–50 mg qd is associated with more rapid resolution of withdrawal symptoms and shorter length of hospital stay.

- Delirium tremens represents a medical emergency best treated in a monitored setting with a continuous intravenous infusion of lorazepam, or 1- to 3-mg boluses of lorazepam given intravenously every 1–3 hours. Severely psychotic or agitated patients may also be treated with haloperidol 3-mg boluses given intravenously every 1–2 hours.

- Wernicke's encephalopathy represents a neurological emergency manifested by the clinical triad of confusion, ataxia, and ocular movement abnormalities (usually horizontal nystagmus).

- For all patients showing signs of Wernicke's encephalopathy, aggressive measures should be undertaken to achieve and maintain abstinence in order to prevent the development of the persisting amnestic disorder.

- Two features helpful in distinguishing alcoholic dementia from Alzheimer's disease are cerebellar atrophy in the former and a language deficit (i.e., anomia) in the latter.

References

Adams WL, Yuan Z, Barboriak JJ, et al: Alcohol-related hospitalizations of elderly people. JAMA 270:1222–1225, 1993

Ashton H: Benzodiazepine withdrawal: outcome in 50 patients. British Journal of Addiction 82:665–671, 1987

Atkinson RM: Substance abuse, in The American Psychiatric Press Textbook of Geriatric Neuropsychiatry. Edited by Coffey CE, Cummings JL. Washington, DC, American Psychiatric Press, 2000, pp 367–400

Atkinson RM, Tolson RL, Turner JA: Late versus early onset problem drinking in older men. Alcohol Clin Exp Res 14:574–579, 1990

Baumgartner GR, Rowen RC: Clonidine vs chlordiazepoxide in the management of acute alcohol withdrawal syndrome. Arch Intern Med 147:1223–1226, 1987

Benzer D, Cushman P: Alcohol and benzodiazepines: withdrawal syndromes. Alcohol Clin Exp Res 4:243–247, 1980

Bjorkqvist SE: Clonidine in alcohol withdrawal. Acta Psychiatr Scand 52: 256–263, 1975

Blow F: Michigan Alcoholism Screening Test—Geriatric Version (MAST-G). Ann Arbor, University of Michigan Alcohol Research Center, 1991

Bonnet U, Banger M, Leweke FM, et al: Treatment of alcohol withdrawal syndrome with gabapentin. Pharmacopsychiatry 32:107–109, 1999

Bradley KA, McDonell MB, Bush K, et al: The AUDIT alcohol consumption questions: reliability, validity, and responsiveness to change in older male primary care patients. Alcohol Clin Exp Res 22:1842–1849, 1998

Brandt J, Butters N, Ryan C, et al: Cognitive loss and recovery in long-term alcohol abusers. Arch Gen Psychiatry 40:435–442, 1983

Bristow MF, Clare AW: Prevalence and characteristics of at-risk drinkers among elderly acute medical in-patients. British Journal of Addiction 87:291–294, 1992

Brown ME, Anton RF, Malcolm R, et al: Alcohol detoxification and withdrawal seizures: clinical support for a kindling hypothesis. Biol Psychiatry 23:507–514, 1988

Brown SA, Schuckit MA: Changes in depression among abstinent alcoholics. J Stud Alcohol 49:412–417, 1988

Bruno F: Buspirone in the treatment of alcoholic patients. Psychopathology 22 (suppl 1):49–59, 1989

Buchsbaum DG, Buchanan RG, Welsh J, et al: Screening for drinking disorders in the elderly using the CAGE questionnaire. J Am Geriatr Soc 40:662–665, 1992

Bullock ML, Culliton PD, Olander RT: Controlled trial of acupuncture for severe recidivist alcoholism. Lancet 1:1435–1439, 1989

Butler D, Messiha FS: Alcohol withdrawal and carbamazepine. Alcohol 3:113–129, 1986

Carlen PL, Worztman G, Holgate RC, et al: Reversible cerebral atrophy in recently abstinent chronic alcoholics measured by computed tomographic scans. Science 200:1076–1078, 1978

Carlen PL, Penn RD, Fornazzari L, et al: Computerized tomographic scan assessment of alcoholic brain damage and its potential reversibility. Alcohol Clin Exp Res 10:226–232, 1986

Carlen PL, McAndrews MP, Weiss RT, et al: Alcohol-related dementia in the institutionalized elderly. Alcohol Clin Exp Res 18:1330–1334, 1994

Chang MM, Kwon J, Hamada RS, et al: Effect of combined substance use on laboratory markers of alcoholism. J Stud Alcohol 51:361–365, 1990

Croop RS, Faulkner EB, Labriola DF: The safety profile of naltrexone in the treatment of alcoholism. Arch Gen Psychiatry 54:1130–1135, 1997

Cushman P: Delirium tremens: update on an old disorder. Postgrad Med 82:117–122, 1987

Cyr MG, Wartman SA: The effectiveness of routine screening questions in the detection of alcoholism. JAMA 259:51–54, 1988

Denney MR, Baugh JL, Hardt HD: Sobriety outcome after alcoholism treatment with biofeedback participation: a pilot inpatient study. International Journal of the Addictions 26:335–341, 1991

D'Onofrio G, Rathlev NK, Ulrich AS, et al: Lorazepam for the prevention of recurrent seizures related to alcohol. N Engl J Med 340:915–919, 1999

Duckert F, Johnsen J: Behavioral use of disulfiram in the treatment of problem drinking. International Journal of the Addictions 22:445–454, 1987

Feuerlein W, Reiser E: Parameters affecting the course and results of delirium tremens treatment. Acta Psychiatr Scand 73:120–123, 1986

Fleming MF, Manwell LB, Barry KL, et al: Brief physician advice for alcohol problems in older adults: a randomized community-based trial. J Fam Pract 48:378–384, 1999

Fuller RK, Neiderhiser DH: Evaluation and application of urinary diethylamine method to measure compliance with disulfiram therapy. J Stud Alcohol 42:202–207, 1980

Fuller RK, Branchey L, Brightwell DR, et al: Disulfiram treatment of alcoholism: a Veterans Administration cooperative study. JAMA 256:1449–1455, 1986

Golombok S, Higgitt A, Fonagy P, et al: A follow-up study of patients treated for benzodiazepine dependence. Br J Med Psychol 60:141–149, 1987

Gorelick DA: Pharmacological treatment, in Recent Developments in Alcoholism, Edited by Galanter M. New York, Plenum, 1993, pp 413–427

Gorelick DA, Paredes A: Effect of fluoxetine on alcohol consumption in male alcoholics. Alcohol Clin Exp Res 16:261–265, 1992

Grant I, Adams KM, Reed R: Aging, abstinence, and medical risk factors in the prediction of neuropsychologic deficit among long-term alcoholics. Arch Gen Psychiatry 41:710–718, 1984

Higgitt AC, Lader MH, Fonagy P: Clinical management of benzodiazepine dependence. BMJ 291:688–690, 1985

Hoey LL, Nahum A, Vance-Bryan K: A retrospective review and assessment of benzodiazepines in the treatment of alcohol withdrawal in hospitalized patients. Pharmacotherapy 14:572–578, 1994

Holroyd S, Duryee JJ: Substance use disorders in a geriatric psychiatry outpatient clinic: prevalence and epidemiologic characteristics. J Nerv Ment Dis 185:627–632, 1997

Horwitz RI, Gottlieb LD, Kraus ML: The efficacy of atenolol in the outpatient management of the alcohol withdrawal syndrome: results of a randomized clinical trial. Arch Intern Med 149:1089–1093, 1989

Hurt RD, Dale LC, Offord KP, et al: Inpatient treatment of severe nicotine dependence. Mayo Clin Proc 67:823–828, 1992

Jernigan TL, Schafer K, Butters N, et al: Magnetic resonance imaging of alcoholic Korsakoff patients. Neuropsychopharmacol 4:175–186, 1991

Johnson BA, Roache JD, Javors MA, et al: Ondansetron for reduction of drinking among biologically predisposed alcoholic patients: a randomized controlled trial. JAMA 284:963–971, 2000

Jorenby DE, Leischow SJ, Nides MA, et al: A controlled trial of sustained-release bupropion, a nicotine patch, or both for smoking cessation. N Engl J Med 340:685–691, 1999

Kraemer KL, Mayo-Smith MF, Calkins DR: Impact of age on the severity, course, and complications of alcohol withdrawal. Arch Intern Med 157:2234–2241, 1997

Kranzler HR, Meyer RE: An open trial of buspirone in alcoholics (letter). J Clin Psychopharmacol 9:379–380, 1989

Kraus ML, Gottlieb LD, Horwitz RI, et al: Randomized clinical trial of atenolol in patients with alcohol withdrawal. N Engl J Med 313:905–909, 1985

Law M, Tang JL: An analysis of the effectiveness of interventions intended to help people stop smoking. Arch Intern Med 155:1933–1941, 1995

Lesch OM, Walter H, Freitag H, et al: Carbohydrate-deficient transferrin as a screening marker for drinking in a general hospital population. Alcohol Alcohol 31:249–256, 1996

Linnoila M, Eckardt M, Durcan M, et al: Interactions of serotonin with ethanol: clinical and animal studies. Psychopharmacol Bull 23:452–457, 1987

Malcolm R, Ballenger JC, Sturgis ET, et al: Double-blind controlled trial comparing carbamazepine to oxazepam treatment of alcohol withdrawal. Am J Psychiatry 146:617–621, 1989

Mant A, Duncan-Jones P, Saltman D, et al: Development of long term use of psychotropic drugs by general practice patients. BMJ 296:251–254, 1988

Mellinger GD, Balter MB, Uhlenhuth EH: Prevalence and correlates of the long-term regular use of anxiolytics. JAMA 251:375–379, 1984

Merry J, Marks V: The effect of alcohol, barbiturate, and diazepam on hypothalamic-pituitary-adrenal function in chronic alcoholics. Lancet 2:990–991, 1972

Moore RD, Bone LR, Geller G, et al: Prevalence, detection, and treatment of alcoholism in hospitalized patients. JAMA 261:403–407, 1989

Mowe M, Bohmer T: Increased levels of alcohol markers (GGT, MCV, ASAT, ALAT) in older patients are not related to high alcohol intake (letter). J Am Geriatr Soc 44:1136–1137, 1996

Nakada T, Knight RT: Alcohol and the central nervous system. Med Clin North Am 68:121–131, 1984

Nakamura CM, Molgaard CA, Stanford EP, et al: A discriminant analysis of severe alcohol consumption among older persons. Alcohol Alcohol 25:75–80, 1990

Naranjo CA, Bremner KE, Lanctot KL: Effects of citalopram and a brief psycho-social intervention on alcohol intake, dependence and problems. Addiction 90:87–99, 1995

Newman JP, Terris DJ, Moore M: Trends in the management of alcohol withdrawal syndrome. Laryngoscope 105:1–7, 1995

Oslin D, Liberto JG, O'Brien J, et al: Naltrexone as an adjunctive treatment for older patients with alcohol dependence. Am J Geriatr Psychiatry 5:324–332, 1997

Oslin DW, Katz IR, Edell WS, et al: Effects of alcohol consumption on the treatment of depression among elderly patients. Am J Geriatr Psychiatry 8:215–220, 2000

Page RD, Linden JD: "Reversible" organic brain syndrome in alcoholics. Quarterly Journal of Studies on Alcohol 35:98–107, 1974

Paille FM, Guelfi JD, Perkins AC, et al: Double-blind randomized multicentre trial of acamprosate in maintaining abstinence from alcohol. Alcohol Alcohol 30:239–247, 1995

Pfefferbaum A, Rosenbloom M, Crusan K, et al: Brain CT changes in alcoholics: effects of age and alcohol consumption. Alcohol Clin Exp Res 12:81–87, 1988

Pfefferbaum A, Sullivan EV, Rosenbloom MJ, et al: Increase in brain cerebrospinal fluid volume is greater in older than in younger alcoholic patients: a replication study and CT/MRI comparison. Psychiatry Res: Neuroimaging 50:257–274, 1993

Poldrugo F: Acamprosate treatment in a long-term community-based alcohol rehabilitation programme. Addiction 92:1537–1546, 1997

Rodrigo EK, King MB, Williams P: Health of long term benzodiazepine users. BMJ 296:603–606, 1988

Ron MA: The alcoholic brain: CT scan and psychological findings. Psychol Med Monogr Suppl 3:1–33, 1983

Rosenbloom A: Emerging treatment options in the alcohol withdrawal syndrome. J Clin Psychiatry 49 (12, suppl):28–31, 1988

Rosse RB, Riggs RL, Dietrich AM, et al: Frontal cortical atrophy and negative symptoms in patients with chronic alcohol dependence. J Neuropsychiatry Clin Neurosci 9:280–282, 1997

Rubino FA: Neurologic complications of alcoholism. Psychiatr Clin North Am 15:359–372, 1992

Salive ME, Cornoni-Huntley J, LaCroix AZ, et al: Predictors of smoking cessation and relapse in older adults. Am J Public Health 82:1268–1271, 1992

Salmon DP, Butters N: The etiology and neuropathology of alcoholic Korsakoff's syndrome: some evidence for the role of the basal forebrain. J Clin Exp Neuropsychol 7:181–210, 1985

Sellers EM, Higgins GA, Sobell MB: 5-HT and alcohol abuse. Trends Pharmacol Sci 13:69–75, 1992

Solomon K, Manepalli J, Ireland GA, et al: Alcoholism and prescription drug abuse in the elderly: St. Louis University grand rounds. J Am Geriatr Soc 41:57–69, 1993

Spies CD, Neuner B, Neumann T, et al: Intercurrent complications in chronic alcoholic men admitted to the intensive care unit following trauma. Intensive Care Med 22:286–293, 1996

Stuppaeck CH, Pycha R, Miller C, et al: Carbamazepine versus oxazepam in the treatment of alcohol withdrawal: a double-blind study. Alcohol Alcohol 27:153–158, 1992

Sullivan JT, Sykora K, Schneiderman J, et al: Assessment of alcohol withdrawal: the revised Clinical Institute Withdrawal Assessment for Alcohol scale (CIWA-Ar). British Journal of Addiction 84:1353–1357, 1989

Swift RM: Pharmacologic treatments for drug and alcohol dependence: experimental and standard therapies. Psychiatric Annals 23:697–702, 1998

Weingartner H, Buchsbaum MS, Linnoila M: Zimelidine effects on memory impairments produced by ethanol. Life Sci 33:2159–2163, 1983

Whitworth AB, Fischer F, Lesch OM, et al: Comparison of acamprosate and placebo in long-term treatment of alcohol dependence. Lancet 347:1438–1442, 1996

Willenbring ML: Organic mental disorders associated with heavy drinking and alcohol dependence. Clin Geriatr Med 4:869–887, 1988

Wojnar M, Bizon Z, Wasilewski D: The role of somatic disorders and physical injury in the development and course of alcohol withdrawal delirium. Alcohol Clin Exp Res 23:209–213, 1999

7

Treatment of Movement Disorders

In this chapter, we focus on clinically relevant information about diagnosis, differential diagnosis, and basic treatment of selected movement disorders in geriatrics. The chapter is intended to assist geriatricians and geriatric psychiatrists in detecting movement abnormalities, making decisions about neurological or neuropsychiatric referral, and evaluating care provided by consultants. We identify medications effective for various movement-related disorders and provide dosing information when appropriate.

Movement Abnormalities

The first step in diagnosis of a movement disorder is careful observation and description of the movement abnormality. The abnormality is then labeled, using one of the terms defined in this section, and a differential diagnosis of etiology is formulated. Most movement abnormalities can represent either idiopathic or secondary disorders.

Akinesia and Bradykinesia

Akinesia is difficulty initiating movement, and *bradykinesia* is slowing of volitional and many involuntary movements. These are among the most disabling of movement difficulties and significantly affect quality of life as well as ability to perform activities of daily living. Akinesia/bradykinesia result in many other symptoms, including masklike facies (decreased blinking), drooling (decreased swallowing), hypophonia, and micrographia.

Athetosis

Athetosis refers to slow, writhing dystonic movements that occur distally (in fingers, for example). Athetosis may be seen in combination with chorea as choreoathetosis.

Chorea

Chorea refers to arrhythmic, jerky, purposeless involuntary movements occurring in a random sequence. The movements can be brisk or slow and involve limbs, face, or trunk. Etiologies of chorea in elderly patients are listed in Table 7–1. Movement disorders in which chorea is prominent include tardive dyskinesia, Huntington's disease, and edentulous dyskinesia.

Dystonia

Involuntary, sustained muscle contraction resulting in twisting, unusual postures or repetitive movements is termed *dystonia*. Dystonia is classified as focal (e.g., blepharospasm, torticollis, writer's cramp), segmental (e.g., Meige's syndrome), hemidystonic (e.g., secondary to stroke or tumor), multifocal, or generalized (Kishore and Calne 1997). Causes of late-onset dystonia are listed in Table 7–2. Dystonia at rest is usually a more severe

Table 7–1. Etiologies of chorea in elderly patients

Hereditary diseases

  Huntington's disease

  Neuroacanthocytosis

  Benign hereditary chorea

Other CNS degenerations

  Olivopontocerebellar atrophy

  Machado-Joseph disease

  Kufs disease

  Dentatorubropallidoluysian atrophy

Aging related

  Spontaneous orofacial dyskinesia

  Edentulous orodyskinesia

  "Senile chorea"

Drug induced

  Neuroleptics, metoclopramide, flunarizine, cinnarizine, antiparkinsonian drugs, lithium, benzodiazepines, TCAs, MAOIs, carbamazepine, amphetamines, methylphenidate, methadone, steroids, estrogens (including vaginal cream), antihistamines, α-methyldopa, anticonvulsants (phenytoin, ethosuximide, carbamazepine, and phenobarbital), digoxin, methadone, toluene, other drugs

Metabolic

  Hyperthyroidism

  Hypoparathyroidism

  Hypo- and hypernatremia, hypomagnesemia, and hypocalcemia

  Hypo- and hyperglycemia

  Acquired hepatocerebral degeneration, Wilson's disease

Infectious

  Encephalitis

  Subacute bacterial endocarditis

  Creutzfeldt-Jakob disease

Table 7–1. Etiologies of chorea in elderly patients *(continued)*

Toxins

    Alcohol intoxication/withdrawal, anoxia, carbon monoxide, manganese, mercury, toluene, thallium

Immunological

    Systemic lupus erythematosus

    Sydenham's chorea (recurrence)

    Primary anticardiolipin antibody syndrome

Vascular

    Infarctions (usually involving striatum, subthalamic nucleus)

    Hemorrhage

    Arteriovenous malformation

    Polycythemia rubra vera

    Migraine

Tumors

Trauma: subdural hematoma

Miscellaneous: including paroxysmal choreoathetosis

Note. CNS = central nervous system; MAOI = monoamine oxidase inhibitor; TCA = tricyclic antidepressant.
Source. Adapted from Jackson GR, Lang AE: "Hyperkinetic Movement Disorders," in *The American Psychiatric Press Textbook of Geriatric Neuropsychiatry,* 2nd Edition. Edited by Coffey CE, Cummings JL. Washington, DC, American Psychiatric Press, 2000, pp. 531–557. Used with permission.

symptom than action dystonia such as writer's cramp. Dystonia is relieved by sleep and rest and worsened by stress, fatigue, and emotional upset (Kishore and Calne 1997). Patients can sometimes suppress dystonias with sensory "tricks" such as touching the skin around a blepharospastic eye (Kishore and Calne 1997). Along with other dystonias, writer's cramp can be effectively treated with periodic injections of botulinum toxin into forearm muscles (Jankovic and Schwartz 1993). Acute and tardive dystonias secondary to neuroleptic drug exposure are discussed later in this section (see "Drug-Induced Syndromes").

Table 7–2. Etiologies of late-onset dystonia

Idiopathic dystonia

Generalized dystonia (rare)

Segmental/multifocal dystonia

Focal dystonias

  Spasmodic torticollis

  Cranial dystonia: blepharospasm, oromandibular dystonia, spasmodic
   dysphonia

  Writer's cramp

Secondary dystonia

Drugs: including neuroleptics (including metoclopramide), dopamine
  receptor agonists, anticonvulsants, antimalarial drugs

Stroke: hemorrhage or infarction

Other focal lesions: vascular malformation, tumor, abscess,
  demyelination

Trauma: head injury or peripheral injury and subdural
  hematoma

Encephalitis

Toxins: manganese, carbon monoxide poisoning, methanol, carbon
  disulfide

Paraneoplastic

Hypoparathyroidism

Central pontine myelinolysis

Degenerative diseases

  Parkinson's disease

  Progressive supranuclear palsy

  Cortical-basal ganglionic degeneration

  Multiple system atrophy

Disorders simulating dystonia

Psychogenic dystonia

Atlantoaxial subluxation

Seizures

Posterior fossa tumor

Oculomotor disturbance

Source. Adapted from Jackson GR, Lang AE: "Hyperkinetic Movement Disorders," in *The American Psychiatric Press Textbook of Geriatric Neuropsychiatry,*
2nd Edition. Edited by Coffey CE, Cummings JL. Washington, DC, American Psychiatric Press, 2000, pp. 531–557. Used with permission.

Hemiballismus

Hemiballismus is a flinging, rotatory movement occurring with infarcts or tumors of the subthalamic nucleus. Symptoms often resolve spontaneously over several weeks. Reserpine, haloperidol, or clozapine may be useful.

Myoclonus

In *myoclonus,* movements are sudden, brief, shocklike, and usually irregular. Myoclonus can be focal, multifocal, segmental, or generalized. It can frequently be triggered by stimuli such as noise, light, touch, or muscle stretch (as with asterixis). Myoclonus can be distinguished from tremor by distinct pauses between jerks. It can be distinguished from tics by suppressibility of the latter. In elderly patients, myoclonus is most commonly secondary to metabolic disorders, infections, drugs, hypoxia, or degenerative disease. A more complete list of etiologies of myoclonus in elderly patients is shown in Table 7–3.

Rigidity

Rigidity is an increase in muscle tone during passive movement, usually more evident around distal joints. Lead-pipe rigidity is smooth, whereas cogwheeling is ratchety because it incorporates a tremor. For examination of rigidity to be carried out, the patient must be capable of relaxing the tested limb. Rigidity secondary to medications or other causes is often (but not always) symmetric; asymmetric rigidity may suggest the presence of Parkinson's disease (Kishore and Calne 1997).

Tics

Tics are involuntary, rapid, repetitive, stereotyped vocalizations or movements. They can be simple (e.g., blinking, shrugging, throat clearing, sniffing) or complex (e.g., touching, obscene gestures, echolalia, coprolalia). They are worsened by stress, anxiety, and fatigue and may be relieved by concentration on another task. Tics are usually multifocal, but they commonly involve the upper

Table 7–3. Etiologies of myoclonus in elderly patients

Physiological myoclonus
Hiccups, sleep starts, exercise-induced, anxiety-induced
Essential myoclonus
Secondary myoclonus
Metabolic causes
  Hepatic failure, renal failure, dialysis syndrome, hyponatremia,
    hypoglycemia, nonketotic hyperglycemia
Viral encephalopathies
  Herpes simplex encephalitis, arbovirus encephalitis, encephalitis
    lethargica, postinfectious encephalomyelitis
Drugs: TCAs, levodopa, MAOIs, antibiotics, lithium, SSRIs
Toxins: bismuth, heavy metal poisons, methyl bromide, DDT
Physical encephalopathies
  Postanoxic (Lance-Adams syndrome)
  Posttraumatic
  Heat stroke
  Electric shock
  Decompression injury
Dementing and degenerative diseases
  Creutzfeldt-Jakob disease
  Alzheimer's disease
  Cortical-basal ganglionic degeneration
  Parkinson's disease
  Huntington's disease
  Multiple system atrophy
  Pallidal degenerations
Focal central nervous system damage
  Poststroke
  Olivodentate lesions (palatal myoclonus)
  Spinal cord lesions (segmental/spinal myoclonus)
  Tumor
  Trauma
  Postthalamotomy (often unilateral asterixis)

Note. DDT = dichlorodiphenyltrichloroethane; MAOI = monoamine oxidase inhibitor; SSRI = selective serotonin reuptake inhibitor; TCA = tricyclic antidepressant.
Source. Adapted from Jackson and Lang 2000 with permission.

body. The subjective experience is one of a buildup of tension, with relief when the movement occurs. Patients may be able to suppress tics temporarily. They occur during all stages of sleep (Kishore and Calne 1997). In elderly patients, tics can be seen after head injury or stroke, with certain medications, or in mentally retarded individuals. A more complete list of etiologies of tics in elderly patients is shown in Table 7–4.

Table 7–4. Etiologies of tics in elderly patients

Idiopathic

  Persistent childhood-onset tic disorder

  Simple tic

  Multiple motor tics

  Tourette's disorder (multiple motor and vocal tics)

  Adult-onset tic disorder

Secondary

  Postencephalitic

  Head injury

  Carbon monoxide poisoning

  Poststroke

  Drugs: stimulants, levodopa, neuroleptics, carbamazepine, phenytoin, phenobarbital

  Mental retardation syndromes (including chromosomal abnormalities)

Source. Adapted from Jackson GR, Lang AE: "Hyperkinetic Movement Disorders," in *The American Psychiatric Press Textbook of Geriatric Neuropsychiatry,* 2nd Edition. Edited by Coffey CE, Cummings JL. Washington, DC, American Psychiatric Press, 2000, pp. 531–557. Used with permission.

Tremor

Tremor is rhythmic oscillation of a body part, often seen in the hands and head. Tremors can be coarse or fine and can vary in frequency. Types of tremor include resting, postural, and kinetic. In some classifications, kinetic is further subdivided into simple kinetic and intentional, the latter present during target-directed movements (Deuschl et al. 1998). Tremor is tested first by observation of the patient sitting, with hands on thighs (resting); after this observation, the patient is asked to extend his or her arms away from the body (kinetic) and hold them out parallel to the floor (postural); the patient is then asked to touch a target, such as the examiner's finger (intentional). Latent resting and postural tremors may be elicited by asking the patient to perform a distracting activity such as drawing a "figure 8" in the air while the examiner observes the other hand. Etiologies of tremor in elderly patients are listed in Table 7–5. Important tremor syndromes discussed in the treatment section include Parkinson's disease, drug-induced tremor, and essential tremor.

Table 7–5. Etiologies of tremor in elderly patients

Resting tremor
  Parkinson's disease
  Secondary parkinsonian syndromes
  Rubral (midbrain) tremor
  Essential tremor (only if severe)
Postural tremor
  Physiological tremor
  Exaggerated physiological tremor
    Endocrine: hypoglycemia, thyrotoxicosis, pheochromocytoma, steroids
    Drugs/toxins: β-adrenergic receptor agonists, dopamine receptor agonists, lithium, TCAs, neuroleptics, theophylline, caffeine, valproate, amphetamines, alcohol withdrawal, mercury, lead, arsenic, and others
  Essential tremor
  Primary writing tremor
  Parkinson's disease
  Other akinetic-rigid syndromes
  Idiopathic dystonia (including focal dystonia)
  Tremor with peripheral neuropathy
  Cerebellar tremor

Table 7–5.   Etiologies of tremor in elderly patients *(continued)*

Kinetic tremor (simple or intentional)

  Disease of cerebellar "outflow" (dentate nucleus and superior cerebellar peduncle)

  Vascular

  Tumor

  Acquired hepatocerebral degeneration

  Drugs/toxins (e.g., mercury)

  Multiple sclerosis

Miscellaneous tremor syndromes

  Psychogenic tremor

  Orthostatic tremor

  Rhythmical myoclonus (e.g., palatal, spinal)

  Asterixis

  Clonus

  Epilepsia partialis continua

Note.   TCA = tricyclic antidepressant.
Source.   Adapted from Jackson GR, Lang AE: "Hyperkinetic Movement Disorders," in *The American Psychiatric Press Textbook of Geriatric Neuropsychiatry*, 2nd Edition. Edited by Coffey CE, Cummings JL. Washington, DC, American Psychiatric Press, 2000, pp. 531–557. Used with permission.

Treatment of Selected Movement Disorders

Degenerative Disorders

Corticobasal Degeneration

Corticobasal degeneration is a progressive disease with motor signs of rigidity, akinesia/bradykinesia, kinetic and postural tremor, dystonia, and myoclonus, as well as cortical impairment (dementia) and an alien hand phenomenon (Watts et al. 1997). It usually has an asymmetric onset, and structural and functional neuroimaging abnormalities may be asymmetric, as shown in Table 7–6. Symptoms are not responsive to levodopa or dopamine agonists. Kinetic tremor and myoclonus may respond to clonazepam, and rigidity may respond to baclofen (Watts et al. 1997). In the early stages of the disease, kinetic tremor may also respond to propranolol. Management largely revolves around physical, occupational, and speech therapy (Watts et al. 1997).

Dementia With Lewy Bodies

Dementia with Lewy bodies presents as if it were a combination of Parkinson's disease and Alzheimer's disease, with prominent motor as well as cortical impairment. Myoclonus and absence of resting tremor are an order of magnitude more likely than in Parkinson's disease (Louis et al. 1997). Motor signs either are poorly responsive to levodopa or may respond partially at extremely low doses (e.g., Sinemet 10/100 mg daily). Clozapine at very low doses (e.g., 12.5 mg daily) is associated with improvement in motor signs for some patients, and other atypical antipsychotics (quetiapine and olanzapine, but not risperidone) may also be helpful. Donepezil and other acetylcholinesterase inhibitors often have positive motor as well as cognitive effects, as noted in the chapter on the treatment of dementia (see Chapter 8).

Huntington's Disease

Huntington's disease, characterized by chorea, personality or mood changes, and dementia, usually has an onset earlier in life. It can be distinguished from tardive dyskinesia by the more prominent appearance in Huntington's disease of forehead chorea, flowing movements, dysarthria, facial apraxia, impersistence of tongue protrusion, oculomotor defects, gait disorder, postural instability, and swallowing difficulties, and the more prominent appearance in tardive dyskinesia of mouth movements and stereotyped movements (Wojcieszek and Lang 1994). When Huntington's disease does appear later in life, it often progresses more slowly and involves less severe cognitive impairment compared with early-onset forms (Myers et al. 1985). Neuroimaging abnormalities in Huntington's disease are listed in Table 7–6.

The movement abnormalities of Huntington's disease sug-

Table 7–6. Neuroimaging in selected movement disorders

Movement disorder	Structural (MRI) findings	Functional (PET) findings
Huntington's disease	Caudate atrophy	Hypometabolism in caudate and frontal lobes
Wilson's disease	Hypo- or hyperintensities in basal ganglia, thalamus, midbrain, and frontal lobes	Hypometabolism in striatum, frontal-parietal cortices, and white matter; reduced fluorodopa uptake
Parkinson's disease	Normal	Reduced fluorodopa uptake in striatum, especially putamen; hypermetabolism in pallidum by FDG scan
Progressive supra-nuclear palsy	Midbrain atrophy	Reduced fluorodopa uptake in striatum
Multisystem atrophy (Shy-Drager syndrome)	Cerebellar and brain stem atrophy; hyperintensity in dorsolateral putamen	Reduced fluorodopa uptake in caudate and putamen; hypometabolism in frontal lobes and striatum by FDG scan
Corticobasal degeneration	Contralateral and later bilateral frontoparietal atrophy	Asymmetric hypometabolism in parietal and frontal lobes by FDG scan; asymmetric reduction of fluorodopa uptake in striatum

Note. FDG = fluorodeoxyglucose; MRI = magnetic resonance imaging; PET = positron emission tomography.
Source. Adapted from Kishore A, Calne DB: "Approach to the Patient With a Movement Disorder and Overview of Movement Disorders," in *Movement Disorders: Neurologic Principles and Practice.* Edited by Watts RL, Koller WC. New York, McGraw-Hill, 1997, pp. 3–14. Copyright 1997, McGraw-Hill Companies. Used with permission.

gest overactivity of the dopaminergic system. In the early stages of the disease, dopamine$_2$ (D$_2$) receptor antagonists active in the dorsal striatum such as haloperidol may be helpful; usual antipsychotic doses are employed. Atypical antipsychotics, with the possible exception of risperidone, are likely much less useful for this indication.

Parkinson's Disease and Parkinsonism

The classic parkinsonian triad consists of rigidity, akinesia, and tremor. Posture is stooped, steps are small and shuffling, balance is unsteady, and the patient exhibits decreased arm swing, en bloc turns, and festination (accelerating, shuffling gait). These features of Parkinson's disease are associated with a greatly increased risk of falls. Parkinson's disease may also be associated with dementia, depression, and generalized anxiety, syndromes discussed in other chapters. Idiopathic Parkinson's disease is distinguished from secondary parkinsonism by the prominence of resting tremor, asymmetry of signs and symptoms, and better response to levodopa therapy (Lang and Lozano 1998a, 1998b). Parkinson's disease is distinguished from other neurodegenerative disorders by clinical examination findings (see below) and neuroimaging features, as shown in Table 7–6.

Anticholinergic medications are not recommended for treatment of Parkinson's disease in elderly patients because of an unfavorable risk-benefit ratio (Lang and Lozano 1998a, 1998b). Amantadine and the selective monoamine oxidase–B (MAO-B) inhibitor selegiline are used but provide moderate benefit at best (Lang and Lozano 1998a, 1998b). With selegiline, it may be advisable to coprescribe pyridoxine (vitamin B$_6$) 100 mg daily to prevent development of peripheral neuropathy.

Levodopa and dopamine agonists are the mainstays of treatment for Parkinson's disease. Levodopa is the most effective therapy and is associated with a better outcome if initiated before severe disability develops (Lang and Lozano 1998a, 1998b). In general, levodopa is more consistently effective for rigidity and akinesia than for tremor.

Carbidopa–levodopa (Sinemet) is initiated in elderly patients at a dose of one-half of a 25/100 tablet bid (25 = mg carbidopa; 100 = mg levodopa); this is increased every week by ½ to 1 tablet (Scharre and Mahler 1994) to an initial target dose of 25/100 tid (Charles and Davis 1996). Further increases are made slowly and titrated to clinical effect, with the goal of alleviating disability rather than eliminating all symptoms. Food affects levodopa absorption significantly, so this medication should be given consistently with respect to meals, preferably on an empty stomach. Immediate-release levodopa effects peak in 1 hour and last 3–8 hours.

After a variable number of years taking levodopa, motor complications often occur (Scharre and Mahler 1994). These include dyskinesias (chorea, dystonia, myoclonus), earlier "wearing off" with time after a dose, and unpredictable periods in which parkinsonian symptoms acutely and transiently recur (known as "on-off" phenomena). Levodopa-induced dyskinesias may respond to a gradual lowering of levodopa dosage or to the addition of low-dose clozapine (25–30 mg daily) (Pierelli et al. 1998). Controlled-release (CR) Sinemet does not alleviate dyskinesias or "on-off" phenomena, but it does reduce "wearing off." Levodopa and other dopamine receptor agonists are tapered on discontinuation because of the risk of inducing neuroleptic malignant syndrome (NMS) when stopped abruptly.

When levodopa at a total daily dose of 1,000 mg is ineffective for controlling symptoms of Parkinson's disease, a dopamine receptor agonist is added (Scharre and Mahler 1994). Drugs currently marketed for this indication include the ergot derivatives bromocriptine (Parlodel) and pergolide (Permax) and the newer, nonergoline agents pramipexole (Mirapex) and ropinirole (ReQuip). In general, the nonergoline drugs have better side-effect profiles than the ergot derivatives, which have been associated with pulmonary infiltrates, skin inflammation, paresthesias, and other adverse effects. All dopaminergic drugs have side effects, however, and since some are shared with levodopa, these medications are best dosed apart in time when used in combination.

Catechol-O-methyltransferase (COMT) inhibitors such as tolcapone and entacapone prolong the action of levodopa and increase brain concentrations of dopamine, thus reducing "wearing off" effects (Gottwald et al. 1997). These agents lack antiparkinsonian activity when administered alone. When these agents are used in combination with levodopa, adverse effects such as hallucinations or increased dyskinesias may necessitate a reduction in levodopa dose (Lang and Lozano 1998a, 1998b).

Pallidotomy is considered for a subset of patients, mainly those with disabling dyskinesias that limit therapy with dopaminergic medications (Samuel et al. 1998). In general, symptoms that are resistant to dopaminergic therapy do not respond to surgical intervention (Lang et al. 1997). Surgery results primarily in contralateral improvement in symptoms and, in many cases, a better response to levodopa. Reported complications have included death, stroke, visual defects, paralysis, speech and swallowing problems, and cognitive impairment ("Pallidotomy for Parkinson's Disease" *The Medical Letter* 1996). Different outcomes reported by different surgical centers may be related to the specific location of the surgical lesion in the globus pallidus (Gross et al. 1999; Ondo et al. 1998).

Deep-brain stimulation with implantable electrodes is increasingly used as an alternative to surgery for Parkinson's disease patients and others with severe tremor syndromes. A recent randomized trial found that continuous thalamic stimulation was as effective as thalamotomy for this indication, resulted in greater functional improvement, and was associated with fewer adverse effects than ablative surgery (Schuurman et al. 2000). ECT may also be useful for motor symptoms of Parkinson's disease.

Progressive Supranuclear Palsy

Progressive supranuclear palsy is characterized by the unusual constellation of impaired vertical gaze, prominent axial rigidity, extensor posturing of the neck, early dysarthria, symmetrical onset of parkinsonism (without prominent tremor), frequent falls, and frontal lobe dementia (Golbe 1997; Kishore and Calne 1997).

Neuroimaging findings for this disorder are listed in Table 7–6. In general, pharmacotherapy is ineffective. Limited benefit is seen for some patients treated with carbidopa–levodopa, amantadine, cholinergic agents, and amitriptyline (Golbe 1997). Botulinum toxin injection may be helpful for certain dystonic symptoms, while ECT has been reported to make motor and cognitive symptoms worse (Golbe 1997).

Drug-Induced Syndromes

Akathisia

Akathisia is a subjective feeling of restlessness, with an irresistible urge to move. It is thus often not classified as a "movement disorder" per se, although the observed behavior consists of pacing, stomping, tapping, running, and crossing and uncrossing of legs. It is often mislabeled as "agitation" in elderly patients. The excessive motor activity of akathisia particularly involves the lower extremities. Akathisia is the most common neurological adverse effect of neuroleptic medications. It can occur acutely, subacutely, or as a tardive syndrome. The preferred treatment for akathisia is a switch to an atypical antipsychotic, although lowering the dose of a typical neuroleptic can be effective. Propranolol 20–80 mg daily or a benzodiazepine such as lorazepam can lessen symptom severity. Anticholinergic medication is generally not helpful. The syndrome of tardive akathisia is especially pernicious and requires treatment with medication such as reserpine (Burke et al. 1989).

Dystonia (Acute)

Acute dystonia is a movement disorder that involves sustained muscle contraction, often affecting the neck and face musculature, that may occur within minutes to hours of neuroleptic exposure. The neck is seen to twist and to pull back (retrocollis), the jaw muscles may lock, and blepharospasm may occur. Other manifestations include oculogyric crisis or opisthotonos. Less commonly, laryngeal musculature is affected, with respiratory compromise.

Dystonia occurs less frequently in elderly than in younger patients but is seen in geriatric populations. The acute disorder is treated with benztropine (Cogentin) 0.5–1 mg or diphenhydramine (Benadryl) 25 mg im or iv. This can be followed up with a oral anticholinergic, given for a temporary period while the dose of neuroleptic is lowered or a switch is made to an atypical antipsychotic. Indefinite continuation of the anticholinergic is often associated with adverse events such as delirium, constipation, and urinary retention in elderly patients.

Neuroleptic Malignant Syndrome

As noted in the chapter on antipsychotic medications (Chapter 2), the central features of NMS include high fever, muscle rigidity of the lead-pipe variety, fluctuating consciousness, and autonomic instability. Laboratory abnormalities typically include elevations in creatine kinase, white blood cell count (often with left shift), and liver function tests. Acute renal failure can occur as a consequence of myoglobinuria. In our experience, formes frustes of NMS may be seen in elderly patients, with less extreme muscle rigidity and temperature elevation, that nonetheless respond to usual treatments for NMS. NMS is often complicated by comorbid medical illness. As noted in the discussion of NMS in Chapter 2, the derangement of dopaminergic neurotransmission in this disorder may be a consequence of neuroleptic use or abrupt withdrawal of medications used for Parkinson's disease, or (more rarely) of lithium or SSRI use.

Neuroleptic malignant syndrome represents a medical emergency that is managed in a monitored setting, with aggressive hydration and cooling, and treatment of comorbid medical illness. These are the mainstays of treatment. ECT can also be very effective as a treatment for NMS. Specific pharmacological interventions may or may not be used; these include amantadine 100 mg orally or via nasogastric (NG) tube bid, titrated up to 200 mg bid as tolerated; bromocriptine 2.5 mg orally or via NG tube tid, titrated up to 10 mg tid as tolerated; and sodium dantrolene 1 mg/kg, repeated up to a cumulative dose of 10 mg/kg/day. When the patient has been stabilized, intravenous dantrolene may be switched to oral dantrolene 4–8 mg/kg/day in four divided doses. For patients who have been administered decanoate medications, very slow clearance is highly problematic when NMS is present; plasmapheresis has been used successfully in some cases (Gaitini et al. 1997).

Parkinsonism

Along with vascular (arteriosclerotic) disease, medications are the most common cause of secondary parkinsonism in elders (Miller and Jankovic 1990; Scharre and Mahler 1994). Other causes are listed in Table 7–7. In contrast to idiopathic parkinsonism, medication-induced parkinsonism is more often characterized by the absence of tremor and the presence of prominent bilateral rigidity and akinesia/bradykinesia. Neuroleptics are most often implicated, although lithium, SSRI antidepressants, and other medications can also underlie this syndrome.

Treatment of drug-induced parkinsonism consists of discontinuation of the offending agent, although the parkinsonism in some cases persists for months to years after the drug is discontinued. Amantadine 50–100 mg bid may be useful in some cases, as may low doses of anticholinergic medications.

Tardive Dyskinesia

A variety of tardive syndromes have been described, including tardive dystonia, tardive akathisia, tardive tremor, and tardive myoclonus. The most prevalent tardive syndrome is tardive stereotypy, often referred to as *tardive dyskinesia* (TD) (Stacy et al. 1993). The clinical appearance is of mouthing, chewing, puckering, smacking, sucking, licking, and other orolingual movements. Choreic movements of fingers, hands, arms, and feet are also seen. Associated speech abnormalities include impaired phonation, intelligibility, and slowed rate of production (Khan et al. 1994). Most cases of TD are not severely debilitating.

A less common manifestation of TD is respiratory dyskinesia, with irregular respiratory movements, dyspnea, grunting, and

Table 7–7. Causes of secondary parkinsonism

Atherosclerosis

Degeneration

  Basal ganglia calcification (Fahr's disease)

  Dementia with Lewy bodies

  Olivopontocerebellar atrophy

  Parkinson-dementia complex of Guam

  Progressive supranuclear palsy

  Shy-Drager syndrome

  Striatonigral degeneration

  Wilson's disease

Drug-induced

  Antipsychotics

  Lithium

  Metoclopramide

  Methyldopa

  Reserpine

Endocrine

  Hypoparathyroidism

  Hypothyroidism

Hydrocephalus, normal pressure

Infection

  AIDS

  Creutzfeldt-Jakob disease

  Postencephalitic (von Economo's) encephalitis

Intoxication

  Carbon monoxide

  Manganese

  MPTP

Traumatic encephalopathy

Tumors or masses, basal ganglia

  Arteriovenous malformations

  Neoplasms

Note. MPTP = 1-methyl-4-phenyl-1,2,5,6-tetrahydropyridin E.

gasping (Kruk et al. 1995). Complications of this syndrome include respiratory alkalosis and aspiration pneumonia. TD has also been reported to present as severe dysphagia as an isolated movement abnormality (Gregory et al. 1992).

Tardive dyskinesia has traditionally been understood as a syndrome of abnormal involuntary movements occurring in association with chronic neuroleptic therapy. In fact, the syndrome can be observed in drug-naive elders. Moreover, in cases in which neuroleptics were used, therapy might not have been chronic; TD has been identified in 3.4% of older patients after 1 month and 5.9% of older patients after 3 months of taking neuroleptics (Jeste et al. 1999b). The elderly are particularly at risk; the prevalence of TD among institutionalized elderly is 60% (Byne et al. 1998). For this population, it is important that assessments for dyskinetic movements be made regularly, with a standardized assessment instrument such as the Abnormal Involuntary Movement Scale (Psychopharmacology Research Branch 1976). For elderly patients on stable antipsychotic doses, these assessments are made every 3–6 months.

Risk factors for TD include longer duration of antipsychotic use, co-administration of anticholinergic drugs, presence of an affective disorder, alcohol abuse/dependence, degenerative brain disease, diabetes (Casey 1997; Jeste et al. 1995), history of interruption of neuroleptic treatment (van Harten et al. 1998), extrapyramidal signs early in treatment (Woerner et al. 1998), presence of "negative" symptoms (Liddle et al. 1993), and high serum ferritin levels (Wirshing et al. 1998). The risk of TD can be reduced by using atypical antipsychotics in preference to conventional neuroleptics (Jeste et al. 1999a; Kane 1999), by minimizing the dose of neuroleptic used (Morgenstern and Glazer 1993), and possibly by avoiding routine use of adjunctive anticholinergic medications (Bergen et al. 1992). When symptoms of TD occur, these same preventive measures may be helpful in halting its progression. Taper and discontinuation of a typical neuroleptic will result in remission of TD in up to one-half of cases. In addition, specific treatments are available that result in variable symptomatic improvement. These include atypical antipsychotics, β-blockers, calcium channel blockers, benzodiazepines, and vitamin E.

Clozapine, risperidone, and olanzapine used at usual geriatric doses (see Chapter 2) have been reported to be associated with symptomatic improvement in TD (Chouinard 1995). Olanzapine has also been used to treat respiratory dyskinesia (Gotto 1999). Anecdotally, propranolol at dosages of up to 30 mg tid is reported to be effective in treating TD in elderly patients. Of calcium channel blockers, nifedipine has been found most effective and diltiazem least effective (Cates et al. 1993; Loonen et al. 1992). With nifedipine, better response was seen in cases of severe TD, among elderly patients, and at higher doses (e.g., 80 mg) (Cates et al. 1993; Kushnir and Ratner 1989). Clonazepam was found to improve TD symptoms in nongeriatric patients, especially dystonic symptoms (Thaker et al. 1990). The dose of clonazepam used for geriatric patients for this purpose should not exceed 2 mg daily.

Data regarding the efficacy of vitamin E in the treatment of TD are conflicting (Adler et al. 1993; Dabiri et al. 1994; Egan et al. 1992; Elkashef et al. 1990; Shriqui et al. 1992). Methodological problems such as excessive dropout rates have plagued even the best studies (Lohr and Caligiuri 1996). Some of the discrepancy in outcomes could be attributed to inadequate vitamin E doses or short follow-up in certain of the studies. It appears that vitamin E is most effective in cases in which symptoms are of fewer than 5 years' duration (Lohr and Caligiuri 1996). Vitamin E is initiated at 400 IU daily, and the dosage is increased by 400 IU each week until a dosage of 800 IU bid is achieved. Side effects are benign and are mostly gastrointestinal in nature. Since it has known antioxidant effects, and given its benign side-effect profile, some clinicians recommend vitamin E routinely for patients who are taking conventional neuroleptics on a long-term basis.

The prognosis for patients with TD (stereotypy) is not as grim as was once believed. Even in older, institutionalized patients, 30% improve over time and 28% recover completely (Cavallaro et al. 1993). In population studies, prevalence is stable over 10 years of treatment, even when conventional neuroleptics continue to be used (Gardos et al. 1994). The problem is that it is impossible to predict which patients will suffer the (probably rare) outcome of relentless disease progression. For this reason, it is recommended that use of conventional antipsychotics be minimized. Tardive akathisia does carry a worse prognosis in that it is often persistent and treatment resistant.

Tardive Dystonia

Tardive dystonia can occur as a consequence of neuroleptic exposure. Like acute dystonia, tardive dystonia is not common in elderly patients, but it has been reported (Kiriakakis et al. 1998). It is usually focal initially, involving the craniocervical region, but is progressive in most cases. It rarely remits completely (Gironell et al. 1999) and causes significant pain and disability (Wojcik et al. 1991). Treatment involves discontinuation of the neuroleptic and a switch to clozapine (or possibly another atypical antipsychotic). Tardive dystonia is the one tardive syndrome for which anticholinergic agents (e.g., benztropine) may be useful. In addition, botulinum toxin injection may be helpful, as it is for other dystonias (Jankovic and Brin 1991).

Tremor

As noted earlier, tremor is a less prominent manifestation of drug-induced parkinsonism than of idiopathic Parkinson's disease. When it occurs with neuroleptic use, it is often symmetric at onset. One tremor variant is the *rabbit syndrome,* which involves muscles of the perinasal and oral region. Drug-induced tremors usually abate when the neuroleptic is discontinued. If ongoing therapy is required, a switch to an atypical antipsychotic or to a less-potent neuroleptic is indicated.

Neuroleptics and a large number of other psychotropic agents can also cause an exaggeration of physiological tremor that is usually postural. Some of these medications are listed in Table 7–5. These tremors often require little intervention, other than reassurance. When these tremors are persistent and disabling, usual management involves withdrawal of the offending drug. It has been observed clinically that fine drug-induced tremors may become more coarse with the development of drug-induced toxicity, as is the case with lithium. When such a progression is seen, toxicity should be suspected and the medication dose should be reduced or withheld until the symptom improves.

Other Movement Abnormalities

Essential Tremor

Essential tremor is a coarse postural tremor that is usually first noticed in older age. It is often familial and has a high prevalence in the general population. Essential tremor is most commonly seen in the hands, involving alternating flexion-extension movements and/or abduction-adduction movements of the fingers (Kishore and Calne 1997). The movements can be severe enough to interfere with writing, eating, drinking, and other activities, or be so mild and intermittent that they pass unnoticed (Louis et al. 1998). In some cases, the tremor progresses slowly over time to involve the tongue, head, voice, or trunk. Many of those with essential tremor note that alcohol markedly reduces the tremor. Effective treatments include propranolol 40 mg tid and gabapentin 400 mg tid (Gironell et al. 1999). Anecdotal reports suggest that mirtazapine 30 mg qhs may also be effective. In refractory cases, deep brain stimulation has been used successfully to reduce this tremor.

Periodic Limb Movements of Sleep and Restless Legs Syndrome

These syndromes and their treatment are discussed in Chapter 5 ("Anxiolytic and Sedative-Hypnotic Medications").

Tourette's Disorder and Other Primary Tic Disorders

Tourette's disorder is a syndrome of multiple motor and vocal tics often associated with obsessive-compulsive behaviors or attention-deficit/hyperactivity disorder. Tourette's disorder is not often highly symptomatic in elderly patients, since most patients experience improvement in their symptoms with age, and residual symptoms of the disorder are usually mild (Bruun 1988; Burd et al. 1986). Tics can, however, change or even worsen in late life (Lang et al. 1983). For disabling symptoms, established treatments include clonidine and haloperidol (Kurlan 1997). Risperidone may be useful for this indication, as it is in younger patients, although this has not been specifically studied in elders. Botulinum toxin injections may also be useful for control of tics (Kwak et al. 2000).

Vascular Parkinsonism

Symptoms of parkinsonism secondary to ischemic brain injury include prominent gait difficulty, postural instability, hyperactive reflexes, incontinence, dementia, and pseudobulbar affect (Winikates and Jankovic 1999). This syndrome is poorly responsive to levodopa and is managed by steps taken to reduce the risk of vascular events, such as antiplatelet therapy and control of hypertension (see Chapter 8: "Treatment of Dementias and Other Cognitive Syndromes").

Chapter Summary

- Akinesia and bradykinesia are among the most disabling of movement difficulties and significantly affect quality of life as well as ability to perform activities of daily living.

- Dementia with Lewy bodies presents as if it were a combination of Parkinson's disease and Alzheimer's disease, with prominent motor as well as cortical impairment.

- The classic parkinsonian triad consists of rigidity, akinesia, and tremor; these features are associated with a greatly increased risk of falls.

- Levodopa is the most effective therapy for Parkinson's disease and, if initiated before severe disability develops, is associated with a better outcome.

- When levodopa at a total dose of 1,000 mg daily is ineffective in controlling symptoms of Parkinson's disease, a dopamine receptor agonist is added.

- Anticholinergic medications are not recommended for treatment of Parkinson's disease in elderly patients because of an unfavorable risk-benefit ratio.

- After a variable number of years on levodopa, motor complications often occur; these include dyskinesias (chorea, dystonia, myoclonus), earlier "wearing off" with time after a dose, and unpredictable periods in which parkinsonian symptoms acutely and transiently recur ("on-off" phenomena).

- Levodopa and other dopamine agonists are tapered on discontinuation because of the risk of inducing neuroleptic malignant syndrome when stopped abruptly.

- Catechol-O-methyltransferase inhibitors (e.g., tolcapone, entacapone) prolong the action of levodopa and increase brain concentrations of dopamine but lack antiparkinsonian activity when administered alone.

- Surgical ablation (pallidotomy) and deep-brain stimulation are treatment alternatives for a subset of patients with Parkinson's disease.

- Akathisia is a common adverse effect of neuroleptics that is often mislabeled as "agitation" in elderly patients.

- In contrast to Parkinson's disease, medication-induced parkinsonism is more often characterized by the absence of tremor and the presence of bilateral rigidity and bradykinesia.

- Treatment of drug-induced parkinsonism consists of discontinuation of the offending agent, although in some cases the parkinsonism persists for months to years after the drug is discontinued.

- When a fine drug-induced tremor becomes more coarse, toxicity should be suspected and the medication dose should be reduced or withheld until the symptom improves.

- The risk of tardive dyskinesia can be reduced by using atypical antipsychotics in preference to conventional neuroleptics, by minimizing the dose of neuroleptic used, and possibly by avoiding routine use of adjunctive anticholinergic medications.

- Specific treatments for tardive dyskinesia—atypical antipsychotics, β-blockers, calcium channel blockers, benzodiazepines, and vitamin E—result in variable symptomatic improvement; many patients improve over time with no specific treatment.

- Essential tremor is a prevalent syndrome in geriatrics and may be highly debilitating; it can be treated effectively with propranolol or gabapentin.

- Tourette's disorder is not often highly symptomatic in elderly patients, since most patients experience improvement in their symptoms with age, and residual symptoms are usually mild.

References

Adler LA, Peselow E, Rotrosen J, et al: Vitamin E treatment of tardive dyskinesia. Am J Psychiatry 150:1405–1407, 1993

Bergen J, Kitchin R, Berry G: Predictors of the course of tardive dyskinesia in patients receiving neuroleptics. Biol Psychiatry 32:580–594, 1992

Bruun RD: The natural history of Tourette's syndrome, in Tourette's Syndrome and Tic Disorders. Edited by Cohen DJ, Bruun RD, Leckman JF. New York, Wiley, 1988, pp 21–40

Burd L, Kerbeshian J, Wilkenheiser M, et al: Prevalence of Gilles de la Tourette's syndrome in North Dakota adults. Am J Psychiatry 143:787–788, 1986

Burke RE, Kang UJ, Jankovic J, et al: Tardive akathisia: an analysis of clinical features and response to open therapeutic trials. Mov Disord 4:157–175, 1989

Byne W, White L, Parella M, et al: Tardive dyskinesia in a chronically institutionalized population of elderly schizophrenic patients: prevalence and association with cognitive impairment. Int J Geriatr Psychiatry 13:473–479, 1998

Casey DE: The relationship of pharmacology to side effects. J Clin Psychiatry 58 (suppl 10):55–62, 1997

Cates M, Lusk K, Wells BG: Are calcium-channel blockers effective in the treatment of tardive dyskinesia? Ann Pharmacother 27:191–196, 1993

Cavallaro R, Regazzetti MG, Mundo E, et al: Tardive dyskinesia outcomes: clinical and pharmacologic correlates of remission and persistence. Neuropsychopharmacology 8:233–239, 1993

Charles PD, Davis TL: Drug therapy for Parkinson's disease. South Med J 89:851–856, 1996

Chouinard G: Effects of risperidone in tardive dyskinesia: an analysis of the Canadian Multicenter Risperidone Study. J Clin Psychopharmacol 15 (1, suppl):36S–44S, 1995

Dabiri LM, Pasta D, Darby JK, et al: Effectiveness of vitamin E for treatment of long-term tardive dyskinesia. Am J Psychiatry 151:925–926, 1994

Deuschl G, Bain P, Brin M: Consensus statement of the Movement Disorder Society on Tremor. Ad Hoc Scientific Committee. Mov Disord 13 (suppl 3):2–23, 1998

Egan MF, Hyde TM, Albers GW, et al: Treatment of tardive dyskinesia with vitamin E. Am J Psychiatry 149:773–777, 1992

Elkashef AM, Ruskin PE, Bacher N, et al: Vitamin E in the treatment of tardive dyskinesia. Am J Psychiatry 147:505–506, 1990

Gaitini L, Fradis M, Vaida S, et al: Plasmapheresis in neuroleptic malignant syndrome. Anaesthesia 52:165–168, 1997

Gardos G, Casey DE, Cole JO, et al: Ten-year outcome of tardive dyskinesia. Am J Psychiatry 151:836–841, 1994

Gironell A, Kulisevsky J, Barbanoj M, et al: A randomized placebo-controlled comparative trial of gabapentin and propranolol in essential tremor. Arch Neurol 56:475–480, 1999

Golbe LI: Progressive supranuclear palsy, in Movement Disorders: Neurologic Principles and Practice. Edited by Watts RL, Koller WC. New York, McGraw-Hill, 1997, pp 279–295

Gotto J: Treatment of respiratory dyskinesia with olanzapine. Psychosomatics 40:257–259, 1999

Gottwald MD, Bainbridge JL, Dowling GA, et al: New pharmacotherapy for Parkinson's disease. Ann Pharmacother 31:1205–1217, 1997

Gregory RP, Smith PT, Rudge P: Tardive dyskinesia presenting as severe dysphagia. J Neurol Neurosurg Psychiatry 55:1203–1204, 1992

Gross RE, Lombardi WJ, Lang AE, et al: Relationship of lesion location to clinical outcome following microelectrode-guided pallidotomy for Parkinson's disease. Brain 122:405–416, 1999

Jankovic J, Brin MF: Therapeutic uses of botulinum toxin. N Engl J Med 324:1186–1194, 1991

Jankovic J, Schwartz K: The use of botulinum toxin in the treatment of hand dystonias. J Hand Surg 18A:883–887, 1993

Jeste DV, Caligiuri MP, Paulsen JS: Risk of tardive dyskinesia in older patients: a prospective longitudinal study of 266 patients. Arch Gen Psychiatry 52:756–765, 1995

Jeste DV, Lacro JP, Bailey A, et al: Lower incidence of tardive dyskinesia with risperidone compared with haloperidol in older patients. J Am Geriatr Soc 47:716–719, 1999a

Jeste DV, Lacro JP, Palmer B, et al: Incidence of tardive dyskinesia in early stages of low-dose treatment with typical neuroleptics in older patients. Am J Psychiatry 156:309–311, 1999b

Kane JM: Tardive dyskinesia in affective disorders. J Clin Psychiatry 60 (suppl 5):43–47, 1999

Khan R, Jampala VC, Dong K, et al: Speech abnormalities in tardive dyskinesia. Am J Psychiatry 151:760–762, 1994

Kiriakakis V, Bhatia KP, Quinn NP, et al: The natural history of tardive dystonia. A long-term follow-up study of 107 cases. Brain 121:2053–2066, 1998

Kishore A, Calne DB: Approach to the patient with a movement disorder and overview of movement disorders, in Movement Disorders: Neurologic Principles and Practice. Edited by Watts RL, Koller WC. New York, McGraw-Hill, 1997, pp 3-14

Kruk J, Sachdev P, Singh S: Neuroleptic-induced respiratory dyskinesia. J Neuropsychiatry Clin Neurosci 7:223–229, 1995

Kurlan RM: Tourette's syndrome, in Movement Disorders: Neurologic Principles and Practice. Edited by Watts RL, Koller WC. New York, McGraw-Hill, 1997, pp 569–575

Kushnir SL, Ratner JT: Calcium channel blockers for tardive dyskinesia in geriatric psychiatric patients. Am J Psychiatry 146:1218–1219, 1989

Kwak CH, Hanna PA, Jankovic J: Botulinum toxin in the treatment of tics. Arch Neurol 57:1190–1193, 2000

Lang AE, Lozano AM: Parkinson's disease, Part 1. N Engl J Med 339:1044–1053, 1998

Lang AE, Lozano AM: Parkinson's disease, Part 2. N Engl J Med 339:1130–1143, 1998

Lang AE, Moldofsky H, Awad AG: Long latency between the onset of motor and vocal tics in Tourette's syndrome. Ann Neurol 14:693–694, 1983

Lang AE, Lozano AM, Montgomery E, et al: Posteroventral medial pallidotomy in advanced Parkinson's disease. N Engl J Med 337:1036–1042, 1997

Liddle PF, Barnes TRE, Speller J, et al: Negative symptoms as a risk factor for tardive dyskinesia in schizophrenia. Br J Psychiatry 163:776–780, 1993

Lohr JB, Caligiuri MP: A double-blind placebo-controlled study of vitamin E treatment of tardive dyskinesia. J Clin Psychiatry 57:167–173, 1996

Loonen AJM, Verwey HA, Roels PR, et al: Is diltiazem effective in treating the symptoms of (tardive) dyskinesia in chronic psychiatric inpatients? A negative, double-blind, placebo- controlled trial. J Clin Psychopharmacol 12:39–42, 1992

Louis ED, Klatka LA, Liu Y, et al: Comparison of extrapyramidal features in 31 pathologically confirmed cases of diffuse Lewy body disease and 34 pathologically confirmed cases of Parkinson's disease. Neurology 48:376–380, 1997

Louis ED, Ford B, Wendt KJ, et al: Clinical characteristics of essential tremor: data from a community-based study. Mov Disord 13:803–808, 1998

Miller LG, Jankovic J: Neurologic approach to drug-induced movement disorders: a study of 125 patients. Southern Med J 83:525–532, 1990

Morgenstern H, Glazer WM: Identifying risk factors for tardive dyskinesia among long-term outpatients maintained with neuroleptic medications. Arch Gen Psychiatry 50:723–733, 1993

Myers RH, Sax DS, Schoenfeld M, et al: Late onset of Huntington's disease. J Neurol Neurosurg Psychiatry 48:530–534, 1985

Ondo WG, Jankovic J, Lai EC, et al: Assessment of motor function after stereotactic pallidotomy. Neurology 50:266–270, 1998

Pallidotomy for Parkinson's disease. The Medical Letter, 38 (December 6):107, 1996

Pierelli F, Adipietro A, Soldati G, et al: Low dosage clozapine effects on L-dopa induced dyskinesias in parkinsonian patients. Acta Neurol Scand 97:295–299, 1998

Psychopharmacology Research Branch, NIMH: Abnormal Involuntary Movement Scale (AIMS), in ECDEU Assessment Manual for Psychopharmacology (DHEW Publ No ADM-76-388). Edited by Guy W. Rockville, MD, National Institute of Mental Health, 1976, pp 534–537

Samuel M, Caputo E, Brooks DJ, et al: A study of medial pallidotomy for Parkinson's disease: clinical outcome, MRI location and complications. Brain 121:59–75, 1998

Scharre DW, Mahler ME: Parkinson's disease: making the diagnosis, selecting drug therapies. Geriatrics 49:14–23, 1994

Schuurman PR, Bosch DA, Bossuyt PM, et al: A comparison of continuous thalamic stimulation and thalamotomy for suppression of severe tremor. N Engl J Med 342:461–468, 2000

Shriqui CL, Bradwejn J, Annable L, et al: Vitamin E in the treatment of tardive dyskinesia: a double-blind placebo-controlled study. Am J Psychiatry 149:391–393, 1992

Stacy M, Cardoso F, Jankovic J: Tardive stereotypy and other movement disorders in tardive dyskinesias. Neurology 43:937–941, 1993

Thaker GK, Nguyen JA, Strauss ME, et al: Clonazepam treatment of tardive dyskinesia: a practical GABAmimetic strategy. Am J Psychiatry 147:445–451, 1990 van Harten PN, Hoek HW, Matroos GE, et al: Intermittent neuroleptic treatment and risk for tardive dyskinesia: Curacao Extrapyramidal Syndromes Study III. Am J Psychiatry 155:565–567, 1998

Watts RL, Brewer RP, Schneider JA, et al: Corticobasal degeneration, in Movement Disorders: Neurologic Principles and Practice. Edited by Watts RL, Koller WC. New York, McGraw-Hill, 1997, pp 611–621

Winikates J, Jankovic J: Clinical correlates of vascular parkinsonism. Arch Neurol 56:98–102, 1999

Wirshing DA, Bartzokis G, Pierre JM, et al: Tardive dyskinesia and serum iron indices. Biol Psychiatry 44:493–498, 1998

Woerner MG, Alvir JMJ, Saltz BL, et al: Prospective study of tardive dyskinesia in the elderly: rates and risk factors. Am J Psychiatry 155:1521–1528, 1998

Wojcieszek JM, Lang AE: Hyperkinetic movement disorders, in The American Psychiatric Press Textbook of Geriatric Neuropsychiatry. Edited by Coffey CE, Cummings JL. Washington, DC, American Psychiatric Press, 1994, pp 405–431

Wojcik JD, Falk WE, Fink JS, et al: A review of 32 cases of tardive dystonia. Am J Psychiatry 148:1055–1059, 1991

Treatment of Dementias and Other Cognitive Syndromes

In this chapter, we focus on specific treatment of individual dementing disorders as well as symptomatic treatment of selected neuropsychiatric syndromes arising in the context of dementia. Delirium, amnestic disorder, and other syndromes of cognitive impairment are also covered.

Specific treatment of dementia is determined by etiology, so it is not sufficient to make a syndromic diagnosis of dementia; it is imperative that dementia etiology be identified. Diagnostic criteria have been formulated for Alzheimer's disease (AD) (McKhann et al. 1984), vascular dementia (Roman et al. 1993), dementia with Lewy bodies (McKeith et al. 1996), frontotemporal dementia (Lund and Manchester Groups 1994), and alcohol-related dementia (Oslin et al. 1998).

Neuropsychiatric disturbances in dementia may be a direct

consequence of degeneration of brain areas involving emotion or behavioral control (Sultzer et al. 1995). There is evidence from a positron emission tomography (PET) study that this degeneration is regionally specific, with agitation and disinhibition associated with frontotemporal hypometabolism, anxiety and depression with parietal hypometabolism, and psychosis with frontal hypometabolism (Sultzer et al. 1995). In addition, there is increasing evidence that behavioral syndromes relate to specific neurotransmitter deficits; for example, serotonergic system dysfunction may be related to aggression in AD, and noradrenergic hypofunction may be related to social withdrawal. Since neurotransmitter deficits are multiple in later disease stages, future treatment may involve pharmacological "cocktails" with multiple therapeutic targets.

Evaluation of the Cognitively Impaired Elder

Initial evaluation of the elderly patient presenting with evidence of cognitive dysfunction includes a history, physical and neurological examination, and mental status examination. Cognitive evaluation using the Mini-Mental State Exam uncovers mainly cortical deficits, and this examination can be supplemented with tests such as Trails A and B, timed naming (e.g., types of animals), clock-drawing, and Luria hand sequences to identify frontal-subcortical dysfunction (Cummings and Benson 1992). Disturbance of consciousness with attentional difficulties helps distinguish delirium from dementia. The electroencephalogram (EEG) can be useful when such disturbance is difficult to assess, as it is extremely sensitive to functional changes in delirium (Chui and Zhang 1997; Jacobson et al. 1993). At this stage of the evaluation, a syndromic diagnosis is made (e.g., delirium, dementia, or single-domain impairment such as amnestic disorder) and a differential diagnosis of etiology is formulated.

Although a detailed history provides the most significant information about etiology, laboratory investigation is required to rule out reversible causes of dementia. Minimally, this includes a complete blood count, chemistries, liver function tests, thyroid function tests (specifically, thyroid-stimulating hormone), vitamin B_{12} and folate levels, and syphilis serology. Neuroimaging study is required for the differential diagnosis of vascular dementia. Although head computed tomography may be sufficient, magnetic resonance imaging (MRI) is superior in detecting white matter lesions. If MRI is used, it is important to avoid overinterpretation of white matter changes seen only on T_2-weighted studies (Small et al. 1997). If the etiological diagnosis of dementia remains unclear, neuropsychological testing should be performed. ApoE (apolipoprotein E) genotyping can help to increase the specificity of diagnosis in the patient who meets clinical diagnostic criteria for AD (Mayeux et al. 1998), but it is not useful in predicting whether the disease will develop in an asymptomatic individual. In addition, ancillary tests such as single photon emission computed tomography, functional MRI, positron emission tomography, lumbar puncture, HIV testing, and heavy metal screening should be considered when the dementia etiology is still unclear.

Treatment of Specific Cognitive Disorders

Alcohol-Related Dementia (Alcohol-Induced Persisting Dementia)

Characteristics of alcohol-related dementia are covered in the chapter on treatment of substance-related disorders (see Chapter 6) and in the proposed diagnostic criteria (Oslin et al. 1998). Currently, no neuropathological criteria exist for definite alcoholic dementia, and validation of criteria remains to be accomplished. Treatment requires abstinence, and any medications that help to maintain abstinence may be of use. In addition, since this disorder may involve a cholinergic deficit (Levy et al. 1999), acetylcholinesterase inhibitors may be of benefit.

Alzheimer's Disease

Existing treatments for AD fall into three categories: cognition-enhancing agents, antioxidants, and drugs associated with a reduced risk of developing AD.

Currently marketed cognition-enhancing agents include tacrine, donepezil, rivastigmine, and galantamine. Tacrine has fallen out of use because of hepatotoxic effects. In our experience, these drugs are associated with moderate to substantial cognitive and functional improvement in some patients with mild to moderate AD, and little improvement in others. These drugs are thought to have disease-modifying effects as well as symptomatic effects. Moreover, these agents can be associated with significant reduction in behavioral disturbances associated with AD, particularly in later stages of the disease. In current practice, cholinesterase inhibitors are initiated as early as possible after the diagnosis of probable AD is made and their use is continued throughout disease progression.

Donepezil is a selective inhibitor of acetylcholinesterase, whereas rivastigmine inhibits both acetylcholinesterase and butylcholinesterase. Galantamine not only inhibits cholinesterase but increases acetylcholine release via nicotinic receptor modulation. The importance of these differences in vivo is unclear, and no comparative studies of these agents have been published to date. The cost of the three drugs is approximately equal.

Tacrine is no longer a drug of choice because of potential hepatotoxic effects and the need for frequent monitoring of liver function tests. A number of other cholinergic drugs are either under investigation or pending FDA approval at this time.

Several randomized, controlled trials have demonstrated functional as well as cognitive improvement with donepezil 5–10 mg po qd (S. L. Rogers and Friedhoff 1996; S. L. Rogers et al. 1998) and with rivastigmine 6–12 mg po qd (Rosler et al. 1999) in patients with mild to moderate AD. These drugs are generally well tolerated when titrated slowly, with expectable but transient cholinergic side effects of nausea, diarrhea, and insomnia. Donepezil is begun at 5 mg qd (usually qhs) and titrated to the target dose of 10 mg qd at 6 weeks. Rivastigmine is begun at 1.5 mg bid, and the dosage is increased by 1.5 mg bid every 2 weeks to the target dose of 6 mg bid. Effects of a cholinesterase inhibitor are usually apparent by 12 weeks, and the drug is continued indefinitely, unless the patient is noncompliant or continues to deteriorate at the pretreatment rate (Flint and Van Reekum 1998).

There is some evidence that estrogen has cognition-enhancing effects (Asthana et al. 1999; Rodriguez and Grossberg 1998), although it is more useful in prevention than in treatment of AD (Mulnard et al. 2000). Estrogen may be recommended for postmenopausal women with or without AD unless specifically contraindicated because of smoking, high breast cancer risk, or risk of vascular event. Estrogen may be administered as transdermal estradiol 0.05 mg/day applied twice weekly in a cyclic regimen for women with an intact uterus (McEvoy et al. 2000). Estrogen may work synergistically with cholinesterase inhibitors (Schneider et al. 1996). Efforts are currently under way to develop nonfeminizing estrogens for use in men (Rodriguez and Grossberg 1998).

An extract of *Ginkgo biloba* (EGb 761) has been shown to be effective in slowing disease progression and, in some cases, improving cognition in a cohort of patients with AD and vascular dementia at a dosage of 40 mg po tid (LeBars et al. 1997). It has been noted elsewhere, however, that the effects of this extract are not as robust as those of donepezil and that the extract is less convenient because of the need for tid dosing (Flint and Van Reekum 1998). In addition, case reports have associated ginkgo with episodes of serious bleeding (hematoma and intracranial hemorrhage), and there are concerns about product purity and potency, since ginkgo is not FDA regulated but is marketed as a dietary supplement ("Ginkgo Biloba for Dementia" *The Medical Letter* 1998).

The antioxidants vitamin E 2,000 IU daily and selegiline 10 mg daily were each found to slow the rate of progression of AD in a 2-year randomized, controlled trial of patients with moderate dementia (Sano et al. 1997). No benefit was found with combined therapy. Since vitamin E has fewer drug interactions and a more benign side-effect profile than selegiline, vitamin E 1,000 IU po bid is recommended for all AD patients except those with vitamin K deficiency; for the vitamin K–deficient patient, dose should be limited to 200–800 IU daily (American Psychiatric Association 1997). In an earlier study, the nonsteroidal anti-inflammatory drug (NSAID) indomethacin 100–150 mg daily was found to slow progression in patients with mild to moderate AD over a 6-month study period, compared with a control group (Rogers et al. 1993). The risks of NSAID use have generally limited this therapeutic option, but this situation is changing now, with the availability of the cyclooxygenase-2 (COX-2) inhibitors, as discussed below.

There is now fairly compelling evidence that long-term use of estrogen and anti-inflammatory drugs reduces the risk of developing AD. Among postmenopausal women, estrogen reduces the risk to as low as one-third that of control groups (Kawas et al. 1997; Tang et al. 1996). With anti-inflammatory drugs, most studies involve ibuprofen, although for various reasons this is not the ideal candidate for prophylactic treatment (Aisen and Davis 1997). Considering new evidence that cyclooxygenase-2 (COX-2) is implicated in neurodegeneration, the COX-2-specific NSAIDs (celecoxib and rofecoxib) may prove particularly useful (Aisen and Davis 1997).

Cholesterol-lowering "statin" drugs have been associated in epidemiological studies with a greatly reduced risk of AD. In animal models, these drugs have been shown to reduce levels of amyloid β peptides implicated in the pathogenesis of AD (Fass-bender et al. 2001). These drugs are likely to have a very important role in AD prevention in the future.

Risk reduction efforts also include the development of a vaccine for AD containing a synthetic form of β-amyloid protein; immunization of Alzheimer-model mice with this protein resulted in reduction of amyloid plaques and other neuropathological changes characteristic of AD (Heemels 2000).

Amnestic Disorder

Isolated memory impairment can be found in association with head trauma, thiamine and other vitamin deficiency states, infections such as herpes encephalitis, cerebrovascular insufficiency, and other medical conditions afflicting the elderly. The primary intervention for an amnestic disorder is timely treatment of the underlying medical condition. Aggressive thiamine replacement or antiviral therapy can be associated with relatively rapid resolution of amnesia. With cerebrovascular insufficiency, one pattern that can be seen is that of transient global amnesia, in which memory impairment occurs in spells lasting minutes to hours. When this pattern is recognized and the underlying cerebrovascular disease is managed effectively, the spells can resolve and stroke can be prevented. With head trauma, amnesia can resolve gradually, over the 2 years following injury.

With any serious cerebral insult, however, persistent amnesia can be seen. Some evidence suggests that pathology of the cholinergic system may represent a final common pathway in these diverse conditions (Siegfried 2000). If so, cholinesterase inhibitor therapy (as described in the specific drug summaries at the end of this chapter) might prove useful.

Delirium

Treatment of delirium is discussed in the chapter on antipsychotic medications (see Chapter 2). It should be noted here that the clinical practice of using the cholinesterase inhibitors (e.g., donepezil) to treat delirium is becoming more common, despite a dearth of evidence from controlled studies. As noted earlier, our experience is that donepezil 5 mg po qd can be effective in controlling symptoms and well tolerated by the delirious patient but may not be as immediately effective as a conventional high-potency typical antipsychotic such as haloperidol.

Dementia of Depression

Major depression can be associated with cognitive impairment characterized by particular difficulty with tasks requiring effort, including timed tasks, and vigilance (attention). When the depression is adequately treated, the dementia syndrome resolves. One special case is the poststroke patient with dementia and depression, in whom treatment with medication such as nortriptyline has been associated with cognitive recovery as well (Kimura et al. 2000).

Frontotemporal Dementia (Frontal Lobe Dementia)

Data from animal studies suggest that the alpha$_2$ (α_2)–adrenergic receptor agonists clonidine and guanfacine may be helpful in patients with certain frontal lobe symptoms, by attenuating the distracting properties of irrelevant stimuli (Coull 1994). A recent study in humans found a distinct difference between the two agents; only guanfacine, at a dose of 29 µg/kg, improved planning and spatial working memory (Jakala et al. 1999). Clinical experience suggests that the dopamine agonists pramipexole and ropinirole may help overcome apathy, increase motor activity and speed, and increase motivation. (These drugs are discussed further in Chapter 7, in the context of the treatment of movement disorders.) Arousal may be optimized with the use of dextroamphetamine or methylphenidate, although these drugs are believed to work better for subcortical than for cortical disease. SSRI antidepressants may be useful for obsessive-compulsive symptoms. Amantadine may be useful for disruptive vocalizations, but this benefit can be short-lived. There is no evidence that cholinergic-enhancing drugs are of any benefit in frontotemporal dementia. Other agents that may be useful include mood stabilizers and stimulating antidepressants such as bupropion and fluoxetine.

Dementia With Lewy Bodies (Lewy Body Dementia)

Dementia with Lewy bodies (Lewy body dementia) is a progressive dementia that presents with cognitive and motor symptoms characteristic of both AD and Parkinson's disease, with genetic relationships to both (Saitoh and Katzman 1996). Psychiatric symptoms are prominent and include vivid visual hallucinations, delusions, and depression (Papka et al. 1998). Unusual features include dramatic fluctuation in symptoms; repeated falls; and frequent, transient episodes of loss of consciousness (McKeith et al. 1996).

Like Alzheimer's disease, dementia with Lewy bodies is associated with markedly reduced levels of choline acetyltransferase, the enzyme that catalyzes synthesis of acetylcholine, particularly in temporal and parietal cortices (Papka et al. 1998). These reductions may be severe for patients with visual hallucinations (Papka et al. 1998). Patients with dementia with Lewy bodies may benefit even more than AD patients from treatment with cholinesterase inhibitors (McKeith et al. 2000; Samuel et al. 2000). In responders, cognitive, behavioral, and functional improvements are seen that are sometimes dramatic.

Treatment of motor symptoms in dementia with Lewy bodies is covered in the chapter on movement disorders (see Chapter 7). It is worth reiterating that patients with dementia with Lewy bodies are exquisitely sensitive to extrapyramidal effects of neuroleptic medication, and conventional neuroleptics should be avoided in this population. This issue is discussed further in Chapter 2 ("Antipsychotic Medications").

Mental Retardation

Increasingly, clinicians caring for geriatric patients are confronted with the complex task of diagnosing neuropsychiatric syndromes in patients with developmental disorders with varying degrees of baseline cognitive impairment. These patients are affected by the same psychiatric and neuropsychiatric disorders as the rest of the population; they are likely to suffer greater degrees of impairment, however, because of their inability to describe subjective feelings and experiences, and because stress may disproportionately disrupt their information-processing abilities (Duffy and Hobbs 2000). Assessment and treatment of the geriatric patient with mental retardation is an area well deserving of further research and training. The reader is directed to an excellent overview of the topic by Duffy and Hobbs (2000).

Mild Cognitive Dysfunction

Various overlapping but nonsynonymous terms have been applied to patients with mild or subclinical cognitive dysfunction. Patients with such dysfunction constitute a highly heterogeneous population with variable prognoses, but, in fact, only a small minority has a benign prognosis (Ritchie et al. 2000). In general, good controlled studies are lacking regarding this syndrome. Some of the same agents useful in the prevention and treatment of AD (see earlier discussion on AD) may also be useful in the treatment of mild cognitive dysfunction: cholinesterase inhibitors, estrogen, and vitamin E. One randomized controlled trial showed that Ginkgo biloba was not effective for this purpose (van Dongen et al. 2000).

Parkinson's Disease With Dementia

A substantial minority of Parkinson's disease patients (up to 40%) develop dementia (Mayeux et al. 1992). In general, dementia is more common in patients with early gait and balance difficulties than in those with tremor-dominant disease (Cummings 1995). There is some evidence that the dementia of Parkinson's disease is associated with a cholinergic deficit (Levy et al. 1999), but the use of cholinergic agents is complicated by the underlying dopaminergic deficit central to the disease. Clear guidelines do not exist regarding treatment of the cognitive deficits per se, although treatments of the motor dysfunction are often associated with perceived cognitive improvement (e.g., on timed tasks). In addition, selegiline, a drug used in the treatment of Parkinson's disease, is an antioxidant with neuroprotective effects (Sano et al. 1997) and should be considered for use in Parkinson's disease patients with emerging cognitive impairment.

Schizophrenia-Related Cognitive Dysfunction

Domains of cognition affected in schizophrenia include serial learning, executive function, vigilance, and attentional ability and distractibility (Friedman et al. 1999). Atypical antipsychotics are associated with improvement in prefrontal functions such as working memory and executive function (Friedman et al. 1999). α_2-Adrenergic receptor agonists such as guanfacine and clonidine are associated with improvements in serial learning, working memory, and attention (Friedman et al. 1999). It may be that guanfacine is superior to clonidine for this indication (Jakala et al. 1999). Cholinergic drugs are associated with improvement in memory, language, and praxis (Friedman et al. 1999).

Vascular Dementia

Treatment of vascular dementia involves modification of stroke risk, optimization of cerebral perfusion, and treatment of associated neuropsychiatric symptoms. Stroke risk is modified by antiplatelet agents, statin drugs, and estrogen and via control of hypertension, embolism, elevated lipid levels, and diabetes. The antiplatelet agent of first choice is aspirin 325 mg, usually prescribed as enteric-coated (e.g., Ecotrin). For those who are unable to tolerate aspirin because of gastrointestinal bleeding or distress or who have evidence of continued ischemia despite aspirin therapy, the antiplatelet agent clopidogrel (Plavix) is used. This agent has replaced ticlopidine, which had problematic hematological side effects. Clopidogrel is slightly more effective than aspirin and is as safe as aspirin; its only significant side effect is skin rash (CAPRIE Steering Committee 1996). The combination drug Aggrenox (aspirin and extended-release dipyridamole) confers greater protection against stroke than aspirin alone for those who have had a transient ischemic attack or ischemic stroke in the past; however, this combination is no better than aspirin alone in lowering mortality in this population and is much more expensive (Hervey and Goa 1999). As noted in the specific drug summary at the end of this chapter, Aggrenox is taken in divided doses (bid).

Statin drugs (e.g., pravastatin, simvastatin) significantly reduce cholesterol levels and lower stroke risk (Hebert et al. 1997) and are an increasingly important component of the prevention and treatment of vascular dementia. The role of estrogen therapy is not yet established, but estrogen is known to have complex effects that may reduce the risk of ischemia and stroke (Konno et al. 1997).

For patients with multi-infarct dementia (a subtype of vascular dementia), systolic blood pressure is lowered to the range of 135 to 150 mm Hg, where both cerebral blood flow and cognitive performance are optimized (Meyer et al. 1986). Embolism secondary to atrial fibrillation is controlled with either warfarin or aspirin, depending on the patient's risk factors for stroke ("Warfarin Versus Aspirin for Prevention of Thromboembolism" 1994), and embolism after myocardial infarction is prevented with warfarin (Azar et al. 1996). In general, anticoagulants are used only when there is an identified source of emboli and when not contraindicated because of risk of falls or intracranial hemorrhage (Cummings 1995). Embolism from complicated carotid plaques may be prevented by endarterectomy (Kistler et al. 1991).

Improvement in cerebral perfusion is correlated with improvement in activities of daily living and cognitive functioning. Many of the interventions designed to lower stroke risk (e.g., lowering lipid levels and controlling diabetes) are also associated with improved perfusion (Desmond et al. 1993). Estrogen is also associated with increased cerebral perfusion in postmenopausal women. In addition, since cigarette smoking has complex effects known to promote ischemia (Wolf 1986), quitting smoking is associated with improved cerebral blood flow and cognition (Rogers et al. 1985). Treatment with pentoxifylline (Trental) 400 mg tid was found in a randomized, controlled trial to result in improved global and cognitive function in patients with large-vessel ischemic disease (multi-infarct dementia) over a 9-month period (Group TEPM-IDS 1996). This drug has also been shown to slow progression in multi-infarct dementia and to decrease the risk of transient ischemic attacks (Frampton and Brogden 1995). Pentoxifylline has an unclear role in treating patients with multi-infarct dementia already taking clopidogrel because it can be as-

sociated with bleeding when used in combination with antiplatelet agents (McEvoy et al. 2000).

Treatment of Behavioral
Disturbances in Dementia

Various neuropsychiatric syndromes associated with dementia
may manifest as problematic or potentially dangerous behaviors.
Specific pharmacological treatments of depression, anxiety, and
psychosis in the context of dementia are discussed in earlier
chapters. It is important to note that problematic behaviors related to treatable dementias may improve with treatment of core
neurotransmitter deficits. For example, patients with AD treated
with donepezil are less likely to be threatening, destroy property,
talk loudly, or be given sedatives than those not treated with this
drug (Cummings et al. 2000). In this section, we focus on three
areas of behavioral disturbance commonly seen in patients with
dementia, regardless of etiology: agitation and aggression, hypersexuality, and sundowning.

Agitation and Aggression

Among patients with dementia, behaviors on this spectrum may
be the most disruptive and problematic. Since "agitation" ranges
broadly, from repetitive vocalization through nonaggressive physical behavior (e.g., pacing) to aggressive physical behavior, a
critical first step is to list and describe target behaviors. An instrument such as the Overt Agitation Severity Scale can facilitate this
task (Yudofsky et al. 1997). Consensus guidelines have been formulated for the management of agitation in dementia (Alexopoulos et al. 1998). The following discussion is based on those
guidelines as well as our own experience.

For all types of agitation, reversible precipitants should be
identified and corrected. Pain, nicotine withdrawal, and having
a disruptive roommate are examples of precipitants indicating
specific interventions. Careful attention should be paid to the

pattern of behavioral disturbance, such as occurrence during shift changes or mealtimes, since stimulation may exacerbate agitation and aggression. Bathing is often the precipitant for impulsive aggressive acts. Environmental interventions (e.g., keeping the shower room and bathwater warm, avoiding waterspray to the face) are strongly recommended for patients who resist bathing (Kovach and Meyer-Arnold 1997; Sloane et al. 1995). Environmental interventions are also often appropriate for pacing, which is sometimes managed simply by creating a hazard-free path, and for repetitive vocalization.

Psychiatric assessment facilitates the subtyping of agitation into one of several categories, with treatment implications as shown in Figure 8–1:

- *Patient is delirious:* underlying cause is treated; antipsychotics are used for symptomatic treatment, if needed.
- *Patient is in pain:* cause is treated, if possible; pharmacological and nonpharmacological analgesics are used, if needed.
- *Patient has signs or symptoms to suggest any of the following medication-responsive syndromes* (whether or not DSM-IV-TR criteria are met):
  - *Psychosis:* suspiciousness, paranoia, hallucinations, delusions
  - *Mania or hypomania:* pressured speech, hyperactivity, decreased sleep
  - *Depression:* negativism, irritability, dysphoria, anxiety

Many cases of agitation will be adequately treated at this point in the algorithm. When agitation persists, further environmental modifications should be implemented and nonspecific pharmacological treatment should be considered.

For persistent, nonspecific agitation/aggression in dementia, trazodone has traditionally been a drug of choice, at a standing dosage ranging from 12.5 mg bid to 100 mg tid. Trazodone can also be used prn, since it has a relatively rapid onset of action.

The use of antipsychotic medications to treat nonpsychotic

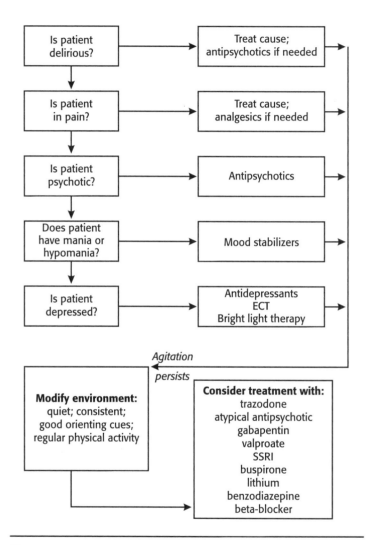

Figure 8–1. Treatment of agitation in patients with dementia. SSRI = selective serotonin reuptake inhibitor.

agitation in the context of dementia in elderly patients is controversial, as discussed in Chapter 2 ("Antipsychotics"). In general, long-term use of conventional antipsychotics is best avoided in patients with dementia, but atypical antipsychotics are emerging as an important treatment option in this population. Risperidone 1 mg daily was shown to be effective in treating aggression and possibly other behavior disturbance in AD, vascular dementia, and mixed dementia, with effects persisting for at least 12 months (Bhana and Spencer 2000). Olanzapine 5–10 mg daily was shown to be effective in treating agitation/aggression in AD patients in a 6-week randomized trial, with side effects of somnolence and gait disturbance (Street et al. 2000).

Gabapentin 600–2,400 mg daily in divided doses (tid) may also helpful for agitation and anxiety in dementia (Hawkins et al. 2000; Herrmann et al. 2000; Roane et al. 2000). Valproate is commonly used for problematic behaviors in patients with dementia. Those with agitation may have a response when serum levels are below 50 µg/mL, while those with aggression may require levels in the usual therapeutic range of 50 to 100 µg/mL. The role of lamotrigine for this indication is not yet characterized, but this drug has been identified as possibly being neuroprotective in AD and so may have multiple benefits.

The SSRI citalopram at doses of 10–30 mg daily has been associated with improvement in irritability, hostility, anxiety, agitation, and disruptive vocalization in patients with AD (Nyth and Gottfries 1990; Pollock et al. 1997). Citalopram's effect on disruptive vocalization deserves further study, because this behavior is generally not responsive to pharmacological intervention (Bourgeois et al. 1997).

β-Blockers may be useful in treating agitation and aggression in the patient with dementia, although effects on blood pressure and pulse dictate caution in using these agents in elderly patients. Propranolol was used to treat impulsive aggression in a small series of patients with dementia at doses up to 80 mg daily (Shankle et al. 1995). In elderly patients, propranolol is started at 10 mg bid, and the dosage is increased every 3–7 days to clinical effect. The dosage range required to treat agitation in elderly patients is not known. Pindolol may be less likely to induce hypotension and bradycardia than propranolol and to have an onset of action within 2 weeks, compared with the 4 weeks seen with propranolol. In geriatric patients, pindolol is started at 5 mg daily, and the dosage is increased very slowly, by 5 mg every 3–4 weeks, to a maximum daily dose of 40–60 mg. β-Blockers are contraindicated in patients with asthma, diabetes, heart failure, cardiogenic shock, sinus bradycardia, or more than first-degree heart block (McEvoy et al. 2000). They should be used with caution in patients with Wolff-Parkinson-White syndrome or hepatic or renal impairment, or those taking catecholamine-depleting drugs or phenothiazines. Significant drug interactions involving β-blockers may occur with monoamine oxidase inhibitors (MAOIs) and general anesthetics.

For persistent aggressive behavior in the patient with dementia, estrogen may be useful. Estrogen 0.625 mg qd was found in one randomized controlled trial to be effective in reducing aggression in women and men with moderate to severe dementia (Kyomen et al. 1999).

Hypersexuality and Inappropriate Sexual Behaviors

Persistent inappropriate sexual behaviors may occur in the patient with dementia and can severely limit placement options. These behaviors can be caused by medications such as parkinsonism drugs, be associated with neurological conditions such as Klüver-Bucy syndrome, be a symptom of mania, or be found as an isolated symptom in the patient with dementia. Little information is available from systematic study to guide clinical practice in treating this problem.

Case report literature and our own experience suggest that treatment for hypersexuality in nonbipolar patients is most appropriately initiated with an SSRI antidepressant. Whether efficacy depends on antiobsessional effects, anti-impulsivity effects, or antilibidinal side effects is unclear. In our experience, positive responses have been noted with fluoxetine 20 mg daily, citalopram 20 mg daily, or paroxetine 20 mg daily. No data are available to guide duration of treatment; patients who respond favorably are often treated indefinitely.

If no response to the SSRI is seen, a trial of estrogen or medroxyprogesterone acetate (MPA) is undertaken. Elderly men, as well as elderly women, have been treated successfully with estrogen, administered as a 0.625-mg conjugated estrogen daily oral dose or a 0.05 to 0.10-mg transdermal estradiol patch (Lothstein et al. 1997). MPA was used successfully in treating hypersexuality in four elderly men with dementia at a dose of 300 mg im weekly for 1 year (Cooper 1987). In that series, behavior improved within 2 weeks, and serum level of testosterone was reduced 90% and serum level of luteinizing hormone was reduced 60%. After the trial ended, testosterone and luteinizing hormone levels returned to baseline, but improvement in sexual behavior continued. No adverse effects of MPA were noted. One other group reported successful use of a smaller dose of MPA (150–200 mg im) every other week (Weiner et al. 1992). There are no case reports detailing use of MPA in elderly women for this indication.

Other anti-androgens that may be useful in the treatment of hypersexuality include cimetidine 600–1,600 mg daily, spironolactone 75 mg daily, or ketoconazole 100–200 mg daily (Wiseman et al. 2000). Caution is advised when ketoconazole is used because of significant cytochrome P450 (CYP) 3A drug interactions, as discussed in Chapter 1 ("Introduction to Geriatric Psychopharmacology"). Amantadine may also be useful in treating sexual inappropriateness and other disinhibited behaviors in dementia at dosages of 25 mg bid to 100 mg bid.

Sundowning

"Sundowning" refers to a specific pattern of agitation in which symptoms worsen acutely in the evening hours. It can occur in delirium or dementia; in some patients with dementia, the development of sundowning can signal the presence of a superimposed delirium. This pattern of agitation is likely related to light exposure, sleep cycles, and the timing of medication use (Martin et al. 2000).

The sleep-inducing hormone melatonin is useful in the treatment of sundowning in some patients (Cohen-Mansfield et al. 2000). Decreased melatonin levels are found in a subset of elderly patients, possibly more often in those with AD (Liu et al. 1999). Evening bright light therapy can also be useful for sundowning, as described in Chapter 3 ("Antidepressants").

Antipsychotic agents, both conventional and atypical, can also be useful in the treatment of sundowning. These medications are best prescribed at low doses on a standing, rather than prn, basis. For sundowning, the antipsychotic can be given 1–2 hours before the time of usual behavioral disturbance to take advantage of sedative effects. For example, a 76-year-old patient with AD with predictable agitation at around 5:00 P.M. was treated successfully with risperidone 0.5 mg po at 3:00 P.M. and 0.5 mg at bedtime. The same caveats about treating patients with dementia with Lewy bodies with antipsychotics, discussed earlier in this chapter (see "Dementia With Lewy Bodies"), apply to the treatment of sundowning.

Chapter Summary

- Specific treatment of dementia is determined by etiology, so it is not sufficient to make a syndromic diagnosis of dementia; it is imperative that the etiology of the dementia be identified.

- Although a detailed history provides the most significant information about dementia etiology, laboratory investigation is necessary to rule out reversible causes of dementia.

- In current practice, cholinesterase inhibitors are initiated as early as possible after the diagnosis of probable AD is made, and their use is continued throughout disease progression.

- Some evidence suggests that estrogen has cognition-enhancing effects, although it may prove more useful in prevention than in treatment of AD.

- Vitamin E 1,000 IU po bid is recommended for all AD patients except those with vitamin K deficiency.

- There is now compelling evidence that statin drugs, estrogen, and anti-inflammatory drugs reduce the risk of developing AD.

- The primary intervention for an amnestic disorder is timely treatment of the underlying medical condition.

- For delirium, anecdotal experience suggests that donepezil 5 mg po qd can be an effective pharmacological intervention that is well tolerated.

- Patients with Lewy body dementia may benefit even more than patients with AD from treatment with cholinesterase inhibitors; conventional neuroleptics should be avoided in the Lewy body dementia population.

- Treatment of vascular dementia involves modification of stroke risk, optimization of cerebral perfusion, and treatment of associated neuropsychiatric symptoms.

- In stroke risk modification, the antiplatelet agent of first choice is aspirin 325 mg qd.

- Statin drugs (e.g., pravastatin, simvastatin) significantly reduce cholesterol levels and clearly lower stroke risk.

- Problematic behaviors related to treatable dementias may improve with treatment of putative core neurotransmitter deficits.

- A critical first step in managing agitation or aggression in dementia is to list and describe target behaviors.

- Environmental interventions (e.g., keeping the shower room and bathwater warm, avoiding waterspray to the face) are strongly recommended for patients with dementia who resist bathing.

- Psychiatric assessment facilitates the subtyping of dementia-associated agitation into one of several categories, with treatment implications as shown in Figure 8–1.

- For persistent, nonspecific agitation/aggression in dementia, a range of treatment alternatives exists, as shown in Figure 8–1.

- Treatment for dementia-related hypersexuality not due to mania is most appropriately initiated with an SSRI antidepressant. If no response to the SSRI is seen, a trial of estrogen or medroxyprogesterone acetate is undertaken.

- Sundowning is likely related to light exposure, sleep cycles, and the timing of medications. Melatonin, bright light therapy, and antipsychotics can be useful in the treatment of sundowning.

References

Aisen PS, Davis KL: Anti-inflammatory therapy for Alzheimer's disease: a status report. International Journal of Geriatric Psychopharmacology 1:2–5, 1997

Alexopoulos GS, Silver JM, Kahn DA, et al: The Expert Consensus Guideline Series: treatment of agitation in older persons with dementia. Postgrad Med (Special Report) April 1998, pp 1–88

American Psychiatric Association: Practice guideline for the treatment of patients with Alzheimer's disease and other dementias of late life. Am J Psychiatry 154 (5, suppl):1–39, 1997

Asthana S, Craft S, Baker LD, et al: Cognitive and neuroendocrine response to transdermal estrogen in postmenopausal women with Alzheimer's disease: results of a placebo-controlled, double-blind, pilot study. Psychoneuroendocrinology 24:657–677, 1999

Azar AJ, Koudstaal PJ, Wintzen AR, et al: Risk of stroke during long-term anticoagulant therapy in patients after myocardial infarction. Ann Neurol 39:301–307, 1996

Bhana N, Spencer CM: Risperidone: a review of its use in the management of the behavioural and psychological symptoms of dementia. Drugs Aging 16:451–471, 2000

Bourgeois MS, Burgio LD, Schulz R, et al: Modifying repetitive verbalizations of community-dwelling patients with AD. The Gerontologist 37:30–39, 1997

CAPRIE Steering Committee: A randomised, blinded trial of clopidogrel versus aspirin in patients at risk of ischaemic events. Lancet 348:1329–1339, 1996

Chui H, Zhang Q: Evaluation of dementia: a systematic study of the usefulness of the American Academy of Neurology's practice parameters. Neurology 49:925–935, 1997

Cohen-Mansfield J, Garfinkel D, Lipson S: Melatonin for treatment of sundowning in elderly persons with dementia—a preliminary study. Archives of Gerontology and Geriatrics 31:65–76, 2000

Cooper AJ: Medroxyprogesterone acetate (MPA) treatment of sexual acting out in men suffering from dementia. J Clin Psychiatry 48:368–370, 1987

Coull JT: Pharmacological manipulations of the alpha$_2$-noradrenergic system. Effects on cognition. Drugs Aging 5:116–126, 1994

Cummings JL: Dementia: the failing brain. Lancet 345:1481–1484, 1995

Cummings JL, Benson DF: Dementia: A Clinical Approach, 2nd Edition. Boston, MA, Butterworth-Heinemann, 1992

Cummings JL, Donohue JA, Brooks RL: The relationship betwen donepezil and behavioral disturbances in patients with Alzheimer's disease. Am J Geriatr Psychiatry 8:134–140, 2000

Desmond DW, Tatemichi TK, Paik M, et al: Risk factors for cerebrovascular disease as correlates of cognitive function in a stroke-free cohort. Arch Neurol 50:162–166, 1993

Duffy JD, Hobbs E: Mental retardation, in Textbook of Geriatric Neuropsychiatry, 2nd Edition. Edited by Coffey CE, Cummings JL. Washington, DC, American Psychiatric Press, 2000, pp 463–476

European Pentoxifylline Multi-Infarct Dementia Study Group: European Pentoxifylline Multi-Infarct Dementia Study. Eur Neurol 36:315–321, 1996

Fassbender K, Simons M, Bergmann C, et al: Simvastatin strongly reduces levels of Alzheimer's disease beta amyloid peptides Abeta 42 and Abeta 40 in vitro and in vivo. Proc Natl Acad Sci U S A 98:5856–5861, 2001

Flint AJ, Van Reekum R: The pharmacologic treatment of Alzheimer's disease: a guide for the general psychiatrist. Can J Psychiatry 43:689–697, 1998

Frampton JE, Brogden RN: Pentoxifylline (Oxpentifylline): a review of its therapeutic efficacy in the management of peripheral vascular and cerebrovascular disorders. Drugs Aging 7:480–503, 1995

Friedman JI, Temporini H, Davis KL: Pharmacologic strategies for augmenting cognitive performance in schizophrenia. Biol Psychiatry 45:1–16, 1999

Ginkgo biloba for dementia. The Medical Letter June 19, 1998, pp 63–64

Hawkins JW, Tinklenberg JR, Sheikh JI, et al: A retrospective chart review of gabapentin for the treatment of aggressive and agitated behavior in patients with dementias. Am J Geriatr Psychiatry 8:221–225, 2000

Hebert PR, Gaziano JM, Chan KS, et al: Cholesterol lowering with statin drugs, risk of stroke, and total mortality. JAMA 178:313–321, 1997

Heemels MT: Alzheimer's disease. Plaque removers and shakers (News). Nature 406(6795):465, 2000

Herrmann N, Lanctot K, Myszak M: Effectiveness of gabapentin for the treatment of behavioral disorders in dementia. J Clin Psychopharmacol 20:90–93, 2000

Hervey PS, Goa KL: Extended-release dipyridamole/aspirin. Drugs 58: 469–475, 1999

Jacobson SA, Leuchter AF, Walter DO: Conventional and quantitative EEG in the diagnosis of delirium among the elderly. J Neurol Neurosurg Psychiatry 56:153–158, 1993

Jakala P, Riekkinen M, Sirvio J, et al: Guanfacine, but not clonidine, improves planning and working memory performance in humans. Neuropsychopharmacology 20:460–470, 1999

Kawas C, Resnick S, Morrison A, et al: A prospective study of estrogen replacement therapy and the risk of developing Alzheimer's disease: the Baltimore Longitudinal Study of Aging. Neurology 48:1517–1521, 1997

Kimura M, Robinson RG, Kosier JT: Treatment of cognitive impairment after poststroke depression: a double-blind treatment trial. Stroke 31:1482–1486, 2000

Kistler JP, Buonanno FS, Gress DR: Carotid endarterectomy: specific therapy based on pathophysiology. N Engl J Med 325:505–507, 1991

Konno S, Meyer JS, Terayama Y, et al: Classification, diagnosis and treatment of vascular dementia. Drugs Aging 11:361–373, 1997

Kovach CR, Meyer-Arnold EA: Preventing agitated behaviors during bath time. Geriatr Nurs 18:112–114, 1997

Kyomen HH, Satlin A, Hennen J, et al: Estrogen therapy and aggressive behavior in elderly patients with moderate-to-severe dementia. Am J Geriatr Psychiatry 7:339–348, 1999

LeBars PL, Katz MM, Berman N, et al: A placebo-controlled, double-blind, randomized trial of an extract of Ginkgo biloba for dementia. JAMA 278:1327–1332, 1997

Levy ML, Cummings JL, Kahn-Rose R: Neuropsychiatric symptoms and cholinergic therapy for Alzheimer's disease. Gerontology 45 (suppl 1): 15–22, 1999

Liu RY, Zhou JN, van Heerikhuize J, et al: Decreased melatonin levels in postmortem cerebrospinal fluid in relation to aging, Alzheimer's disease, and apolipoprotein E–epsilon 4/4 genotype. J Clin Endocrinol Metab 84:323–327, 1999

Lothstein LM, Fogg-Waberski J, Reynolds P: Risk management and treatment of sexual disinhibition in geriatric patients. Conn Med 61:609–618, 1997

Lund and Manchester Groups: Clinical and neuropathological criteria for frontotemporal dementia. J Neurol Neurosurg Psychiatry 57:416–418, 1994

Martin J, Marler M, Shochat T, et al: Circadian rhythms of agitation in institutionalized patients with Alzheimer's disease. Chronobiol Int 17:405–418, 2000

Mayeux R, Denaro J, Hemenegildo N, et al: A population-based investigation of Parkinson's disease with and without dementia. Relationship to age and gender. Arch Neurol 49:492–497, 1992

Mayeux R, Saunders AM, Shea S, et al: Utility of the apolipoprotein E genotype in the diagnosis of Alzheimer's disease. N Engl J Med 338:506–511, 1998

McEvoy GK, Litvak K, Welsh OH, et al: AHFS Drug Information. Bethesda, MD, American Society of Health-System Pharmacists, 2000

McKeith IG, Galasko D, Kosaka K, et al: Consensus guidelines for the clinical and pathologic diagnosis of dementia with Lewy bodies (DLB): report of the Consortium on DLB International Workshop. Neurology 47:1113–1124, 1996

McKeith IG, Grace JB, Walker Z, et al: Rivastigmine in the treatment of dementia with Lewy bodies: preliminary findings from an open trial. Int J Geriatr Psychiatry 15:387–392, 2000

McKhann G, Drachman D, Folstein M, et al: Clinical diagnosis of Alzheimer's disease: report of the NINCDS-ADRDA Work Group under the auspices of Department of Health and Human Services Task Force on Alzheimer's Disease. Neurology 34:939–944, 1984

Meyer JS, Judd BW, Tawakina T, et al: Improved cognition after control of risk factors for multi-infarct dementia. JAMA 256:2203–2209, 1986

Mulnard RA, Cotman CW, Kawas C, et al: Estrogen replacement therapy for treatment of mild to moderate Alzheimer disease: a randomized controlled trial. JAMA 283:1007–1015, 2000

Nyth AL, Gottfries CG: The clinical efficacy of citalopram in treatment of emotional disturbances in dementia disorders. Br J Psychiatry 157:894–901, 1990

Oslin D, Atkinson RM, Smith DM, et al: Alcohol related dementia: proposed clinical criteria. Int J Geriatr Psychiatry 13:203–212, 1998

Papka M, Rubio A, Schiffer RB: A review of Lewy body disease, an emerging concept of cortical dementia. J Neuropsychiatry Clin Neurosci 10:267–279, 1998

Pollock BG, Mulsant BH, Sweet R, et al: An open pilot study of citalopram for behavioral disturbances of dementia. Am J Geriatr Psychiatry 5: 70–78, 1997

Ritchie K, Ledesert B, Touchon J: Subclinical cognitive impairment: epidemiology and clinical characteristics. Compr Psychiatry 41:61–65, 2000

Roane DM, Feinberg TE, Meckler L, et al: Treatment of dementia-associated agitation with gabapentin. J Neuropsychiatry Clin Neurosci 12:40–43, 2000

Rodriguez MM, Grossberg GT: Estrogen as a psychotherapeutic agent. Clin Geriatr Med 14:177–189, 1998

Rogers J, Kirby LC, Hempelman SR, et al: Clinical trial of indomethacin in Alzheimer's disease. Neurology 43:1609–1611, 1993

Rogers RL, Meyer JS, Judd BW, et al: Abstention from cigarette smoking improves cerebral perfusion among elderly chronic smokers. JAMA 253:2970–2974, 1985

Rogers SL, Friedhoff LT: The efficacy and safety of donepezil in patients with Alzheimer's disease: results of a US multicentre, randomized, double-blind, placebo-controlled trial. The Donepezil Study Group. Dementia 7:293–303, 1996

Rogers SL, Farlow MR, Doody RS, et al: A 24-week, double-blind, placebo-controlled trial of donepezil in patients with Alzheimer's disease. Neurology 50:136–145, 1998

Roman GC, Tatemichi TK, Erkinjuntti T, et al: Vascular dementia: diagnostic criteria for research studies. Report of the NINDS-AIREN International Work Group. Neurology 43:250–260, 1993

Rosler M, Anand R, Cicin-Sain A, et al: Efficacy and safety of rivastigmine in patients with Alzheimer's disease: International Randomised Controlled Trial. BMJ 318:633–640, 1999

Saitoh T, Katzman R: Genetic correlations in Lewy body disease, in Dementia With Lewy Bodies. Edited by Perry R, McKeith I, Perry E. Cambridge, UK, Cambridge University Press, 1996, pp 336–349

Samuel W, Caligiuri M, Galasko D, et al: Better cognitive and psychopathologic response to donepezil in patients prospectively diagnosed as dementia with Lewy bodies: a preliminary study. Int J Geriatr Psychiatry 15:794–802, 2000

Sano M, Ernesto C, Thomas RG, et al: A controlled trial of selegiline, alpha-tocopherol, or both as treatment for Alzheimer's disease. N Engl J Med 336:1216–1222, 1997

Schneider LS, Farlow M, Henderson VW, et al: Effects of estrogen replacement therapy on repsonse to tacrine in patients with Alzheimer's disease. Neurology 46:1580–1584, 1996

Shankle WR, Nielson KA, Cotman CW: Low-dose propranolol reduces aggression and agitation resembling that associated with orbitofrontal dysfunction in elderly demented patients. Alzheimer Dis Assoc Disord 9:233–237, 1995

Siegfried KR: Cholinergic approaches to cognition and dementia, in Pharmacotherapy for Mood, Anxiety, and Cognitive Disorders. Edited by Halbreich U, Montgomery SA. Washington, DC, American Psychiatric Press, 2000, pp 519–533

Sloane PD, Rader J, Barrick AL, et al: Bathing persons with dementia. The Gerontologist 35:672–678, 1995

Small GW, Rabins PV, Barry PP, et al: Diagnosis and treatment of Alzheimer disease and related disorders. JAMA 278:1363–1371, 1997

Street JS, Clark WS, Gannon KS, et al: Olanzapine treatment of psychotic and behavioral symptoms in patients with Alzheimer disease in nursing care facilities: a double-blind, randomized, placebo-controlled trial. Arch Gen Psychiatry 57:968–976, 2000

Sultzer DL, Mahler ME, Mandelkern MA, et al: The relationship between psychiatric symptoms and regional cortical metabolism in Alzheimer's disease. J Neuropsychiatry Clin Neurosci 7:476–484, 1995

Tang MX, Jacobs D, Stern Y, et al: Effect of oestrogen during menopause on risk and age at onset of Alzheimer's disease. Lancet 348:429–432, 1996

van Dongen MC, van Rossum E, Kessels AG, et al: The efficacy of ginkgo for elderly people with dementia and age-associated memory impairment: new results of a randomized clinical trial. J Am Geriatr Soc 48:1183–1194, 2000

Warfarin versus aspirin for prevention of thromboembolism in atrial fibrillation: Stroke Prevention in Atrial Fibrillation II Study. Lancet 343:687–691, 1994

Weiner MF, Denke M, Williams K, et al: Intramuscular medroxyprogesterone acetate for sexual aggression in elderly men. Lancet 339: 1121–1122, 1992

Wiseman SV, McAuley JW, Freidenberg GR, et al: Hypersexuality in patients with dementia: possible response to cimetidine. Neurology 54:2024, 2000

Wolf PA: Cigarettes, alcohol and stroke. N Engl J Med 315:1087–1089, 1986

Yudofsky SC, Kopecky HJ, Kunik M, et al: The Overt Agitation Severity Scale for the objective rating of agitation. J Neuropsychiatry Clin Neurosci 9:541–548, 1997

Generic name	clonidine
Trade name	Catapres
Class	Alpha$_2$-adrenergic receptor agonist
Half-life	6–20 hours (longer in renal impairment)
Mechanism of action	Stimulates α_2 receptors, resulting in reduced sympathetic (noradrenergic) outflow
Available formulation	Tablets: 0.1, 0.2, 0.3 mg (also available as transdermal patch)
Starting dose	0.1 mg po qhs
Titration	Increase gradually as needed
Typical daily dose	0.1 mg po bid
Dosage range	0.2–1.0 mg daily (divided bid, tid, or qid)
Therapeutic serum level	Not established

Comments: Not well established as a therapy, but may be useful in treating cognitive and behavioral dysfunction in patients with frontal lobe dementia or dementia of schizophrenia (both off-label uses). Metabolized in liver to inactive metabolites. Excreted in urine and feces. Onset in 30–60 minutes, peak effect in 2–4 hours, and duration 6–10 hours. Drug interactions: β-blockers, other hypotensive agents potentiate hemodynamic effects; TCAs antagonize effects. Adverse effects: hypotension, bradycardia, palpitations, tachycardia, congestive heart failure, drowsiness, headache, dizziness, fatigue, insomnia, anxiety, nightmares, hallucinations, delirium, nervousness, depression, sodium and water retention, constipation, dry mouth, and anorexia. Rebound hypertension on sudden discontinuation.

Generic name	clopidogrel
Trade name	Plavix
Class	Antiplatelet agent
Half-life	7–8 hours
Mechanism of action	Inhibits ADP [adenosine diphosphate]–induced platelet aggregation
Available formulation	Tablet: 75 mg
Starting dose	75 mg qd
Titration	None
Typical daily dose	75 mg
Dosage range	None (reduced dosage in hepatic impairment)
Therapeutic serum level	Not established

Comments: Second-line antiplatelet agent for patients with an intolerance to aspirin because of gastrointestinal bleeding or distress or who have evidence of continued ischemia despite aspirin therapy. Slightly more effective than aspirin and as safe as aspirin; its only significant side effect is skin rash. Much more expensive than aspirin. Well absorbed; metabolized in liver via the CYP1A enzyme to an active metabolite. At high concentrations in vitro, inhibits CYP2C9; in vivo significance of this inhibition is not known. *Adverse effects:* intracranial bleeding, rash, urticaria, diarrhea, nausea, vomiting, gastrointestinal bleeding, neutropenia, prolonged bleeding time, and increased liver function test values.

Generic name	dipyridamole (extended release) and aspirin
Trade name	Aggrenox
Class	Antiplatelet agent
Half-life	Dipyridamole: 13.6 hours Aspirin: 1.71 hours
Mechanism of action	Dipyridamole inhibits uptake of adenosine, and aspirin inhibits platelet cyclo-oxygenase; additive antiplatelet effects
Available formulation	Fixed-dose capsules: 200 mg dipyridamole XR/25 mg aspirin
Starting dose	One capsule bid
Titration	None
Typical daily dose	One capsule bid
Dosage range	None
Therapeutic serum level	Peak steady-state plasma concentrations: Dipyridamole, 1.9 µg/mL Aspirin, 319 ng/mL

Comments: Combination drug is possibly more effective than low-dose aspirin alone in preventing stroke in patients who have had a transient ischemic attack or an ischemic event. Capsule must be swallowed whole, without chewing or crushing. Dipyridamole undergoes glucuronidation in the liver, and the metabolite is excreted mainly via bile into the feces; aspirin undergoes hydrolysis to salicylic acid, then undergoes conjugation in the liver and is excreted in the urine. Avoid use in patients with significant hepatic or renal impairment, those who drink three or more alcoholic drinks daily, those with vitamin K deficiency or inherited bleeding disorders, and those with peptic ulcer disease. *Drug interactions:* increased risk of bleeding with verapamil, anticoagulants, or other antiplatelet agents; aspirin increases methotrexate toxicity and increases concentrations of valproate, phenytoin, and acetazolamide; aspirin diminishes the effect of ACE inhibitors, diuretics, probenecid, and sulfinpyrazone. *Adverse effects:* headache, dyspepsia, abdominal pain, anorexia, nausea, vomiting, diarrhea, seizures, fatigue, malaise, syncope, amnesia, confusion, somnolence, cardiac failure, purpura, bleeding (no more than with aspirin alone), rectal bleeding, hemorrhoids, hemorrhage, epistaxis, anemia, weakness, back pain, and arthralgia.

Generic name	donepezil
Trade name	Aricept
Class	Acetylcholinesterase inhibitor
Half-life	70 hours
Mechanism of action	Increases concentration of acetylcholine via noncompetitive, reversible inhibition of acetylcholinesterase
Available formulation	Tablets: 5, 10 mg
Starting dose	5 mg qhs
Titration	Increase to 10 mg qhs after 6 weeks if indicated
Typical daily dose	5–10 mg hs
Dosage range	5–10 mg qhs
Therapeutic serum level	Not established

Comments: A drug of choice for cognition enhancement and treatment of behavioral disturbance in AD and in dementia with Lewy bodies. In certain patients at some stages of disease, may be associated with worsening of behavior. Well absorbed. Metabolized in liver via the CYP2D6 and CYP3A4 enzymes and by glucuronidation. Several active metabolites. Eliminated in urine. Use with caution in patients with sick sinus syndrome or other supraventricular conduction problems, peptic ulcer disease, bladder outflow obstruction, seizures, or chronic obstructive pulmonary disease. *Drug interactions:* synergistic effects with other cholinergic agents and antagonistic effects with anticholinergic agents. *Adverse effects:* syncope, insomnia, fatigue, headache, dizziness, depression, abnormal dreams, bruising, nausea, diarrhea, vomiting, anorexia, polyuria, muscle cramps, and arthritis.

Generic name	galantamine
Trade name	Reminyl
Class	Acetylcholinesterase inhibitor
Half-life	8–10 hours
Mechanism of action	Reversible, competitive cholinesterase inhibitor; also increases acetylcholine release via modulation of nicotinic receptors
Available formulation	Tablets: 4, 8, 12 mg
Starting dose	4 mg bid with meals
Titration	Increase after 4 weeks to 8 mg bid; if needed, increase again after 4 weeks to 12 mg bid
Typical daily dose	8 mg bid with meals
Dosage range	8–24 mg daily (divided bid)
Therapeutic serum level	Not established

Comments: A newly approved drug that is potentially a drug of choice for cognition enhancement and treatment of behavioral disturbances in AD and in dementia with Lewy bodies. Rapidly and completely absorbed, with bioavailability over 80%; linear pharmacokinetics, protein binding 18%, low clearance, and moderate volume of distribution. Dose in patients with moderate renal or hepatic impairment should be ≤16 mg daily. Several metabolic pathways, including oxidation (CYP2D6, CYP3A4), demethylation, and glucuronidation. *Adverse effects:* nausea, vomiting, diarrhea, anorexia, weight loss, bradycardia, and tremor. Adverse effects minimized by very slow titration, as noted.

Generic name	guanfacine
Trade name	Tenex
Class	Alpha$_2$-adrenergic receptor agonist
Half-life	17 hours
Mechanism of action	Stimulates α_2 receptors, resulting in reduced sympathetic (noradrenergic) outflow
Available formulation	Tablets: 1, 2 mg
Starting dose	1 mg qhs
Titration	Increase at 3- to 4-week intervals, if needed and as tolerated
Typical daily dose	1 mg hs
Dosage range	1–3 mg qhs
Therapeutic serum level	Not established

Comments: Not well established as a therapy, but may be associated with improvement in executive dyscontrol, serial learning, working memory, and attention in schizophrenia and certain other frontal lobe dementia syndromes (off-label use). 80%–100% bioavailable, 20%–30% protein bound. Undergoes glucuronidation and sulfation in the liver; excreted renally. *Drug interactions:* increased hypotensive effects when used with TCAs or other hypotensive agents. *Adverse effects:* drowsiness, dizziness, headache, nausea, xerostomia, constipation, leg cramps, weakness, and dyspnea.

Generic name	pentoxifylline
Trade name	Trental
Class	Cerebral perfusion enhancer
Half-life	Parent drug: 24–48 minutes Metabolites: 60–96 minutes
Mechanism of action	Unclear; apparently alters rheology of red blood cells to reduce viscosity of blood
Available formulation	CR tablet: 400 mg
Starting dose	400 mg tid with meals
Titration	May reduce dose to bid if side effects occur
Typical daily dose	400 mg tid
Dosage range	400 mg bid to 400 mg tid
Therapeutic serum level	Not established

Comments: Not well established as a therapy, but may be associated with improved global and cognitive function and slower progression of dementia in patients with large-vessel ischemic disease (multi-infarct dementia), and decreased risk of transient ischemic attacks (all off-label uses). Well absorbed; undergoes first-pass metabolism. Metabolized in liver and excreted in urine. *Drug interactions:* enhances anticoagulant effects of warfarin; bleeding when used in combination with other antiplatelet agents, including clopidogrel. *Adverse effects:* mild hypotension, angina, arrhythmias, agitation, dizziness, headache, nausea, dyspepsia, vomiting, blurred vision, and earache.

Generic name	rivastigmine
Trade name	Exelon
Class	Cholinesterase inhibitor
Half-life	1.5 hours
Mechanism of action	Noncompetitive acetylcholinesterase and butylcholinesterase inhibitor
Available formulation	Capsules: 1.5, 3, 4.5, 6 mg
Starting dose	1.5 mg bid
Titration	Increase by 1.5 mg bid every 2 weeks, as tolerated
Typical daily dose	6 mg bid
Dosage range	6–12 mg daily (divided bid)
Therapeutic serum level	Not established

Comments: A drug of choice in the treatment of conditions involving reduced cholinergic function, including AD and dementia with Lewy bodies. Rapidly absorbed, with peak concentrations in 1 hour; absorption delayed by food. Widely distributed (V_d = 1.8–2.7 L/kg). 40% protein bound. Metabolized primarily via hydrolysis, with decarbamylate metabolite excreted in urine. Minimal role of CYP enzymes in metabolism. Duration of cholinesterase inhibition is about 10 hours after a single dose. *Drug interactions:* no significant drug interactions identified. *Adverse effects:* nausea, vomiting, diarrhea, anorexia, abdominal pain, dizziness, headache, fatigue, and malaise.

Generic name	selegiline
Trade names	Eldepryl, Deprenyl, L-Deprenyl
Class	MAOI
Half-life	9 minutes
Mechanism of action	Selective MAO-B inhibitor (at doses < 10 mg daily); psychostimulant (metabolized to amphetamine and methamphetamine)
Available formulations	Capsule: 5 mg Tablet: 5 mg
Starting dose	5 mg with breakfast
Titration	Increase in 1–3 days by 5 mg, as tolerated
Typical daily dose	5 mg bid, with breakfast and lunch
Dosage range	5–10 mg daily
Therapeutic serum level	Not established

Comments: May be useful by virtue of its antioxidant and neuroprotective effects for patients with AD as well as Parkinson's disease with cognitive impairment (both off-label uses). Onset of effect within 1 hour; duration 24–72 hours. Metabolized in liver to amphetamine and methamphetamine. *Drug interactions:* fluoxetine and other selective serotonin reuptake inhibitors, serotonergic antidepressants such as nefazodone and venlafaxine, meperidine and other opioids, nonselective MAOIs. Substrate for CYP2D6. Avoid high-tyramine-content foods. *Adverse effects:* orthostasis, arrhythmias, hypertension, hallucinations, confusion, depression, insomnia, agitation, loss of balance, nausea, vomiting, xerostomia, increased involuntary movements, and bradykinesia.

Generic name	vitamin E (α-tocopherol)
Trade name	Various
Class	Fat-soluble vitamin
Half-life	
Mechanism of action	Prevents oxidation of vitamins A and C; protects polyunsaturated fatty acids in membranes from attack by free radicals and protects red blood cells against hemolysis
Available formulations	Capsules: 100, 200, 330, 400, 500, 600, 1,000 IU Tablets: 200, 400 IU
Starting dose	400–500 IU qd
Titration	Increase by 400–500 IU every 7 days, as tolerated
Typical daily dose	1,000 IU bid (for AD)
Dosage range	800–2,000 IU daily
Therapeutic serum level	Not established

Comments: Found to slow the rate of progression of AD in patients with moderate dementia; may also be useful in those with mild cognitive dysfunction, although not established for that indication. Capsules must be swallowed whole. Oral absorption depends on presence of bile. Distributes to all tissues, especially adipose, where it is stored. Undergoes glucuronidation in the liver and is eliminated in feces and bile. *Drug interactions:* may interfere with response to iron and alter the effects of vitamin K (and warfarin). Toxicity appears as blurred vision, diarrhea, dizziness, flulike symptoms, nausea, and headache.

Index

*Page numbers printed in **boldface** type refer to tables or figures.*

417